Dr. Murray's
Total Body Tune-Up

MICHAEL T. MURRAY, N.D.

Dr. Murray's
Total Body
Tune-Up

Slow Down the Aging Process,
Keep Your System Running Smoothly,
Help Your Body Heal Itself
—for Life!

BANTAM BOOKS

NEW YORK TORONTO LONDON SYDNEY AUCKLAND

Library of Congress Cataloging-in-Publication Data

Murray, Michael T.
[Total body tune-up]
Dr. Murray's total body tune-up : slow down the aging process, keep your system running smoothly, help your body heal itself—for life! / Michael T. Murray.
p.   cm.
Includes bibliographical references and index.
ISBN 0-553-10789-5
1. Health.   2. Longevity.   3. Aging.   4. Self-care, Health.   I. Title
RA776.5M87   2000

613—dc21   00-024599

Published simultaneously in the United States and Canada

PRINTED IN THE UNITED STATES OF AMERICA

BVG   10   9   8   7   6   5   4   3   2   1

To Gina, my wife.
Her love, support, and true friendship
are the major blessings in my life along with
our two wonderful children, Alexa and Zachary.

Contents

Introduction: A New Approach to Health

I am a doctor of naturopathy—an N.D. Naturopathy is the science that harnesses the power of nature to prevent illness and achieve the highest level of health possible. My particular area of focus is clinical nutrition—the use of diet and nutritional support—and herbal medicine.

When people refer to me as an expert in alternative medicine, I usually correct them. I am a proponent of what I like to refer to as *rational* medicine, which combines the best of both conventional medicine and alternative methods. We have all been helped by the wonders of modern high-tech medicine. It can make a life-or-death difference when heroic measures are needed. As far as improving our general level of health, however, I believe it is woefully deficient. Modern medicine fails us most in the treatment of chronic degenerative diseases such as heart disease, high blood pressure, arthritis, and diabetes. In many diseases, the natural approach is simply much more rational. Rather than relying on drugs and surgery to suppress symptoms, I believe it makes more sense to use natural, noninvasive techniques whenever possible to promote health and healing.

My interest in, and commitment to, natural medicine resulted from personal experience. Years ago, when I was a freshman at the University of Oregon, I underwent a four-hour knee operation for a long-standing injury. The orthopedic surgeon told me that I'd be lucky if I walked without a limp. When the cast was removed three months later, I did everything I could to rehabilitate my knee. I wanted to have a full and physically active life, and that meant taking part in basketball games, racquet sports, and jogging. But after a year and a half I was still unable to put any significant stress on my knee. At the suggestion of my father, I went to see Ralph Weiss, N.D., a doctor of natural medicine.

I was skeptical. I knew that Dr. Weiss had helped a lot of people, including members of my family, but I had been treated by one of the top knee specialists in the world. What could Dr. Weiss do that conventional medicine couldn't?

I soon learned. In our first meeting, Dr. Weiss expressed concern not just about my knee but about my diet and lifestyle. He explained things in terms I could understand. He spoke with confidence and wonder about the body's tremendous ability to heal itself. All we had to do, he said, was remove the obstacles that were preventing my knee from healing properly. His technique was to use electro-acupuncture. As soon as the treatment began I could literally feel my leg come alive again. Within minutes it was almost as strong as my healthy leg. That evening, I played basketball again—without pain—for the first time in years.

It was a life-changing experience. I changed my major from history (I had planned to go on to law school) to pre-med and soon fulfilled the entrance requirements to attend Bastyr College (now a university) to pursue a degree in naturopathic medicine.

This book is the culmination of my years of work in the field. Over the past two decades I have treated thousands of patients in my private practice near Seattle, Washington. I teach medical students at Bastyr University, have published many books and articles on natural medicine, and travel widely, speaking to audiences of doctors and lay people. One of my greatest sources of satisfaction is sharing with listeners and readers my excitement about the results of the latest scientific research in the field. I maintain an ever-growing database of more than fifty thousand articles published in medical journals. This body of scientific research now enables us to better confirm which natural medicines are the most safe and effective—as well as telling us which popular remedies *don't* work. The information you find in these pages is based on this research and on my personal experience with patients.

Working with the Body

My purpose in writing this book is to convey the splendor of the human body and motivate you to take the steps necessary to keep it running at its best. My *Total Body Tune-Up* provides a step-by-step program to improve the function of the vehicle that will carry you through life. By tuning up each key body system, you will achieve better health, greater vitality, and renewed zest for living. Just as taking your car in for routine maintenance can improve its mileage and performance, a body tune-up can help slow down the aging process, get rid of "rust," and keep your systems running smoothly for as long as you live.

Several themes, or threads, run through this book. Here are some of the main ideas you will encounter in the chapters ahead.

- *The health of the body depends on the health of its smallest parts: the cells.* These very complex living factories connect to form tissues and organs. In order to function at their peak, cells require a steady stream of chemical building blocks. Cells use these chemical building blocks to build larger molecules just as we use letters of the alphabet to make words, sentences, paragraphs, and books. We truly become what we eat, as the cells utilize the nutrients and energy provided by food to form these larger molecules. Cells are constantly remodeling and reproducing themselves. In fact, that process is the whole basis of healing.

- *Life is the result of chemical and electrical activity.* All the cells of the body are interconnected through an amazingly complex information highway that makes the Internet look primitive by comparison. System failures and disease are often the result of the failure to provide the basic chemical building blocks required for crucial communication links. Even our own thoughts and emotions are translated into chemicals. We are not only what we eat, but also what we think and feel. That is how the mind plays its role as both healer and slayer—through chemical messages. One of the real keys to optimal health is flooding the body with the chemicals of good health by meeting all of your nutritional needs and harnessing the healing power of the mind.

- *Balance is the key to health.* Your body works very hard to keep its internal environment—temperature, fluid levels, and so on—at steady levels. We also depend on various cycles to keep our bodies working: we wake and sleep, we breathe in and breathe out, one hormone switches on a body process and another switches it off. Overall balance is the optimal state for healthy body function. Disease is usually a sign of an imbalance somewhere in the system.

- *The body strives to be healthy.* Health is our natural state. Your body tells you when something is wrong and takes steps to correct the problem. To give a simple example, if you are running low on fluid, your body causes you to feel thirsty. By listening to the body, we can sense when we have fallen out of balance. Just as important, we often know instinctively what to do to restore balance if we know how to listen. One of my primary goals is to encourage my patients to listen more closely, so that the body doesn't have to shout (in the form of pain or disease) in order to get their attention.

- *Each human being is biologically unique.* We all share the same basic structure. But our individual combinations of genes make us unlike anyone else who has ever lived. We all have our own biological needs and our own responses to the world around us. What works for one person may not work for another. That is exactly why this book has so many self-assessment questionnaires that can help you pinpoint your personal needs.

CAUTION Although this book discusses numerous health conditions and offers ideas for preventing or managing them, it is not intended as a substitute for appropriate medical care. Please keep the following in mind as you read:

- Do not self-diagnose. Proper medical care is critical to good health. If you have symptoms that suggest an illness described in this book, please consult a physician, preferably a naturopathic doctor (N.D.), holistic medical doctor (M.D.), doctor of osteopathy (D.O.), chiropractor, or other natural health care specialist.
- If you are currently taking prescription medications, you absolutely must work with your doctor before discontinuing any drug or altering any drug regimen. Make your physician aware of all the nutritional supplements or herbal products you are currently taking.
- If you wish to try a nutritional supplement or herbal product as a therapeutic measure, discuss it with your physician first, especially if you are taking any prescription medication. Doing so can help avoid potential side effects and adverse interactions.
- Many nutritional supplements and herbal products are effective on their own, but they work best when they are used as part of a comprehensive natural approach to health that incorporates diet and lifestyle factors.

It is my sincere hope that you—or someone you care about—will use the information provided in the following pages to achieve greater health and happiness.

Live in good health with passion and joy!

Michael T. Murray, N.D.
Issaquah, Washington

CHAPTER 1

Do You Need a Tune-Up?

Nature is doing her best each moment to make us well.
She exists for no other end. Do not resist. With the least inclination to be well,
we should not be sick.

—*Henry David Thoreau*

O f all nature's miracles, the human body is most amazing. As Thoreau realized, nature works constantly to ensure that your body functions well. Health is our natural state.

But the body is complex and intricate—a collection of interwoven systems, each dependent on the others. Through one system we take in food and break it down into tiny nutrients that the body can use. Another system carries those nutrients to the cells, which use them as fuel. Meanwhile there's a system that carries away waste, recycling when possible and removing the rest. All this activity—and much more—is regulated by constant streams of chemical and electric signals under the control of the brain.

Although we sometimes talk about the "parts" of our bodies, we are closer to the truth when we think of the body as a whole. All those different systems must work as one to achieve their common goal: to keep us alive.

In some ways your body is like a car. Both require fuel, fluids, pumps, valves, lubricants, and an electric spark to run. Both filter and remove wastes. All these systems need to operate with split-second timing.

But there's another similarity that we often overlook. To run at its best, every vehicle requires periodic maintenance. The simplest steps— changing the oil, replacing spark plugs, tightening connections, cleaning out the sludge—make all the difference in how the car performs. We're not talking here about major overhauls, just a few routine steps to keep things humming. A tune-up.

Many people treat their cars better than their bodies. They wouldn't dream of missing the three-thousand-mile oil change. They winterize their vehicle at the first sign of cold weather, rotate the tires, and use fuel additives to keep the engine purring. From experience, they know that routine upkeep will prevent major disasters. A timely tankful of high-octane gasoline, a buck's worth of oil, or a bottle of transmission fluid will avoid a $2,000 engine burnout down the road. As the mechanic in the TV ad says, "You can pay me now . . . or you can pay me later."

A car is designed to last maybe a dozen years at most, and it's pretty easy to replace worn-out parts or repair major damage. But you get only one body in your lifetime. That precious body needs careful attention if you want it to last as long as possible and function at its best. Usually it doesn't take much to produce results. As Thoreau realized, if we have the least inclination to be well, we can avoid serious trouble. Yet many of us neglect to take the basic steps that would keep our organs and tissues working at their peak.

At each moment, the body tries to maintain the ideal conditions needed to carry out its many tasks. The technical term for this is *homeostasis,* which means "same standing." If the temperature rises too high, special systems kick in to cool things back down to normal. If a poisonous substance enters the body, the cells try to destroy or eliminate it before it can cause permanent damage. Every organism on the planet, from the simplest single-celled amoeba to the human being, relies on this internal mechanism, homeostasis, to sustain life.

Often, though, we subject our bodies to severe stress. If the homeostatic mechanism cannot overcome the forces that threaten it, then the system falls out of balance. In the worst cases, it fails completely. The result is disease—a disruption in the ability of a body system or part to carry out its normal function. By keeping our systems finely tuned, we can protect ourselves against disease and enjoy the benefits of health.

No matter how old you are or what your current state of health is, you can take steps to help your body function better. You can work better, feel better, look better—all by taking some basic steps to help your body maintain its optimal homeostasis.

In the chapters to follow, I'll outline a program that will help you do just that. I call it the Total Body Tune-Up.

Time for a Tune-Up?

For starters, read through the following set of questions. The more yes answers you give, the greater your need for a tune-up.

- Do you feel that you are not as healthy and vibrant as other people your age?
- Do you want to have more energy?
- Do you want greater mental clarity?
- Do you often feel blue or depressed?
- Do you get more than one or two colds a year?
- Do you struggle with your weight?
- Do you suffer from lack of libido or impotence?
- Do you have digestive disturbances?
- Do you have weak, brittle, or cracked nails?
- Is your hair dry and lifeless?
- Do you have dark circles under your eyes?
- Are you constantly hungry?
- Do you have trouble getting to sleep, or do you want to sleep all of the time?
- Do you have high cholesterol levels or high blood pressure?
- Do you feel anxious or stressed out most of the time?
- Do you suffer from premenstrual syndrome, fibrocystic breast disease, or uterine fibroids?
- Do you crave sweets?
- Do you suffer from allergies?
- Do you lose your temper easily?
- Do you have bad breath or body odor?
- Do you suffer from chronic postnasal drip or hay fever–like symptoms?

What You Can Expect from Your Tune-Up

Can a tune-up really help with all of these symptoms? Absolutely. These symptoms often indicate nothing more than a squeaky wheel in need of maintenance. Taking the appropriate tune-up step can pay huge dividends in clearing up the immediate symptom. Even more important, a tune-up can ensure better long-term health and avoid the progression of minor problems to more serious conditions. Here are some specific benefits your tune-up can offer.

Increased energy. The quality of your life is often directly related to your energy level. The greatest improvement most people notice with a tune-up is a higher energy level. A tune-up can give you the power to live with more passion and joy.

Improved protection against disease. Everyone wants to be well and stay well. Your body does its best to fight illness. But you must provide the nutrients your body needs to build strong tissues and vigorous immune cells.

Rejuvenation and slower aging. No one can live forever, but everyone wants to live as long as possible. Just as important as the quantity of your years is their quality. No matter how old you get, you want your body always to function at its best. The human body is naturally programmed to make that happen. Most cells in the body reproduce many times during your lifespan. By tuning up, you can make sure that each new generation of cells is as fit and robust as its ancestors. You'll slow down the aging process and start to feel "young before your time."

Better moods and mental function. When you feel better physically, you feel better emotionally too. The body and mind are interconnected. When one is affected, so is the other. After a tune-up you will find your mood elevated and your mind enhanced. You will think more clearly, with more focus.

Better appearance. It's not vain to want to look your best. It's a sign of self-respect. The same strategies for keeping your internal systems humming also work on the external ones—skin, hair, nails.

Greater ability to deal with stress. In today's society, pressure comes from all directions. The demands of work, family, and society all take their toll. Constant stress wears you down both mentally and physically, putting you at risk of serious illness. Some of the most groundbreaking research over the last forty years has documented how stress causes or contributes to a wide range of health problems, from infections to infertility. Your tune-up will show you how to reduce your stress and keep it low. You'll also find out how to energize every one of your body's millions of cells—those tiny biological dynamos.

Better sex. It's natural and normal to enjoy an active sex life for as long as you choose. But if your body isn't functioning right, both your interest in sex and your ability to engage in it can plummet. Besides helping you replenish your energy reserves, a tune-up can increase muscle strength and improve circulation. When your electrical and chemical systems are working at their peak and when your emotions are in healthy balance, you are more responsive to sexual stimulation and better able to express your most intimate feelings with your partner.

Weight control. Your car's mileage drops when it's carrying a heavy load. It's the same with your body. Unnecessary pounds burn up the limited supply of energy all the more quickly. If you have unsuccessfully tried to lose weight, you are not alone. Diet and exercise alone are often not enough. A total body tune-up can help you bring your weight under control—and keep it there—by resetting your metabolism to burn fat rather than storing it.

Quick results. The moment your tune-up begins, your entire system will receive a boost. You may not notice the difference right away, but your body will. Even a change that affects only a few cells can sometimes dramatically correct a big problem. Most of the techniques I describe in this book are simple things you can begin doing today. Depending on your goals, you'll see results within a few days or weeks. Once you experience how good you can feel, you will be naturally motivated to stay on a maintenance program that will help you continue with your positive results.

A happier attitude. Your attitude is like your physical body—it needs to be conditioned. It is easy for people to fall into the trap of a negative attitude if they are too tired, stressed, or unhappy. Your tune-up can help you see the world differently. Your attitude is like a lens through which you filter your life's experiences. Your tune-up will adjust the lens properly and help you see life as a rainbow of miracles and possibilities. Such awareness will naturally make you want to live as well and as long as possible—if for no other reason than just to see what happens next!

Where Should You Start?

No doubt your car has a set of warning systems to let you know if trouble is brewing. The oil light will flash, or a beeper will sound to indicate that the brakes need attention. More advanced models have special computers that tell you if a backup light is out or a door is ajar.

Your body works somewhat the same way. It sends signals to let you know when things aren't quite up to par. Often, though, you may misread those signals or, worse, ignore them entirely. To take just one example: If your fingernails are weak, brittle, or cracked, you may not be consuming enough protein or certain types of fats in your diet, you may not be absorbing key minerals, or your thyroid gland may not be producing adequate supplies of essential hormones. A trip to the nail salon may make your nails look better, but a manicure won't do anything to fix the underlying problem.

When your car isn't running just right, you take it to the garage for service. If you're like most people, you'll describe the problem to the mechanic as best you can: "It goes *grrr—grrr—clunk* when I try to start it in cold weather" or "It makes this funny little *ping-click* noise." The mechanic will then hook the engine up to a device that analyzes performance. The readout might show that the mixture of gas and oxygen is too rich, or that too much exhaust is being produced, or that a frayed electrical connection fails to work every once in a while. Based on these findings (and your budget), you then make your choice about what steps to take and in what order.

Tuning up the body works pretty much the same way. The first step is to identify the chief trouble spots. Then you learn about the options available for addressing the problem and choose the remedy that offers the best results. Once the problem is under control, you can focus on the next area of concern.

As human beings, we all have in common a basic physical makeup—the same internal organs, wiring system, and body parts. The same chemicals flow through our blood vessels, triggering countless metabolic processes. Even our senses work in more or less the same fashion. There may be variations in degree, but normally humans everywhere are able to taste sweet or salty foods, hear the rhythms of music, and see the scarlet hues of a summer sunset.

At the same time, in many critical ways, each person is unique. One of the leading biologists of the twentieth century, Roger Williams, coined the term "biochemical individuality." Our unique biochemical traits determine who we are and how we interact with the world around us. Biochemical individuality results from a combination of our genes and our environment—nature and nurture. These factors play a big role in determining how healthy we are and what ailments we are likely to experience.

In my years of practice, I've found that most of my patients are very good at knowing when something isn't quite right with their bodies. But often they feel discouraged because they have visited doctors who tell them that there is "nothing wrong." Often what that means is that their doctors have been unable to diagnose a specific disease, something they can look up in their textbooks or point to under a microscope. My perspective is different. I practice what is called *functional medicine,* an approach pioneered by the nutritional biochemist Jeffrey Bland, Ph.D. As Dr. Bland put it:

> In functional medicine, the presence or absence of a disease is of secondary consideration to an understanding of the function or dysfunction which prevents or allows a disease to occur. . . . Functional medicine does not focus on the isolated entity called disease, but rather on the specifics of structural and functional mechanisms which comprise the whole person at any particular point in his or her life.

I listen carefully to my patients and regard their comments and complaints as valuable clues. We then work together to discover exactly where their particular problem lies. That involves more than just asking about the specific complaint. When I first meet a patient, I spend most of our session finding out everything I can about that person as an individual. I ask not just "How do you feel?" but "Who are you? What makes you tick? How do you envision your future?" Just as important, I listen carefully to the answers. My goal is to discover what makes each person unique.

In this crucial way, I am *not* like a mechanic who restores your car to good working order. Mechanics know that each Ford Taurus they put up on the rack will be the same as the next one. But as a physician, I know that each person has special needs. My task is to do all I can to discover what those needs are and to design a unique program that has the best chance of resolving those specific problems.

Your Personal Profile

If you were a patient coming to my office for the first time, you would bring with you a completed questionnaire sent to you at the time you made the appointment. Rather than having you take the time to complete the questionnaire all at once, I have placed parts of the questionnaire throughout the book to correspond to the body system discussed in that chapter. The more you understand how your body should work, the better we will be able to find real solutions. In essence, I will be guiding you through the process—from assessment to remedy—just as if you actually were my patient. By completing those questionnaires, you will discover areas that need attention and develop specific strategies to get things back on track.

A word of caution: The questionnaires are tools to help you identify areas of priority. They are not intended as a diagnostic tool in place of a checkup by a physician. After completing various assessments in this book, you may need to discuss the results with your medical doctor, who may decide to order further tests. It's important to realize that you may need medical treatment to address a specific problem before you can gain from a tune-up of a particular system. For example, perhaps the assessment for blood sugar control in Chapter 4, "Tuning Up Your Metabolism," indicates that you may be suffering from diabetes. If so, you must see a doctor immediately for proper diagnosis and treatment. Remember that my *Total Body Tune-Up* is not a treatment program for specific medical illnesses per se. Instead it outlines a program that will help you improve your level of health and maintain that level for a lifetime.

The Tools of My Trade

The tools that I use in my clinical practice to help people get well are primarily natural medicines—vitamins, minerals, other nutritional supplements, and herbal products. The recommendations that I give on how to use these medicines are based upon the patient's need and the appropriateness of long-term supplementation. Some supplements and herbal products are best used in times of need only. Most, however, are suitable for long-term use if necessary or perceived as beneficial. Unlike many drugs, most nutritional supplements and herbal medicines take a little time to work, so be sure to give them a fair trial. However, don't waste your money on a supplement unless you are quite sure that it is providing benefit. Also, remember that your best assurance of success with natural medicines is achieved if you use high quality products.

Most major-brand vitamins and mineral formulas reliably deliver the quantities listed on the label.

With herbal supplements, however, there is often tremendous variation in quality and potency. When several forms of a mineral (such as calcium) are available, I specify which form is most effective. Commercial herbal preparations are available as bulk herbs, teas, tinctures, fluid extracts, and tablets or capsules. In the past, the quality of the extract produced often was difficult to determine because many of the active principles of the herbs were unknown. Today, advances in extraction processes along with improved analytical methods have reduced this problem.

Standardized extracts, also referred to as guaranteed potency extracts, are guaranteed to contain a specified level of active compounds or key biological marker. Stating the content of active compounds or key marker allows for more accurate dosages to be made. Standardization is the only real assurance that you are getting an effective dosage, and I have based all my recommendations on such standardized products.

All in the Family

One of the first sections of the questionnaire explores your family's medical history. Certain medical conditions tend to occur among related individuals. This is what we mean when we say that a disease "runs in the family." In simple terms, a damaged or defective gene can make a person vulnerable to a certain ailment. If that gene gets passed on from parent to child, the child may also be susceptible. The key word here is *susceptibility,* not *destiny.* In most cases, inheriting a defective gene does not mean that the condition will inevitably develop; the problem gene from one parent may be canceled out by a normal gene from the other parent. This self-correcting mechanism is one reason why we humans, like most other species, reproduce sexually. The constant reshuffling of the genetic deck gives the next generation a better chance to survive and reproduce. Still, some defective genes are powerful enough to overcome the normal genes. When they do, trouble strikes.

For example, cancer of the colon, or large intestine, tends to run in families. Relatives tend to share the gene that causes small growths, known as polyps, to develop on the inner lining of the bowel. These growths resemble tiny mushrooms, and some people have hundreds of them. A certain percentage of the polyps will eventually become cancerous. The more polyps present, the greater the risk. You can't change your genes, but you can control to an extent how they are expressed. If you know that others in your family have (or had) colon cancer, you can take action to reduce the chances of developing the disease yourself. For example, you can maintain a diet shown to be protective against colon cancer (low in fat, high in fiber, and carotene-rich) and take nutritional supplements such as extra calcium to reduce your risk. Meanwhile, you and your medical caregivers can monitor the situation through regular examinations. (For more information on preventing colon cancer, see Chapter 2.) The result from this combined approach of maximum protection and proper surveillance is that even if you have a family history of colon cancer, you can dramatically reduce your risk. The same is true for many other conditions.

Table 1: Your Family Medical History Assessment

If one or more close blood relatives (grandparents, parents, aunts and uncles, siblings) suffer from any of the conditions given below, you can take steps to tune up the relevant body systems and reduce your risk of developing the condition.

Alzheimer's disease (see Chapter 7)

Anxiety (see Chapter 7)

Asthma (see Chapter 5)

Cancer

    Breast (see Chapter 10)

    Colon (see Chapter 2)

    Prostate (see Chapter 11)

Depression (see Chapter 7)

Diabetes (see Chapter 4)

Eczema (see Chapter 9)

Gallstones (see Chapter 3)

Glaucoma (see Chapter 7)

Gout (see Chapter 8)

Heart disease (see Chapter 6)

High blood pressure (see Chapter 6)

High cholesterol levels (see Chapter 6)

Obesity (see Chapter 4)

Osteoarthritis (see Chapter 8)

Osteoporosis (see Chapter 8)

Parkinson's disease (see Chapter 7)

Psoriasis (see Chapter 9)

Rheumatoid arthritis (see Chapter 5)

Thyroid problems (see Chapter 4)

Stroke (see Chapter 6)

Key Steps to a Successful Tune-Up

When people come to see me as a physician, I have an advantage in helping them make changes, since I can work with patients to help them bite off no more than they can chew. Since I cannot help you in person, I end this first chapter by giving you the key to a successful tune-up: *Every journey begins with a small step.* Don't be overwhelmed by the recommendations and advice presented in this book. Break things down into steps that you feel comfortable taking, no matter how small they may be. At the end of each chapter there will be a list of key steps for that particular chapter. If, at the very least, you simply follow these key steps, you will definitely experience a successful tune-up.

Lifestyle Tune-Up #1: Cultivate a Positive Attitude

After each chapter I will introduce an important general lifestyle tune-up recommendation. I start with attitude because I feel it is really the most critical factor not only for optimal health, but for an optimal quality of life as well.

As I have seen over and over in my patients' lives (and my own), it is not what happens in our lives that determines our direction; it is our *response* to those challenges that shapes the quality of our life and determines our destiny. Surprisingly, it is often true that hardship, heartbreak, disappointment, and failure serve as the spark for joy, ecstasy, compassion, and success. If you can condition your attitude to be positive, I can promise that you will be happier, more successful, and healthier.

Become an optimist. We humans, by nature, are optimists. The term comes from the Latin word *optimum*, meaning "the greatest good." Optimism is the attitude that looks for the best possible outcome and focuses on the most hopeful aspects of a situation. Some studies have found that people who adopt a positive outlook live longer and suffer from fewer and less severe diseases.

Improve the way you talk to yourself. We all conduct a constant running dialogue in our heads. In time the things we say to ourselves percolate down into our subconscious mind. Those inner thoughts, in turn, affect the way we think and feel. Naturally, if you feed yourself a steady stream of negative thoughts—"I'm no good, I hate myself, I hate the world"—your subconscious will respond in kind. Become aware of your self-talk, and then consciously work to feed positive self-talk messages to your subconscious mind.

Ask better questions. An expert in motivation, Anthony Robbins, believes that the quality of your life is equal to the quality of the questions you habitually ask yourself. For example, if you experience a setback, do you think, "Why am I so stupid? Why do bad things always happen to me?" Or do you think, "Okay, what can I learn from this so that it never happens again? What can I do to make the situation better?" Clearly, the latter response is healthier. Regardless of the specific situation, asking better questions is bound to improve your attitude. Here are some questions to start you off:

- What am I most happy about in my life right now?
- What am I most excited about in my life right now?
- What am I most grateful about in my life right now?
- What am I enjoying most in my life right now?
- What am I committed to in my life right now?
- Whom do I love? Who loves me?
- What must I do today to achieve my long-term goal?

Set positive goals. Learning to set achievable goals is a powerful method for building a positive attitude and raising self-esteem. Achieving goals creates a success cycle: You feel better about yourself, and the better you feel about yourself, the more likely you are to succeed. Here are some guidelines for setting health goals:

- State the goal in positive terms and in the present tense; avoid negative words. It's better to say "I enjoy eating healthy, low-calorie, nutritious foods" than to say "I will not eat sugar, candy, ice cream, and other fattening foods."
- Make your goal attainable and realistic. Start out with goals that are easily attainable, such as drinking six glasses of water a day and switching from white bread to whole wheat. By initially choosing easily attainable goals, you create a success cycle that helps build a positive self-image. Little things add up to make a major difference in the way you feel about yourself.
- Be specific. The more clearly you define your goal, the more likely you are to reach it. For example, if you want to lose weight, what is the weight you desire? What body fat percentage or measurements do you want to achieve?

CHAPTER 2

Tuning Up Your Digestive System

Your car won't go very far if you don't keep it supplied with fuel. The same is true of your body. But your metabolic "engine" is much more complex than even the most sophisticated imported roadster. That's because your body acts as its own refinery, producing energy from the raw materials you eat at each meal.

Your body digests food by breaking it into smaller particles. However, digestion is only part of the story. Before those small particles can reach the cells, they must pass from the intestines into the bloodstream. That process is called absorption.

Damage to delicate cells that line the digestive tract can prevent proper absorption. In some cases a defective intestine allows passage of particles that are too big. Like bulls in the biological china shop, these "macromolecules" can wreak all kinds of havoc in your body. Also, to digest food properly, your body needs the right mix of enzymes, fluids, and bacteria. If the balance among these is out of whack—for example, if too many of the wrong kinds of bacteria are present—all kinds of problems can develop, from inflammation of the bowels to cancer. Tuning up your digestion is among the most important steps you can take to improve your overall health.

How We Digest Food

The process of digestion actually begins a short time before your meal even enters your body. Odors from food tickle your nose. In response, the brain sends signals to your digestive organs, telling them to get ready for the incoming food. For example, the brain tells the glands in your mouth to release saliva. The production of other digestive juices also begins. You don't actually need to smell food to begin the process. Often the mere thought of a meal is enough to literally get the juices flowing.

The act of chewing your food sends another batch of signals to your digestive organs. Chewing mixes the food with saliva. Saliva contains enzymes that immediately kick off the breakdown process. For example, the enzyme salivary amylase whittles molecules of starch into smaller sugar molecules. Fat enzymes (lipases) also go to work. Chewing thoroughly is important for getting the most nutrition out of the food you eat. As part of your tune-up, make an effort to chew each bite completely before swallowing. You'll be doing your stomach a favor.

CASE HISTORY: Something to Chew Over

For a year I'd been working with Trevor, a forty-five-year-old real estate developer, trying to find a way to relieve his feelings of bloating after meals. He was also bothered by frequent burping and belching. I suspected a deficiency of stomach acid (hydrochloric acid) or perhaps an insufficient supply of digestive enzymes. Nothing I tried worked.

Then one day I happened to go out to lunch with him. It wasn't a pretty sight. Trevor talked nonstop while eating. He took huge bites and barely chewed before swallowing. And he ate too fast. He was looking at the dessert menu while I was still finishing my salad.

Watching him eat, I knew I had missed the diagnosis. (Sometimes we doctors make things more difficult than they need to be.) Trevor's problem was aerophagia—a fancy name for swallowing air while eating. When I called this to his attention, he didn't believe me. I insisted he take it seriously, and that he try eating more slowly and chewing each bite thoroughly—and *not* talk during the meal.

To make a long story short, Trevor's cured. Now that's food for thought.

The chewed food (called a bolus) then passes through the esophagus, a muscular tube running from the mouth to the stomach. The muscles are important, because they contract to squeeze the food along. At the juncture with the stomach, the muscles become even stronger, forming a valve called a sphincter. This structure helps prevent food from passing back out of the stomach and up the throat. However, this safety feature doesn't always work, as I'll explain a little later. The top of the esophagus and its neighboring tube, the trachea (your windpipe), are both protected by a muscular structure called the glottis. When you swallow, the glottis closes to prevent food from entering the windpipe. As you know, sometimes the glottis fails to close in time, causing you to cough in an effort to expel the food that "went down the wrong pipe." Things really start getting more interesting when the bolus of food reaches the stomach.

The Stomach

Once food enters the stomach, digestion kicks into high gear. The food gets broken down in two ways: physically and chemically. Muscle motions churn the food so it mixes with digestive juices. At the same time, these motions trigger release of a hormone, gastrin, that "switches on" glands in the stomach lining. These, in turn, release the digestive juices.

The digestive juice you're probably most familiar with is stomach acid, technically known as hydrochloric acid. Sitting by itself in a test tube, this stuff is pretty potent. Inside your stomach, though, it's diluted with saliva, water, and other substances.

The main function of hydrochloric acid is to provide the right environment to produce the real workhorse of stomach digestion, an enzyme called *pepsin,* which breaks down proteins. Without enough hydrochloric acid, proper protein digestion will not occur. Too much of the stuff, and you're at risk of heartburn (esophageal reflux), ulcers, and other tummy troubles. The acid environment of the stomach also prevents the growth of bacteria and yeast.

Stomach glands also produce a thick, sticky fluid called mucin. Mucin forms a layer that protects the cells of the stomach lining from exposure to acid and pepsin. Good thing it does, too, because without mucin, pepsin would quickly eat a hole in your stomach. (Sometimes that happens anyway, causing a condition called peptic ulcer. More about that below.)

The glands also produce fat-digesting enzymes (gastric lipases) and a substance called intrinsic factor, which plays a vital role in helping you absorb vitamin B_{12} in the small intestine. People who don't produce enough intrinsic factor are vulnerable to the problems of vitamin B_{12} deficiency.

Your stomach is busy pumping out digestive fluid all the time, but the rate of production varies. Once the food passes out of the stomach and into the small intestine, other nerve impulses tell the stomach to ease up until the next meal comes along. Food usually remains in the stomach until it is reduced to a semiliquid. Depending on the types of food you eat, that process lasts between forty-five minutes and four hours. Liquids and carbohydrates are the first to move on. Generally, the more fat or fiber in the food, the longer it stays in the stomach.

The stomach phase of digestion is largely a warm-up act. Only small amounts of water, glucose, salts, alcohol, and certain drugs are absorbed in the stomach. Most digestion and absorption actually occur in the small intestine.

Low Acidity

The problem of excess stomach acid gets most of the publicity. Surprisingly, however, the more common cause of indigestion is a *lack* of stomach acid, or hypoacidity. Without acid, enzymes can't break down food into small particles for absorption. In addition, low acid levels can lead to bacterial overgrowth, which can interfere with fat digestion and irritate the mucous membranes that line the intestines. A wide range of medical conditions can result from, or be worsened by, low gastric acidity (see Table 2-1).

Table 2-1: Problems Associated with Low Acidity

Addison's disease	Food allergies
Asthma	Gallbladder disease
Celiac disease	Gastric cancer
Chronic autoimmune disorders	Graves' disease
Dermatitis	Hepatitis
Diabetes mellitus	Lupus erythematosus
Eczema	Osteoporosis

Table 2-1: Problems Associated with Low Acidity

Pernicious anemia	Thyrotoxicosis
Psoriasis	Urticaria
Rosacea	Vitiligo

As a rule, your ability to produce adequate acid declines with age. It may be that certain cells or tissues in the stomach die or lose their ability to function. Most of your nerve cells never regenerate, so loss of these nerves (which control cell activity) may be a factor. Also, chronic problems such as poor diet or chronic use of certain medications may contribute to the decline of cell activity. This helps explain why so many elderly people suffer from such digestive complications as malabsorption. About half of my patients over age sixty have low stomach acid.

Physicians can detect low levels of acid by having you swallow an electronic sensor attached to a string. But there's a simpler method: Complete Part A of the Digestive Assessment, below.

DIGESTIVE ASSESSMENT • PART A
Ruling Out Lack of Stomach Acid Secretion (Hypoacidity)

Circle the number that best describes the intensity of your symptoms on the following scale:

> *0 = I do not experience this symptom*
> *1 = Mild*
> *2 = Moderate*
> *3 = Severe*

Bloating, belching, burning, and flatulence immediately after meals	0	1	2	3
A sense of fullness after eating	0	1	2	3
Indigestion, diarrhea, or constipation	0	1	2	3
Multiple food allergies	0	1	2	3
Nausea after taking supplements	0	1	2	3
Itching around the rectum	0	1	2	3
Weak, peeling, and cracked fingernails	0	1	2	3
Dilated blood vessels in the cheeks and nose	0	1	2	3

Acne	o	I	2	3
Iron deficiency	o	I	2	3
Undigested food in stool	o	I	2	3
Chronic candida infections	o	I	2	3

Add the numbers circled and enter that subtotal here: _____

Circle the number of the answer that applies to you:
Have you ever had a diagnosis of

Asthma	NO = o	YES = 3
Eczema	NO = o	YES = 3
Hepatitis	NO = o	YES = 3
Chronic hives	NO = o	YES = 3
Osteoporosis	NO = o	YES = 3
Psoriasis	NO = o	YES = 3
Rheumatoid arthritis	NO = o	YES = 3
Rosacea	NO = o	YES = 3
Vitiligo	NO = o	YES = 3

Add the numbers circled and enter that subtotal here: _____
Add the two subtotals and enter that total here: _____

Scoring   *9 or more:* **High priority**
             5–8: **Moderate priority**
             1–4: **Low priority**

Interpreting Your Score

A score of 9 or higher indicates a possible deficiency of hydrochloric acid secretion. Low acid means food doesn't break down as quickly, so it remains in the stomach longer than is normal. Feeling full for a long time after meals is a sign of low acid. Poor appetite may indicate that hunger signals are not being generated, which normally happens after the stomach has been empty for a while. The question about fingernails may have surprised you. But people who have slow digestion may not be able to absorb certain fats at the right rate. Without these nutrients, the nails can weaken and dry out.

To deal with low acid levels, follow these steps. **Caution:** *Consult your physician before following this protocol.*

Begin by taking one tablet or capsule containing 10 grains (600 mg) of hydrochloric acid at your next large meal. Hydrochloric acid products are available at your local health food store. If taking one tablet does not aggravate your symptoms, at every meal of the same size after that take that amount plus one additional tablet or capsule. (In other words, take one at the next meal, two at the meal after that, then three at the next meal. Space the tablets evenly during the meal: one at the beginning, the next a few minutes later, and so on.) If taking the tablet aggravates your symptoms, follow the recommendations for peptic ulcers for one month and try again (see pages 30–31). If it still aggravates your symptoms, it is unlikely that low hydrochloric acid is responsible for your indigestion.

Continue to increase the dose until you reach seven tablets per meal, or until you feel a warmth in your stomach, whichever occurs first. A feeling of warmth in the stomach means that you have taken too many tablets for that meal and next time you need to take one less tablet for that meal size. It is a good idea to try the larger dose again at another meal to make sure that it was the supplement that caused the warmth and not something else.

After you have found the largest dose that you can take at your large meals without feeling any warmth, maintain that dose at all meals of similar size. Take less at smaller meals. Remember to take the tablets one at a time at separate points throughout the meal.

As your stomach begins to regain the ability to produce the amount of acid needed to digest your food properly, you will notice the warm feeling again. At that point simply reduce the number of tablets.

High Acidity (Heartburn)

On the opposite end of the spectrum is excess acid, or hyperacidity. Too much acid will often produce the symptom we call heartburn. The name is misleading, because the heart is not involved. Instead, the burning sensation comes from the fact that the acidic contents of the stomach flow back up (reflux) into the esophagus. The esophagus does not have the same protective layers as the stomach, and so it senses pain. The medical term often used to label heartburn is *reflux esophagitis*. If the heartburn is chronic, it is referred to as *gastroesophageal reflux disease,* or GERD for short.

Heartburn can result from having a stomach that's too full. (Remember the old Alka-Seltzer ad? A man with a miserable look on his face moaned, "I can't believe I ate the whole thing!") It also arises due to a weakness of the muscular valve (sphincter) that normally prevents the stomach contents from entering the esophagus. The problem tends to occur when you are lying down, and so is more likely to strike at night.

Other common causes include obesity, cigarette smoking, and consumption of chocolate, fried foods, soft drinks, alcohol, and coffee. Many people produce acid when they become emotionally upset. This is one reason why it is so important to get your stress levels under control (see Lifestyle Tune-Up #2, following this chapter).

To help you pin down the cause of hyperacidity, complete Part B of the assessment.

DIGESTIVE ASSESSMENT • PART B

Ruling Out Ulcers
or Excess Stomach Acid Secretion (Hyperacidity)

Circle the number that best describes the intensity of your symptoms on the following scale:

   0 = I do not experience this symptom
   1 = Mild
   2 = Moderate
   3 = Severe

Stomach pains	0	1	2	3
Stomach pains just before and/or after meals	0	1	2	3
Dependency on antacids	0	1	2	3
Chronic abdominal pain	0	1	2	3
Butterfly sensations in stomach	0	1	2	3
Stomach pain when emotionally upset	0	1	2	3
Sudden, acute indigestion or heartburn	0	1	2	3
Relief of symptoms by carbonated beverages	0	1	2	3
Relief of stomach pain by drinking cream/milk	0	1	2	3
History of ulcer or gastritis	0	1	2	3
Black stool (not caused by taking iron supplements)	0	1	2	3

Add the numbers circled and enter that subtotal here: _____

Circle the number of the answer that applies to you:
   Do you currently have an ulcer?   NO = 0   YES = 10

Is the pain improved with antacids?   NO = 0   YES = 10

Add the numbers circled and enter that subtotal here: _____
Add the two subtotals and enter that total here: _____

Scoring   *9 or more: High priority*
5–8: Moderate priority
1–4: Low priority

Interpreting Your Score

An occasional bout of heartburn (reflux) should not be a cause for concern. However, if the problem is frequent, complications can emerge, including difficulty swallowing, bleeding ulcers, or even cancer of the esophagus. Chronic heartburn may be a sign of a hiatal hernia, an abnormal outpouching of the stomach above the diaphragm. However, while 50 percent of people over the age of fifty have hiatal hernias, only 5 percent of patients with hiatal hernias actually experience reflux esophagitis.

Consuming products that neutralize acid, such as antacid tablets, dairy foods, or carbonated beverages, usually relieves symptoms of hyperacidity. Normally the stomach produces thick mucus that protects its own cells from the corrosive effects of acid. In some people, though, this protective layer is insufficient, allowing the acid to inflame or even destroy the lining of the stomach, resulting in an ulcer.

A score above 9 in this section may indicate an ulcer. To be on the safe side, you must consult a physician for further evaluation if you think you have an ulcer.

WARNING   *Peptic ulcers are potentially serious disorders.* Left untreated, severe complications can develop, including bleeding, perforation (a hole penetrating completely through the stomach, causing leakage of stomach contents), and obstruction. These medical emergencies require immediate hospitalization. Patients with peptic ulcer should be monitored by physicians, even if they are taking any natural remedies.

When dealing with hyperacidity, prevention is always the best approach. In most cases this means identifying and eliminating any causative factors listed above. Perhaps the most effective treatment of chronic reflux esophagitis due to a hiatal hernia is good old-fashioned gravity. Try elevating your upper body when you sleep by placing four-inch blocks under the legs at the head of the bed.

Use antacids with caution. Such products are usually safe and effective when taken occasionally to treat acute heartburn. I usually advise my patients with hyperacidity to take preparations that contain both calcium carbonate and a special licorice extract known as DGL (see page 32) that helps heal and soothe an irritated esophagus and stomach. Calcium carbonate is the acid neutralizer in Tums. Although fast-acting and potent, calcium carbonate can produce what is known as acid rebound three or four hours after use. This means that the body will try to overcompensate for the neutralization of gastric acid by secreting even more acid. While this may not be a problem when treating indigestion, it may play a role in delaying ulcer healing. Be careful not to abuse antacids. Regular use can lead to such side effects as malabsorption of nutrients, bowel irregularities, and kidney stones.

Limit the use of sodium bicarbonate. Many people take sodium bicarbonate (baking soda) for relief of acid indigestion. (Alka-Seltzer is simply ordinary baking soda in a fizzy form.) Although sodium bicarbonate can be useful in the short term, using it often or regularly can increase your sodium intake to unnecessarily high levels. Long-term administration can cause systemic alkalosis (excessively high pH levels throughout the body), leading to such complications as the formation of kidney stones, nausea, vomiting, headache, and mental confusion.

Avoid antacids that contain aluminum. These products (such as Maalox, Rolaids, Di-Gel, Mylanta, and Riopan) are potent and effective, but their aluminum content raises concerns about their long-term safety. Aluminum may play a role in impairing mental function as well as in diseases of the nervous system including Alzheimer's disease, Parkinson's disease, and Lou Gehrig's disease (amyotrophic lateral sclerosis). Absorption of aluminum is made worse if the meal contains any source of citric acid, including citrus fruit, juice, or soda pop. I see no reason to use the aluminum-containing antacids, because the potential risks far outweigh the short-term benefit.

Magnesium salts such as magnesium oxide, magnesium hydroxide, or magnesium carbonate are often found in antacids containing aluminum. Phillips' milk of magnesia is the only major brand I'm aware of that contains only magnesium salts (as magnesium hydroxide) with no other ingredients. Besides acting as a mild antacid, magnesium hydroxide exerts a laxative effect. It is a safe and effective product for people with normal kidney function, though diarrhea is a definite risk.

Avoid the use of such drugs as Tagamet (cimetidine), Zantac (ranitidine), Pepcid (famotidine), and Axid (nizatidine). These drugs were once available only by prescription but are now available over the counter. They work by blocking the action of histamine, a chemical produced by cells that triggers secretion of stomach acid. However, overuse of these products commonly results in digestive disturbances, including nausea, constipation, and diarrhea. Nutrient deficiencies can appear as a result of impaired digestion. Other possible side effects include bacterial overgrowth (including overgrowth of *Helicobacter pylori [H. pylori]*, the organism that causes ulcers), liver damage, allergic reactions, headaches, breast enlargement in men, hair loss, osteoporosis, dizziness, depression, insomnia, and impotence.

Non-Ulcer Dyspepsia

Hyperacidity may also be responsible for a common condition labeled *non-ulcer dyspepsia,* or NUD. Basically, this is a catchall term that means "tummy trouble not caused by an ulcer." NUD—sometimes called irritated stomach syndrome—is a kind of wastebasket diagnosis doctors use when they cannot find any real reason for a patient's upper GI dysfunction, just as irritable bowel syndrome (IBS) is used as a wastebasket diagnosis for lower GI dysfunction.

Symptoms of NUD include heartburn as well as difficulty swallowing, feelings of pressure or heaviness after eating, sensations of bloating after eating, stomach or abdominal pains and cramps, as well as all of the symptoms of IBS. About three out of ten patients with NUD also meet the criteria for IBS.

For NUD, I recommend trying an herbal product by the name of Iberogast. This product, which since 1968 has been Germany's number one natural remedy for digestive disturbance, has recently been introduced into the United States. Iberogast is a formula containing nine herbal extracts. The main ingredient in the formula is clown's mustard (*Iberis amara*). This herb contains mildly bitter compounds known as cucurbitacins. The use of bitter herbs to enhance digestion is a very old therapy. (This is one of the reasons why parsley appears on your plate at restaurants.) Stimulating the bitter receptors on the tongue sets in motion the entire digestive process. For NUD, try Iberogast at a dosage of 20 drops in 4 ounces of water three times daily before meals.

CASE HISTORY: Gut Feelings

Marilee is a forty-four-year-old teacher in a Seattle elementary school. She resembles Sally Jessy Raphael, complete with red glasses. If Marilee were to appear as a guest on Sally's show, the episode might be called "I Can't Stomach This Any Longer!"

For as long as Marilee can remember, she's been plagued by vague but painful digestive disturbances: heartburn, difficulty swallowing, feelings of pressure or heaviness and bloating after eating. Sometimes the cramps were so severe she was out of commission for days on end. Over the years she'd visited scores of doctors. She'd been through every diagnostic test known— barium enemas, endoscopy, sigmoidoscopy, ultrasound. Nothing ever showed up on the resulting images. The best the doctors could come up with as a diagnosis was non-ulcer dyspepsia. No drugs worked to relieve her pain.

Curious about alternative methods, she came to see me. I asked her to undergo a comprehensive digestive stool analysis (a thorough analysis of feces) and food allergy tests. Meanwhile I recommended enteric-coated peppermint oil and pancreatic enzymes (Mega-Zyme, two tablets before meals). I also suggested she avoid all sources of dairy and gluten (that is, avoid all grains except rice).

I was shocked when the test results came back. They failed to reveal any abnormalities or allergies. Nor did the regimen I suggested seem to be helping much. Puzzled, I suggested we try a new approach using Iberogast. Marilee was the first patient for whom I recommended Iberogast, so I really did not know what to expect, but based on the studies I had read, I was quite optimistic.

Her response to the Iberogast was nothing short of astounding. Within a few weeks, she reported complete resolution of the problem that had bothered her for her entire life. Once she felt better, I suggested she try tapering off the Iberogast, but as soon as she cut back on the dose the symptoms began to recur. She'll probably need to keep taking it indefinitely, but she's perfectly happy to do so. I also referred her for acupuncture treatment, since acupuncture can work to stimulate the flow of energy in the digestive tract.

At our last visit she told me how happy she was. As she put it: "Now I can eat, drink, and be Marilee!"

Peptic Ulcer

A peptic ulcer is a hole that develops in the lining of the digestive tract resulting from the corrosive action of acid and the enzyme pepsin. In up to 90 percent of cases, a corkscrew-shaped bacterium known as *Helicobacter pylori*—*H. pylori* for short—appears to be a significant factor. The bug, one of the few that manages to survive in the acidic environment of the upper digestive tract, seems to burrow under the mucus layer and attach itself to the underlying cells. This weakens the protective layer and exposes the cells to acid juices. The bacteria also produce ammonia and other toxic substances, which may further reduce mucus production and trigger inflammatory reactions in the cells and thus lead to ulcer formation.

There are two main types of peptic ulcer. Ulcers in the stomach are called *gastric ulcers;* those that develop in the first segment of the small intestine are called *duodenal ulcers.* People who secrete high amounts of stomach acid tend to develop peptic ulcers more frequently. The chronic use of aspirin or other nonsteroidal anti-inflammatory drugs (NSAIDs) can cause ulcers. Smoking cigarettes or eating certain foods may also contribute to the problem.

Some people may experience no symptoms from a peptic ulcer. Others feel pain or abdominal discomfort forty-five to sixty minutes after a meal or during the night. My patients typically tell me that the pain is gnawing, burning, cramplike, or aching. Sometimes they describe it as "heartburn," but that's a different problem. Usually taking antacids relieves symptoms in a short time. However, antacids won't kill *H. pylori*.

Ulcers are a common problem, affecting over ten million Americans. They tend to occur in later life. Duodenal ulcers affect men four times as often as women.

To detect the presence of *H. pylori,* it is possible to measure the levels of antibodies your body produces in response to the bacteria in the blood or saliva. I prefer these methods to a procedure called endoscopy that involves inserting a flexible tube into the stomach and collecting samples of material, which can then be cultured in a lab to see if *H. pylori* is present.

The natural approach to dealing with peptic ulcers is first to identify and then to eliminate or reduce any factors that may contribute to their development. These include food allergies, a low-fiber diet, cigarette smoking, stress, alcohol, coffee, and drugs, especially NSAIDs (aspirin, ibuprofen, and related drugs). Try eating more slowly and chewing food thoroughly. You might see some improvement if you eat smaller meals more frequently. Once these factors have been controlled or eliminated, we then take steps to heal the ulcer and promote tissue resistance.

These steps also seem to help to eliminate *H. pylori:*

- Eliminate sugar and refined carbohydrates such as white flour from your diet.
- Eliminate milk and eggs.
- Increase the consumption of whole grains, legumes, and vegetables.
- Drink 16 to 24 ounces of vegetable juice per day, including cabbage juice on a regular basis.
- Take a high-potency multiple vitamin and mineral formula with meals.
- Take two to four chewable tablets of deglycyrrhizinated licorice (DGL) twenty minutes before meals. Continue DGL for eight to sixteen weeks after symptoms abate to ensure complete healing. (See Tune-Up Tip on page 32 for information on DGL.)

If symptoms do not disappear or significantly improve after two months, consider using bismuth preparations. Bismuth is a naturally oc-curring mineral that can act as an antacid as well as exert activity against *H. pylori*. The best-known and most widely used bismuth preparation is bismuth subsalicylate (Pepto-Bismol). However, bismuth subcitrate has produced the best results against *H. pylori* and in the treatment of non-ulcer-related indigestion, as well as peptic ulcers. (Bismuth subcitrate is available by prescription through compounding pharmacies. Call 1-800-331-2498 for a referral.) One of the key advantages of bismuth prepara-tions over standard antibiotic approaches is that while *H. pylori* may develop resistance to various antibiotics, it is very unlikely to develop re-sistance to bismuth.

WARNING Bismuth preparations should not be used for more than eight weeks and should not be taken by people with severe kidney disease. They should also not be taken at the same time as antacids or drugs that in-hibit stomach acid output, such as Pepcid, Axid, Tagamet, and Zantac.

The usual dosage for bismuth subcitrate is 240 mg twice daily be-fore meals for a period of four weeks, extended to eight weeks if nec-essary. Do not use bismuth preparations for more than eight weeks. Bismuth is essentially nontoxic in ordinary amounts, but prolonged or ex-cessive use may lead to toxicity. Long-term use or excessive dosages may cause mental confusion, memory loss, incoordination, slurred speech, joint pain, or muscle twitching and spasm.

Tune-Up Tip: Cabbage Juice May Be Right for "U"

Back in the 1950s, physicians at Stanford University showed that cabbage juice could be an effective treatment for peptic ulcers. The lead researcher, Garnett Cheney, believed that cabbage juice contained a substance he called "vitamin U" (for "ulcer"). Although this factor was never identified, Cheney clearly demonstrated that fresh cabbage juice relieved peptic ulcers, usually in less than seven days. Here's one of Dr. Cheney's favorite juice recipes:

> ½ head or 2 cups of green cabbage (green cabbage is best, but red cabbage is also useful)
>
> 2 tomatoes
>
> 4 ribs of celery
>
> 2 carrots

Cut the cabbage into long wedges and feed through the juicer, followed by the tomatoes, then the celery and carrots. Drink up!

Tune-Up Tip: Darn Good Licorice

My all-time favorite natural medicine is a special extract of licorice root known as DGL (it is short for "deglycyrrhizinated licorice," but I tell my patients that it stands for "darn good licorice"). DGL is produced by treating concentrated licorice root juice to remove glycyrrhetinic acid, a compound that can cause elevations in blood pressure due to sodium and water retention. (Yes, eating too much naturally flavored licorice candy can raise blood pressure.) Because the glycyrrhetinic acid has been removed, DGL does not raise blood pressure.

My fondness for DGL is the result of having used it effectively in treating even the most severe peptic ulcers. In fact, I cannot think of a case where DGL did not work. Rather than inhibit the release of acid, DGL stimulates the normal defense mechanisms that prevent ulcer formation. It improves both the quality and quantity of the protective substances that line the intestinal tract, increases the lifespan of the intestinal cell, and improves blood supply to the intestinal lining. There is also some evidence that it inhibits the growth of *H. pylori*.

Numerous clinical studies over the years support my experience. In several head-to-head studies, DGL has been shown to be more effective than

Tagamet, Zantac, or antacids in both short-term treatment and maintenance therapy of peptic ulcers.

The standard dosage for DGL is two to four chewable 380 mg tablets
taken between meals or twenty minutes before meals. Taking DGL after
meals is associated with poor results. DGL therapy should be continued for
at least eight to sixteen weeks after there is a full therapeutic response.

CASE HISTORY: An Acquired Taste Produces Dramatic Results

Tom, a forty-eight-year-old car salesman, did not come to see me for help
with his chronic ulcer. After battling the ulcer for more than eleven years, he
had given up hope. Instead, Tom wanted help for the excruciating pain in his
upper back. All that his medical doctor could offer were NSAIDs such as aspirin and ibuprofen, but Tom could not take these drugs because they aggravated his ulcer too much. After taking his medical history and performing an
exam, I suspected osteopenia—the lack of mineralization of the bone. An
X ray confirmed my suspicion: The severe pain in Tom's upper back resulted
from weakened vertebrae that were collapsing and pressing down on the
nerve roots.

Since being diagnosed with an ulcer more than a decade earlier, Tom
had been taking high doses of prescription Tagamet and over-the-counter
Maalox. This double whammy reduced hydrochloric acid secretion and his
symptoms, but it also blocked the absorption of calcium and other minerals
important for bone health. I told him that our goal was to get him off these
medications and on to a more natural (and rational) approach.

I prescribed a high-potency multiple vitamin and mineral formula along
with extra minerals. We would also use DGL, a special licorice extract, in the
form of chewable tablets. But Tom made a face and told me that he *hated*
licorice. "Can't I just swallow the tablets instead of chewing them?" he asked.
I explained that to be effective in healing peptic ulcers, DGL apparently
must mix with saliva so it can stimulate the growth and regeneration of stomach and intestinal cells. DGL in capsule form has not been shown to be
effective. Well, I guess Tom was desperate, because he agreed to give the
DGL a try.

I instructed him to discontinue Maalox but to continue with his current
dosage of Tagamet and take four tablets of DGL twenty minutes before
meals three times daily. He stocked up on enough DGL to last him till his
next appointment six weeks later.

But in just two weeks I was surprised to see Tom back in the waiting
room. He sheepishly told me that he was picking up some more DGL. He

had acquired a real taste for the stuff and had started eating it like candy. I had told him that DGL was completely safe with no side effects, but I was a little curious if maybe he was experiencing any adverse reactions from taking such high doses. "No," he answered with a smile. "The only 'side effect' I've noticed is that my back pain went away." The gnawing, burning pain that he had been experiencing almost nonstop for the past eleven years was a thing of the past. And he also told me that, despite my warning, he was so upset with the Tagamet that he had discontinued its use.

Tom is hardly a model patient. I told him—and I emphasize the point here—*not to discontinue any prescription medication without talking to a medical doctor first.* And even though something is considered safe, do not run the risk of side effects by exceeding the recommended dosage.

After three months of use, we dropped the DGL to two tablets three times daily. After a total of six months of use, we discontinued the DGL altogether. That was a dozen years ago. Tom has been free of all ulcer symptoms since that time.

The Small Intestine and Associated Organs

Let's return now to our tour of the digestive system. Once the stomach has done its part, muscular contractions of the stomach force the digested material (now called *chyme*, pronounced "kime") out of the stomach and into the small intestine. This narrow, muscular tube is about twenty-one feet long and has three sections, each of which plays a somewhat different role. The *duodenum*, the first ten to twelve inches, is where most of the minerals in your food get absorbed. The *jejunum*, about eight feet long, is the middle section, and is responsible for absorbing water-soluble vitamins, carbohydrates, and proteins. The *ileum* is the last and longest section, measuring about twelve feet, and handles absorption of fat-soluble vitamins, fat, cholesterol, and bile salts.

The inner lining of the small intestine contains thousands of tiny fingerlike projections called *villi* (plural of *villus*). These projections, which form a velvety surface, absorb the nutrients as they flow by. If the entire absorptive area of the small intestine were laid flat, it would be the size of a tennis court. Disorders of the small intestine often lead to malabsorption and various nutritional deficiencies.

Lactose Intolerance

After childhood, much of the world's population loses the ability to produce lactase, the enzyme responsible for digesting the sugar (lactose) found in dairy products. In addition to maturation of the intestine, a temporary lactase deficiency can be the result of infection or irritation, which strips the enzyme away from the surface of the intestinal lining. A primary defiency due to lacking the necessary genes to make the enzyme is quite rare.) Symptoms of lactose intolerance range from minor abdominal discomfort and bloating to severe diarrhea in response to even small amounts of lactose. Perhaps 70 to 90 percent of adults of Asian, African, Native American, and Mediterranean descent are lactase deficient. The deficiency occurs among only 10 to 15 percent of people of northern and western European descent.

Laboratory tests can determine if you are lactose intolerant, but these tests usually just tell patients what they already know: Milk gives them trouble. If you are lactose intolerant, you can buy lactose-free milk. There is also a product, Lactaid, that provides lactase in capsule form. But my recommendation is to stay away from milk and dairy products. You can find soy- or rice-based alternatives now that taste just like the real thing.

It's also a good idea to temporarily avoid milk products if you are suffering from intestinal infection, irritation, or inflammation, which, as I've noted, can cause many people to become lactose intolerant for a short while.

Celiac Disease

Celiac disease is an inherited disorder that causes people to become sensitive to a protein called gluten, a substance found in wheat and rye, and to a lesser extent in barley and oats. Many foods, including commercial soups, sauces, ice creams, and hot dogs, contain gluten to act as a thickening agent. People with celiac disease apparently lack the enzyme needed to digest gluten (or more specifically, a portion of gluten called gliadin). Instead, during digestion, part of the gluten molecule latches on to antibodies in the small intestine. As a result, the lining of the intestine—normally covered with tiny villi—flattens out and becomes smooth, and the intestine loses a lot of its ability to absorb nutrients. People with celiac disease (sometimes called nontropical sprue, gluten-sensitivity enteropathy, or celiac sprue) usually experience mild intestinal pain and indigestion, and they pass stools that are bulky, pale, frothy, greasy, and foul-smelling.

In the past, a biopsy (lab analysis of a tissue sample) was necessary to verify the presence of celiac disease. Today a simple blood test can detect the characteristic antibodies associated with the condition.

Once the diagnosis is established, the treatment is straightforward: Don't eat gluten! Avoid any products containing wheat, rye, barley, and oats, and do not consume milk products until you have been following a gluten-free diet for at least one month, as chronic inflammation due to celiac disease will strip the lactase enzyme away from the surface of the intestinal tract. Once gluten is removed from the diet, the villi of the small intestine usually spring back to life.

Supplementation with pancreatic enzymes (discussed below) may add to the clinical benefits of a gluten-free diet, especially during the first month of treatment. Also, taking 500 to 1,000 mg of papain, the protein-digesting enzyme from papaya, helps some people with celiac disease digest wheat gluten.

—— Bacterial Overgrowth in the Small Intestine ——

The upper portion of the human small intestine should be relatively free of bacteria. That's because bacteria compete with the body's cells for nutrition. When bacteria (or yeast) get to the food first, problems can occur (see Table 2–2). The organisms ferment carbohydrates, producing excessive gas, bloating, and abdominal distention. In a process called putrefaction, they also break down proteins and amino acids into smaller particles called vasoactive amines, which act on the smooth muscle in blood vessels. In the intestinal tract, excessive vasoactive amine synthesis can lead to increased gut permeability ("leaky gut" syndrome; see page 38), abdominal pain, slower passage of food through the intestine (decreased motility), and pain.

Table 2-2: Problems Resulting from Bacterial Overgrowth
            of the Small Intestine

- "Leaky gut" syndrome
- Vitamin deficiency
- Irritable bowel syndrome
- Inflammatory bowel disease (Crohn's disease and ulcerative colitis)
- Autoimmune conditions (for example, rheumatoid arthritis)
- Colon cancer
- Breast cancer
- Skin conditions (psoriasis, eczema, cystic acne)
- Chronic fatigue

Symptoms of bacterial overgrowth in the small intestine are similar to those generally attributed to low stomach acid or pancreatic insufficiency—that is, indigestion and a sense of fullness (bloating). Nausea and diarrhea can occur. Other symptoms are those generally associated with candida overgrowth (see page 56). Many people experience symptoms of arthritis.

Several factors can contribute to the problem of bacterial overgrowth.

- *A weak ileocecal valve.* The ileocecal valve separates the bacteria-rich colon from the ileum, the final segment of the small intestine. Weakness in the ileocecal valve usually results from a low-fiber diet, which can cause long-term constipation or straining excessively at defecation. Increasing dietary fiber may gradually strengthen the ileocecal valve.
- *Inadequate levels of digestive secretions, especially hydrochloric acid, bile, and pancreatic enzymes.* Strategies for dealing with decreased pancreatic enzyme levels and bile secretion are discussed on pages 40–45. See page 21 for information on low acidity in the stomach.
- *Decreased motility (peristalsis) in the small intestine.* Decreased motility most often results from a meal that is too high in sugar. The mechanism is simple. When blood sugar levels rise too rapidly, the brain signals the gastrointestinal tract to slow down. Since glucose is primarily absorbed in the duodenum and jejunum, the message most strongly affects these portions of the gastrointestinal tract. As a result, the duodenum and jejunum become "atonic"—they stop propelling chyme through the intestinal tract. Reducing sugar consumption may be helpful.
- *Low immune function, food allergies, stress, and other factors associated with a reduced level of secretory IgA, the antibody that protects mucous*

membranes. Restoring secretory IgA levels to normal involves eliminating food allergies and enhancing immune function (see pages
165–167). Stress is particularly detrimental to secretory IgA levels.
This explains in part why stressful events tend to worsen gastrointestinal function and food allergies. Tips for dealing with stress
more effectively are discussed in Lifestyle Tune-Up #2, following this
chapter.

"Leaky Gut" Syndrome

The mucous membrane that lines the entire small intestine functions
somewhat like a bouncer at a fancy nightclub. Its job is to let only the
"right" stuff get through to the bloodstream while blocking the "wrong"
stuff from gaining admittance. Normally the membrane is tightly struc-
tured so that only very small molecules, such as amino acids, can pass
through. But when problems such as bacterial overgrowth cause the
membrane to become more permeable, larger, incompletely digested
molecules can force their way into your circulation. The term for this
general condition is *intestinal permeability,* more colloquially known as
"leaky gut."

Large, unwanted molecules floating around in the body can act as toxins that trigger a whole spectrum of problems. Among the symptoms of
leaky gut are allergies, inflammation, rashes, diarrhea, and joint pain.
More serious complications include chronic and debilitating conditions
such as asthma, inflammatory joint diseases such as rheumatoid arthritis,
inflammatory bowel diseases such as Crohn's disease, and skin conditions including psoriasis. Some evidence even suggests that leaky gut may
be a factor in schizophrenia.

Possible causes of leaky gut include use of NSAIDs; infections with
bacteria, yeast, or viruses (including human immunodeficiency virus, or
HIV); or the presence of parasitic organisms such as giardia (sometimes
found in polluted water). Other causes include alcoholism, food allergies,
and poisons in the environment. As cells age, the spaces around them can
widen; consequently, leaky gut is a common complication of aging.

As you can imagine, the presence of toxins due to leaky gut can cause
your detoxification system to work overtime. I'll say more about that in
Chapter 3.

A simple clinical test can indicate whether you have leaky gut. During
the test, you drink a solution containing specific amounts of certain small
and large sugar molecules (mannitol and lactulose, respectively). Six

hours later you give a urine sample for lab analysis. The amounts of sugar in the urine indicate the rate at which the specific molecules enter your circulation. High levels of both sugars indicate leaky gut.

The first step in managing leaky gut syndrome is to determine what may be causing it, such as overuse of NSAIDs. Once those factors are under control, there are other natural steps you can take. Here are some natural strategies for bringing a leaky gut under control:

Identify and eliminate food allergies. See Chapter 5 for more information.

Take amino acids such as glutamine and arginine to reverse intestinal permeability and prevent further damage to the mucous membrane. Glutamine is an important nutrient that the cells of the small intestine need to thrive. Your body also needs glutamine to produce glutathione, an important compound for detoxification. One of the best natural sources of glutamine is whey protein. High-quality glutamine-enhanced whey products such as UniPro's Perfect Protein, Twin Lab's Whey Fuel, and Next Nutrition's Designer Whey Protein can be used to boost glutamine levels as long as you are not allergic to milk (though whey protein is less allergenic than casein, another milk protein). The dosage for glutamine is 3 to 5 g per day; for whey protein 25 to 30 g.

Eat plenty of fiber. In the large intestine, bacteria partially break down fiber to produce a short-chain fatty acid called butyrate. Butyrate is a crucial source of energy for cells in the intestine and is important for regeneration and repair of damaged cells.

Drink 12 to 16 ounces of fresh vegetable juice daily. Fresh vegetable juices are a good source of chlorophyll, which helps heal the intestines. You can also use one of the "green drinks" now on the market. Green drinks such as Barley Green, Kyo-Green, Greens +, Green Magma, and Pro Greens come in powder form, mix easily with water or juice, and are a convenient way to gain the healing benefits of chlorophyll. Drink two servings daily.

Take antioxidants. Antioxidants such as vitamins C and E, beta-carotene, zinc, and selenium can help repair or prevent damage to intestinal cells caused by free radicals. See Lifestyle Tune-Ups # 3 and 4 for dosage recommendations.

Take flaxseed oil. This oil contains key essential fatty acids, which your body uses to make prostaglandins. These hormonelike substances protect the intestinal lining. Take one tablespoon daily.

Be patient. It may take a few months for leaky gut syndrome to respond to dietary strategies.

The Pancreas, Liver, and Gallbladder

For intestinal digestion to proceed smoothly, your body needs to continue producing the right mix of fluids at the right time. As the chyme enters the duodenum, its presence triggers the release of secretions from the other key digestive organs: the pancreas, the liver, and the gallbladder.

Pancreatic Enzymes

The pancreas produces about a quart and a half of digestive juice each day. The juice flows through a duct leading directly into the duodenum. Pancreatic juice is packed with enzymes needed to digest each of the main types of nutrients: proteases (pronounced "PRO-tee-aces"), which are in charge of proteins; lipases, which handle fats; and amylases, which deal with starches and sugars. (As you've probably noticed, the names of many enzymes end in the suffix -ase.) The pancreas also is responsible for producing insulin and glucagon, two hormones that are responsible for controlling blood sugar. Unlike the enzymes that are released into the gastrointestinal tract, insulin and glucagon are secreted into the bloodstream.

There are three kinds of pancreatic proteases: trypsin, chymotrypsin, and carboxypeptidase. You need all three enzymes to handle the hundreds of kinds of proteins found in the diet. If there is a problem with the pancreas, such as a blockage in the duct, incomplete digestion of proteins can result, leading to such complications as allergies or the buildup of toxic substances.

Proteases serve other functions as well. They are responsible for keeping the small intestine free from unwanted critters, including bacteria, yeast, and parasites. (You have zillions of bacteria in your large intestine, but the small intestine is supposed to stay virtually bug-free.) Low levels of proteases can increase the risk of intestinal infection, such as chronic yeast (candida) infections.

While proteases handle proteins, amylases are busy attacking the sugars. Lactase, maltase, and sucrase break down specific complex sugar molecules (lactose, maltose, and sucrose; the suffix -ose indicates a sugar).

The lipases (fat enzymes) from the pancreas break down triglycerides into fatty acids and monoglycerides. Before these fat molecules can be absorbed, however, they need to mix with another digestive substance called bile.

Insufficient pancreatic enzymes can cause a range of digestive problems, including cramps, belching and gas, and diarrhea.

DIGESTIVE ASSESSMENT • PART C
Ruling Out Lack of Pancreatic Enzymes

Circle the number that best describes the intensity of your symptoms on the following scale:

  o = I do not experience this symptom
  1 = Mild
  2 = Moderate
  3 = Severe

Abdominal cramps	o	1	2	3
Indigestion or belching 1–3 hours after eating	o	1	2	3
Fatigue after eating	o	1	2	3
Gas in the lower bowel	o	1	2	3
Alternating constipation and diarrhea	o	1	2	3
Diarrhea	o	1	2	3
Large, greasy (shiny) stools	o	1	2	3
Stool poorly formed	o	1	2	3
Three or more large bowel movements daily	o	1	2	3
Foul-smelling stool or flatulence	o	1	2	3
Dry, flaky skin and/or dry, brittle hair	o	1	2	3
Pain in left side under rib cage	o	1	2	3
Acne	o	1	2	3
Food allergies	o	1	2	3

Add the numbers circled and enter that total here: _____

Scoring   *9 or more: High priority*
        5–8: Moderate priority
        1–4: Low priority

Interpreting Your Score

If you scored higher than 9 in this part of the Digestive Assessment, consider taking extra doses of pancreatic enzymes. In my experience, this is a very effective strategy for pancreatic insufficiency. Make sure you select a product that offers the right degree of enzyme activity for you (see the Tune-Up Tip). Most commercial preparations are derived from enzymes (pancreatin) found in hog pancreases.

Caution: *If you do not experience adequate results with pancreatic enzymes, you should consult a physician.*

Tune-Up Tip: Pancreatic Enzymes

The dosage of pancreatic enzymes is based on the level of enzyme activity in a given product as defined by the United States Pharmacopoeia (USP). Products classified as 1X have at least 25 USP units of amylase activity, at least 2 USP units of lipase activity, and 25 USP units of protease activity. Products of higher potency are labeled accordingly; for example, a 10X product would be ten times as strong as a 1X product. I recommend full-strength products, 8X to 10X, since those at lower strength may be diluted with ingredients such as salt, lactose, or galactose.

Enzyme products are often enteric-coated. This means the pill is coated with a substance that prevents it from breaking down in the stomach, thus delaying the release of enzymes until the pill passes into the small intestine. If you take a 10X USP pancreatic enzyme product, a typical dosage is 350 to 700 mg three times per day immediately before meals as a digestive aid. For anti-inflammatory effects, take the dose on an empty stomach.

Vegetarians or people who observe kosher diets may not want to consume animal-derived products such as pancreatin. They may take protein-digesting enzymes derived from pineapple (bromelain) or papaya (papain). The typical dosage for either is 100 to 200 mg before each meal.

Bile

The liver continuously manufactures bile, a thick, greenish yellow fluid. Bile is essential for the absorption of fats and fatty acids, oils, and fat-soluble vitamins. Bile also aids the action of enzymes. Bile works by breaking up large clumps of fats into smaller droplets and mixing them with water. They also bring water into the picture. This process, called emulsification, gives enzymes a head start in digesting fat molecules more effectively.

Like the proteases, bile helps keep the intestine free from microorganisms. Bile also makes the feces soft by promoting the binding of water into the stool. Constipation, or passage of hard, dry stools, may be the result of insufficient bile.

The liver secretes some bile through ducts that lead directly into the duodenum. The rest of the bile is carried over to the gallbladder, which stores bile until it is needed. Each day the intestine receives about a quart of bile; nearly all of the bile is reabsorbed and returned to the liver when it has completed its work.

DIGESTIVE ASSESSMENT • PART D
Ruling Out Lack of Bile Output

Circle the number that best describes the intensity of your symptoms on the following scale:

  0 = I do not experience this symptom
  1 = Mild
  2 = Moderate
  3 = Severe

Constipation	0	1	2	3
Small, hard, difficult-to-pass stools	0	1	2	3
Gray, shiny, soft stools	0	1	2	3
Pain in right side under rib cage	0	1	2	3
Voluminous flatulence	0	1	2	3
Roughage (fiber) causes constipation	0	1	2	3
Dry, flaky skin and/or dry, brittle hair	0	1	2	3
Indigestion 1–2 hours after eating	0	1	2	3

Add the numbers circled and enter that total here: _____

Scoring   *8 or more: High priority*
       4–7: Moderate priority
       1–3: Low priority

Interpreting Your Score

Some of the signs and symptoms of insufficient bile output can be due to other factors. For example, dry, flaky skin may be a sign of vitamin A or essential fatty acid deficiency. Since bile is required to absorb these fatty substances, insufficient bile output may result in deficiency of these and other nutrients even if dietary intake is adequate. What you take in is not as important as what you actually absorb. A score of 8 or more on this questionnaire indicates that you may benefit greatly from measures designed to increase bile output. A score of 4 to 7 indicates that you need to devote some attention to improving bile output while a score of 3 or less indicates that you may only need to follow the most basic recommendations below.

A sound diet, adequate water intake, and good overall health are usually all you need to produce adequate bile. However, if you have low bile output, it is possible to increase your levels by taking nutritional supplements containing choline (1,000 mg daily) and methionine (500 mg daily) or by taking the extract of artichoke leaves (see the Tune-Up Tip). Because bile can exert a mild laxative effect, increasing the output of bile is usually quite beneficial in treating constipation.

Tune-Up Tip: Artichoke Extract Improves Digestion

The globe artichoke *(Cynara scolymus)* is delicious and nutritious—and it also is good for the tummy. Artichokes have long been used as a folk remedy, but the value of artichoke extract in treating digestive problems is being validated by scientific studies. The secret ingredients are plant compounds known as caffeoylquinic acids.

An extract of the leaves of artichoke was shown to increase the flow of bile by up to 150 percent. Bile attracts water, and so the more bile you produce, the better your colon is able to produce soft, easily passed stools. Bile also helps keep the small intestine free from unwanted organisms.

In one study, patients who had suffered from digestive problems for an average of three years took one or two capsules of artichoke extract three times a day. After six weeks, over 70 percent of them reported significant improvement in their constipation. The treatment also relieved other problems, including vomiting, nausea, abdominal pain, and flatulence. Look for artichoke extracts standardized to contain 15 to 18 percent caffeoylquinic acids. Take 150 to 300 mg three times daily with meals.

CASE HISTORY: This Too Shall Pass

Jean, twenty-five years old, works at the cosmetic counter of a department store. She's a very attractive lady—I am sure many people ask her if she is a model.

For years Jean was bothered by chronic constipation. Her stools were small, hard, and difficult to pass, and her bowel movements—which occurred only every three days or so—were painful. "I don't understand," she said during our office visit. "When I take fiber supplements like Metamucil, it doesn't seem to help—it just makes things much worse."

She was right—it wasn't helping. In fact, it was hurting. Fiber is important, but your liver also has to produce enough bile, and the gallbladder must pump the bile into the small intestine. Without bile, fecal material is unable to hold water. Fiber is supposed to act like a sponge, but unless you have adequate bile, the sponge is dry and hard.

The solution for Jean was artichoke extract, two capsules (320 mg) twice a day, plus eight glasses of water per day. Once the extract got her bile flowing, her movements returned to normal. Now she feels as great on the inside as she looks on the outside.

The Large Intestine

The large intestine, also called the colon, is only about one-fourth the length of the small intestine, about 5 feet, but is considerably bigger in diameter (about 2½ inches, compared to about 1½ inches for the small intestine). By the time the chyme enters the large intestine, virtually all of the nutrients from the food have been absorbed. However, the large intestine absorbs much of the water, salts, and a few other particles. The large intestine is home to countless microbes, most of which are beneficial or harmless. Some of these bacteria help in the final breakdown of food particles. However, illness or poor diet can cause an overgrowth of unfriendly bacteria, a problem called dysbiosis. Your tune-up may involve taking steps to restore the proper balance of "good bugs."

There are basically two kinds of bacteria. Those that need oxygen are called aerobic bacteria; those that thrive without it are known as anaerobic. There is very little oxygen in your intestine (although, as you are well aware, you may produce other kinds of gas). Thus most of the normal bacteria present are anaerobes.

These bacteria act like enzymes in that they break down complex particles into smaller ones, a process known as fermentation. For example, some bacteria change complex sugars into carbon dioxide and alcohol. Other bacteria in your gut partially break down fiber to produce butyrate and other short-chain fatty acids. The cells that line your large intestine directly absorb these fatty acids and use them as one of their key sources of energy. In other words, the fats don't have to circulate in the bloodstream first. If your bacterial population is out of balance, you may not produce enough energy for your intestinal cells to stay healthy and function properly.

The last segment of the colon, about six to eight inches long, is the rectum, which serves as temporary storage for waste products until they can be excreted at the appropriate time. However, this material should be passed along promptly. If the feces remain too long, damage to the cells lining the intestine may occur, leading to a number of potentially serious health problems. A high-fiber diet and plenty of water are essential for maintaining the health of the large intestine. Such a diet increases the frequency and quantity of bowel movements, decreases the time it takes to move stool through the intestine, and decreases the absorption of toxins from the stool. Consuming adequate fiber helps prevent colon problems, including constipation, cancer, diverticulitis, hemorrhoids, and irritable bowel syndrome.

Typically, most people have one bowel movement a day. I think that's a reasonable goal and a good sign of healthy colon activity. But each person is different. Some people might normally have two or three movements a day, while others have one movement every other day. While you should aim for at least one movement a day, what's probably most important is that you have *regular* movements, which means that you have them with a fairly predictable pattern of frequency and at approximately the same time of day. Any change in bowel habits can be a sign of trouble somewhere along the digestive tract.

DIGESTIVE ASSESSMENT • PART E
Colon Function

Circle the number that best describes the intensity of your symptoms on the following scale:

0 = *I do not experience this symptom*
1 = *Mild*
2 = *Moderate*
3 = *Severe*

Alternating diarrhea and constipation	0	1	2	3
Lower abdominal pain or cramps	0	1	2	3
Abdominal distention or bloating	0	1	2	3
Straining at defecation	0	1	2	3
History of use of laxatives	0	1	2	3
Occasional diarrhea	0	1	2	3
Frequent and recurrent infections (colds)	0	1	2	3
Bladder and kidney infections	0	1	2	3
Rectal itching	0	1	2	3
Excessive gas	0	1	2	3

Add the numbers circled and enter that subtotal here: _____

Circle the number of the answer that applies to you:
Have you ever had a diagnosis of

Irritable bowel syndrome	NO = 0	YES = 3
Diverticulitis	NO = 0	YES = 3
Colon polyps	NO = 0	YES = 3
Ulcerative colitis	NO = 0	YES = 3
Hemorrhoids	NO = 0	YES = 3

Do you have bowel movements less than once
a day?   NO = 0   YES = 3

Add the numbers circled and enter that subtotal here: _____
Add the two subtotals and enter that total here: _____

Scoring   *9 or more: High priority*
             5–8: Moderate priority
             1–4: Low priority

Interpreting Your Score

A score of 9 or more means that you will definitely need to make tuning up your large intestine a high priority. If you suffer from a specific condition of the large intestine, focusing on the recommendations for that particular situation is the best choice. A score of 5 to 8 indicates that you need to devote some attention to improving colon function, while a score of 4 or less indicates that you may only need to follow the most basic recommendations to maintain proper functioning.

Constipation

One of the most common problems associated with the large intestine is constipation, which means the infrequent or difficult passage of hard, dry stools. Constipation is a problem for more than four million Americans. It occurs when stool remains in the bowel too long. The "transit time"—the time it takes for food to complete its passage through the digestive system—depends primarily on having adequate amounts of fiber in the diet. Without enough dietary fiber, waste material accumulates and the wrong type of bacteria overgrow. Among people who consume a very high-fiber diet (100 to 170 g of fiber a day), transit time is about thirty hours, producing about a pound of stool. Among Americans, who usually consume only about 20 g of fiber per day, transit time is forty-eight hours or more; typically, stools weigh only about a third of a pound. Besides low fiber, other possible causes of constipation include:

- Use of diuretics (water pills), which reduce body fluid levels
- Use of medications containing codeine, which slows down the muscle and nerve activity needed to pass stools
- Hypothyroidism
- Bowel obstruction (for example, from a polyp or tumor)

To prevent constipation, I recommend a diet that provides at least 25 to 30 g of fiber per day. Each year people in this country consume $400 million worth of commercial laxatives and stool softeners. A lot of that money would be better spent on high-fiber foods containing bran and other fiber-rich ingredients, such as pectin (see the Tune-Up Tip).

WARNING   There is a very good reason why there are warnings on the labels of stimulant laxatives such as senna and cascara preparations. Excessive use leads to dependence on them for a bowel movement. There is also significant concern regarding long-term safety, as long-term laxative use carries with it a threefold increase in colon cancer risk. Do not use stimulant laxatives for more than one week.

The other key strategies for preventing constipation are to drink plenty of water and get some regular exercise. Moving the body keeps all the systems humming, including the bowels. People who are sedentary often have transit times of seventy-two hours or more; in the elderly the time can be even longer.

Tune-Up Tip: Pears for Pectin

One of the best foods to help tune up the gastrointestinal tract is the humble pear. Pears are an excellent source of soluble fiber, including pectin. In fact, pears are actually higher in pectin that apples. This also makes them quite useful in helping to lower cholesterol levels.

I grew up in southern Oregon, some of the best pear-growing country in the world. There are many varieties of pears. My favorites are Anjou, Bartlett, and Comice. Fresh pears are best when they yield to pressure similar to an avocado. Unripe pears will ripen at home if stored at room temperature. Once ripe, they should be refrigerated.

Bowel Retraining

Some people develop unhealthy habits that actually "train" the bowel to become constipated. For example, they ignore the "call of nature" and do not visit the toilet as soon as the urge strikes. Other people become dependent on laxatives to produce a bowel movement. Fortunately, it is possible to retrain your body and develop a more regular pattern of bowel movements.

- Eat a high-fiber diet, particularly fruits and vegetables.
- Drink six to eight glasses of fluids per day.
- Identify known causes of constipation—for example, not enough fiber in the diet or the use of drugs such as diuretics.

- Do not repress an urge to defecate, but visit the toilet as soon as you can.
- Sit on the toilet at the same time every day (even when the urge to defecate is not present), preferably immediately after breakfast or exercise.
- Exercise at least twenty minutes three times per week.
- Take 3 to 5 g of a gel-forming fiber supplement (such as Metamucil or other psyllium preparations) at night before retiring.
- Do not take enemas.
- Taper off using laxatives. In the first week, take a stimulant laxative containing either cascara or senna every night before bed. Take the lowest amount necessary to reliably ensure a bowel movement every morning. Each week thereafter, decrease the dosage by half. If constipation recurs, go back to the previous week's dosage. Decrease dosage if diarrhea occurs.

Tune-Up Tip: If Your Child Is Constipated

For children with a history of constipation, the first thing I recommend is eliminating milk and other dairy products from the diet. It is well accepted that intolerance to cow's milk (the result of either an allergy or lactose intolerance) can produce diarrhea. What is not as well known is the fact that cow's milk intolerance can also lead to constipation. A study published in the *New England Journal of Medicine* in 1998 provides ample evidence of this association. The study involved sixty-five children with chronic constipation (defined as having one bowel movement every three to fifteen days). All of the children had been referred to a pediatric gastroenterology clinic and had previously been treated with laxatives without success. After fifteen days of observation, the patients received cow's milk or soy milk for two weeks. After a one-week period with no milk of any kind, the feedings were reversed. A positive response was defined as eight or more bowel movements during a treatment period. Forty-four of the sixty-five children (68 percent) had a positive response while receiving soy milk. None of the children who received cow's milk had a positive response. In all forty-four children with a positive response, the response was confirmed with a double-blind challenge with cow's milk. When the children were given cow's milk, they also had a higher frequency of allergy symptoms, including runny nose, eczema, and asthma.

If your child is constipated, start by eliminating cow's milk and other dairy products while increasing the intake of high-fiber foods, especially pears, apples, and other whole fruit. If this approach is not successful, try Maltsupex (a barley malt extract available at any drugstore). Avoid mineral oil as well as stimulant laxatives such as cascara unless absolutely necessary.

Irritable Bowel Syndrome

Irritable bowel syndrome (IBS) is a very common condition in which the large intestine fails to function properly. IBS has also been known as nervous indigestion, spastic colitis, mucous colitis, and intestinal neurosis. Approximately 15 percent of the population suffers from IBS at some time in their lives. Characteristic symptoms of IBS include:

- Abdominal pain and distension
- More frequent bowel movements
- Pain during bowel movements or relief of abdominal pain with movements
- Constipation or diarrhea
- Excessive production of mucus in the colon
- Flatulence
- Nausea
- Loss of appetite
- Anxiety
- Depression

Stress is a major component of IBS, as well as most other gastrointestinal disorders (be sure to read Lifestyle Tune-Up #2, following this chapter).

The main dietary causes of IBS are lack of dietary fiber or food allergies, or both. Simply increasing the intake of plant food in the diet is effective in many cases. Try to eat foods containing soluble fiber, such as vegetables, fruits, oat bran, and legumes (beans, peas, and so on). This kind of fiber produces a softer stool, which is easier to pass during a movement. (The fiber found in wheat bran is insoluble.) As a bonus, soluble fiber is better at lowering cholesterol levels.

You may want to take a supplement rich in soluble fiber. Choose formulas that contain one or more of these fiber sources: psyllium seed husks, pectin, oat bran, guar gum, beet fiber, carrot fiber. For best results, I recommend that you take enough of the formula to provide 3 to 5 g of fiber. Take your dose at night, an hour or so before going to bed. The goal is to trigger an easy bowel movement in the morning.

Avoid white table sugar, or sucrose. Sugar has a very detrimental effect on bowel function, particularly in patients with IBS.

Nearly two out of three patients with IBS have allergies to one or more foods. The most common foods causing problems in IBS are milk and dairy products, corn, wheat, eggs, peanuts, and chocolate. I recommend eliminating all of these foods for at least a week in order to determine if a food allergy is the problem. After a week, if symptoms improve, slowly add one food back every three or four days. If symptoms return, you are likely allergic to that food.

If you have followed the above steps but still have symptoms of IBS, you may want to try peppermint oil (see the Tune-Up Tip).

Tune-Up Tip: Mint Condition

For relief of irritable bowel syndrome (IBS), try peppermint oil. Select an enteric-coated preparation, which prevents the oil from being released in the stomach; this allows it to reach the small and large intestines, where it relaxes intestinal muscles. (Without enteric coating, peppermint oil tends to produce heartburn.) Several double-blind studies have shown enteric-coated peppermint oil capsules to be a very effective treatment of irritable bowel syndrome, with roughly eight out of ten people gaining significant relief or complete elimination of their symptoms.

Enteric-coated peppermint oil is thought to work by improving the rhythmic contractions of the intestinal tract and relieving intestinal spasm. An additional benefit is its effectiveness against *Candida albicans* (an overgrowth of *C. albicans* may be an underlying factor in IBS, especially in cases that do not respond to dietary advice and for those who consume large amounts of sugar).

Peppermint oil usually does the job. If after a month results are less than satisfactory, you might consider trying artichoke extract (see page 44), which relieves a wide range of digestive symptoms.

———— Dysbiosis: Bugs out of Balance ————

Right now you have more bacteria milling about in your intestinal tract than you have cells in your body. We're talking trillions here. And there are more than four hundred different species present at any given time.

We couldn't survive for long without these little creatures. They inhibit diseases (including cancer), control the acid levels in the intestine, reduce cholesterol, and help your body incorporate vitamins so it can make the necessary enzymes.

The most important good bugs are *Lactobacillus acidophilus* and *Bifi-*

dobacterium bifidum. Foods fermented with lactobacilli—yogurt, cheese, miso, and tempeh—are of great importance in the diets of many cultures around the world. It's possible to supplement the diet with additional doses of acidophilus (see the Tune-Up Tip). This strategy helps prevent and treat such conditions as antibiotic-induced diarrhea, yeast overgrowth, and urinary tract infections.

Tune-Up Tip: Billions of Bugs

Probiotics—which, literally translated, means "for life"—is a term used to signify the health-promoting effects of "friendly" bacteria as well as substances that promote their growth. Doses of probiotic bacteria are measured in terms of the number of bacteria contained in the product. If you are suffering from an intestinal disorder, I recommend a probiotic supplement that provides at least five to ten billion live organisms daily. Less than that may be ineffective; conversely, if you take too much more, you may feel some mild gastrointestinal disturbance. However, if you are currently taking a prescription antibiotic, you may need to take doses of up to twenty billion organisms to counteract its effects.

Consider taking additional doses of FOS (fructooligosaccharides) along with your probiotic bacteria. These sugars are fuel that bacteria need to grow but that your body does not metabolize. A typical dosage is 1,000 to 3,000 mg daily.

You don't need to keep taking such a regimen forever. Once your bacterial balance is restored after a month or so, you can taper off.

Sometimes the numbers of unfriendly bacteria rise, crowding out the friendly species. A popular term for this condition is *dysbiosis*. There are different patterns of dysbiosis (see page 54), and the potential consequences are many and serious (see Table 2-2, on page 37).

THE STRAIGHT POOP

By rummaging through your trash barrel, a nosy person might learn a lot about the way you live. Similarly, it is possible to learn a great deal of information about what's going in your body by analyzing what you "throw away"—that is, your feces.

In my practice, I ask most of my patients with digestive disturbances to undergo a test called the comprehensive digestive stool analysis (CDSA). The test involves collecting a stool sample and sending it to a laboratory for study and interpretation. By studying the results, I can tell how well your digestive system is working—if you are absorbing nutrients properly, whether you have the correct balance of bacteria and yeast, and whether your immune function is up to par. There are three laboratories that I am familiar with that provide this often necessary battery of tests. These labs will happily send your doctor information on the CDSA.

- Great Smokies Diagnostic Laboratory (1-800-522-4762)
- Diagnost-Techs (1-800-87-TESTS)
- Meridian Valley Clinical Laboratory (1-253-859-8700)

According to Leo Galland, M.D., a leading expert in dysbiosis, abnormal bacterial overgrowth occurs in four interconnected patterns: putrefaction, deficiency, fermentation excess, and sensitization.

Putrefaction is common among people who consume a diet high in fat and low in fiber. Such a diet causes bugs called *Bacteroides* to flourish. The presence of these bacteria stimulates activity by certain enzymes that break down bile, causing an increase in both tumor-causing particles and in estrogen levels. In turn, high hormone levels can stimulate the growth of cancer in the colon and breast. Diets low in fat and high in fiber reverse the problem. Treatment with probiotics can help.

Deficiency arises when the numbers of friendly bacteria (bifidobacteria, lactobacilli, and *Escherichia coli*) dwindle. This pattern is common among people with irritable bowel syndrome or food intolerance. Deficiency and putrefaction often occur in the same person and are addressed in the same way.

Fermentation excess occurs when normally friendly bacteria go into overdrive. One result is excess production of gas, leading to abdominal distention, flatulence, diarrhea or constipation, and an overall blah feeling. This condition is usually seen in people who consume high levels of carbohydrates. Cutting back on carbohydrates and fiber can help.

Sensitization basically means that your body is allergic to bacteria that are harmless to most people. The presence of the bacteria triggers an immune response, involving the release of substances that are designed to fight infection. The longer the bacteria persist, and the more of them there are, the more your body tries to eradicate them. The result may be inflammatory bowel disease, connective tissue diseases, on skin disorders. Supplementation with probiotics and an increase in dietary fiber can help.

CASE HISTORY: Fighting Bugs with Bugs

A patient I'll call Marty is a thirty-eight-year-old stockbroker. He's in good health and is athletic. If you saw him on the street, you might think he looks a bit like the actor Robert Downey Jr. He has that same sort of manic energy at times as well.

Marty came to me for help with a problem that he found pretty embarrassing: He was passing huge amounts of gas throughout the day, and his rectum itched like mad all the time. I asked him a personal question: "Is the gas odorous?" He was a little surprised by his own answer: "You know, thank goodness, it's really not."

The lack of smell was a clue. From Marty's history I learned that his symptoms had begun three months before, after he had visited Thailand. He returned from his trip with some beautiful souvenir silks and a whopping case of diarrhea. His doctor did not identify any parasite, so the most likely diagnosis was traveler's diarrhea, caused by exposure to different strains of normal gut inhabitants.

The doctor prescribed several courses of an antibiotic. The drug worked for a few days, but soon Marty developed symptoms of a condition called pseudomembranous enterocolitis (PME), also known as antibiotic-associated colitis. The name tells the tale: His colitis, or inflammation of the colon, was the result of his antibiotic therapy. The drug killed the friendly bacteria and promoted the overgrowth of toxin-producing microbes. The toxins were irritating his intestine. They were also generating gas. Results from Marty's lab test (the comprehensive stool and digestive analysis) confirmed my suspicions. He had an overgrowth of yeast (*Candida albicans*); also, some bacteria that shouldn't have been there showed up on the culture.

Rather than give Marty more antibiotics, I placed him on a regimen of probiotics. To replace his missing "good bugs," I recommended doses of three billion *Lactobacillus acidophilus* and *Bifidobacterium bifidum* organisms at breakfast. I also suggested use of enteric-coated oregano oil to help control the yeast overgrowth. Oregano oil is quite toxic to the yeast, and the enteric coating helps the oregano oil get to the small and large intestine. For good measure, I asked Marty to take 3 g of psyllium seed husks with 12 ounces of apple juice at night to make sure he got enough fiber to feed the good bugs as well as to help bind some of the toxins being formed as the yeast was dying off. He also avoided refined sugar and dairy products.

After a month of this treatment, Marty's problem resolved. I told him that when he is planning to travel to a third world country or an area where there is poor water quality or sanitation, he should supplement with two billion live *L. acidophilus* and *B. bifidum* daily at least one week prior to his trip, during his stay, and one week after visiting. He told me that he plans to return to Thailand—but that he won't be returning to the doctor who prescribed antibiotics.

Yeast Overgrowth

In addition to dysbiosis, an overgrowth of the usually benign yeast *Candida albicans* in the large intestine causes the complex medical syndrome known as chronic candidiasis or "yeast syndrome." Overgrowth with candida may cause a wide variety of symptoms not just in the gastrointestinal tract but in virtually every system of the body, including the genitourinary, endocrine, nervous, and immune systems.

As is true of all yeasts (which are fungi), *Candida albicans* normally lives harmoniously in the creases and crevices of the digestive tract (and the vaginal tract in women). However, when this yeast overgrows, and if immune system mechanisms are depleted or if the normal lining of the intestinal tract is damaged, the body can absorb yeast cells, particles of yeast cells, and various toxins they produce. If this happens, numerous body processes may be disrupted. Yeast syndrome is characterized by malaise, which is a general feeling of being sick all over—kind of like a mild but nagging flu. Fatigue, allergies, immune system malfunction, depression, chemical sensitivities, and digestive disturbances are just some of the symptoms you may experience if you have yeast syndrome.

Women are eight times more likely than men to experience yeast syndrome. This is because the yeast balance can be disturbed due to the effects of estrogen, birth control pills, and the more frequent use of antibiotics by women. A profile of a typical patient with candidiasis appears in Table 2-3.

Table 2-3: Candidiasis Patient Profile

Sex: Female
Age: 15–50
General symptoms:
- Chronic fatigue
- Loss of energy
- General malaise

- Decreased libido
Gastrointestinal symptoms:
- Thrush
- Bloating, gas
- Intestinal cramps
- Rectal itch

- Altered bowel function

Genitourinary system complaints:
- Vaginal yeast infection
- Frequent bladder infections

Endocrine system complaints:
- Primarily menstrual complaints

Nervous system complaints:
- Depression
- Irritability
- Inability to concentrate

Immune system complaints:
- Allergies
- Chemical sensitivities
- Low immune function

History:
- Chronic vaginal yeast infections

- Chronic antibiotic use for infections or acne
- Oral birth control usage
- Oral steroid hormone usage

Associated conditions:
- Premenstrual syndrome
- Sensitivity to foods, chemicals, and other allergens
- Endocrine disturbances
- Eczema
- Psoriasis
- Irritable bowel syndrome

Other:
- Craving for foods rich in carbohydrates or yeast

Here is a seven-step plan for dealing with yeast overgrowth.

Step 1: Identify and address predisposing factors. Eliminate the use of antibiotics, steroids, immune-suppressing drugs, and birth control pills (unless there is an absolutely necessary medical reason; check with your doctor). Determine if decreased digestive secretions may be contributing to the problem (see pages 22–23, 41 and 43). Seek treatment for problems such as diabetes, impaired immunity, or impaired liver function, all of which can predispose you to yeast overgrowth.

Step 2: Follow a candida control diet. This means eliminating from your diet refined sugar and other simple sugars, milk or other dairy products (because of trace levels of antibiotics), and foods with a high content of yeast or mold, including alcoholic beverages, cheeses, dried fruits, melons, and peanuts. Also, avoid all known or suspected food allergies.

Step 3: Provide nutritional support. Take a high-potency multiple vitamin and mineral formula, additional antioxidants, and 1 tbsp of flaxseed oil daily.

Step 4: Support immune function. Deal with stress by using positive stress-coping techniques (see Lifestyle Tune-Up #2, following this chapter). Avoid factors that can impair immune function, such as alcohol, sugar, smoking, and elevated cholesterol levels. Make sure that you get plenty of rest and good-quality sleep as well. Another measure you can take is to support your thymus gland function by taking 750 mg of crude polypeptide fractions daily (see page 160).

Step 5: Promote detoxification and elimination. Help your body cleanse itself by taking 3 to 5 grams of a soluble fiber source such as guar gum, psyllium seed, or pectin at night.

Step 6: Take probiotics. Ingest five to ten billion viable *L. acidophilus* and *B. bifidum* cells daily.

Step 7: Use appropriate antiyeast therapy. My approach in the past few years has been to use an enteric-coated volatile oil preparation (such as Candida Formula from Enzymatic Therapy or, previous to this product's introduction, Peppermint Plus from Enzymatic Therapy or ADP from Biotics Research Laboratories) at a dosage of two capsules twice daily between meals with a glass of water, along with one tablet of an enteric-coated fresh garlic preparation (for example, Garlinase, Garlipure, Garlique, or Garlicin). I have found this approach to be effective in eliminating the overgrowth of *Candida albicans* in most cases. Use for at least one month.

These simple steps should take care of most cases of chronic candidiasis. If you don't notice significant improvement or complete resolution within one month, find a physician in your area who is knowledgeable about yeast syndrome. A prescription antiyeast drug may be appropriate.

——— Preventing Colon and Rectal Cancer ———

The cells in your large intestine are exposed to many types of substances that result from digestion and the activity of microorganisms. What's more, the cells have a high turnover rate—your intestinal lining completely replaces its cells every week or so. All this metabolic activity makes the cells particularly vulnerable to damage. In some cases, that damage can result in cancer of the colon or rectum.

Not counting skin cancer, colon and rectal (colorectal) cancers are the fourth most common form of cancer. Approximately fifty-six thousand people in the United States will die this year because of the disease, accounting for about 3 percent of all deaths.

While scientists do not know the exact cause of colorectal cancer, we do know that it is among the most preventable forms of cancer, even in people with a positive family history of this disease. Clearly diet plays a huge role. The typical American diet—high in fat, low in fiber from fruits and vegetables—is largely to blame. Fat takes longer to digest than other nutrients. Breaking down fat can cause a kind of residue to form in the intestine. This residue irritates cells and can cause them to become abnormal. What's more, as I've explained, fat triggers production of bile, and bile acids may further irritate and damage cells. Lack of fiber means all this bad stuff isn't able to pass out of the intestine as fast as it should.

Colorectal cancer often begins when a polyp grows on the intestinal lining. A polyp is a mushroom-shaped clump of tissue. Most polyps are harmless, but a small percentage of them can become cancerous. Colorectal cancer may or may not cause symptoms (see box).

POSSIBLE SYMPTOMS OF COLORECTAL CANCER

- Change in bowel habits
  - Diarrhea
  - Constipation
  - Narrow stools
- Blood in the stool
- Weakness or fatigue
- Cramping or gnawing abdominal pain
- Loss of appetite or nausea
- Weight loss
- Straining during a bowel movement (especially common in rectal cancer)

Your doctor can detect polyps through a procedure called a sigmoidoscopy, which uses a viewing scope to examine the lower part of the intestine, or a colonoscopy, which explores the whole organ. Often the polyp can be removed by snipping it off at the base. However, if many polyps are present, or if some of them appear to be progressing into cancer, it may be necessary to remove a section of the intestine through surgery.

Obviously, preventing colorectal cancer is the best way to go. The best strategy is to eat a healthy diet. Cut down on meat, protein, and animal fat. Avoid meat that has been fried, charcoal-grilled, or cooked at high temperatures; these forms of preparation produce high levels of cancer-causing compounds. Increase fiber intake by eating fruits, vegetables, and whole grains. Foods rich in calcium, vitamin C, and folate appear to offer protection.

Calcium is of special interest, because it readily binds with irritants in the colon and blocks their ability to stimulate cell proliferation. A recent study found that when people who had had polyps removed supplemented their diet with 1,200 mg of calcium a day, cell growth in the colon returned to normal.

A healthy lifestyle helps too. Drinking more than one or two alcoholic beverages—especially beer—a day appears to increase the risk, perhaps by encouraging cells to reproduce more rapidly and by damaging the new cells. Cigarette smoking may cause a high risk of polyps; in smokers, polyps are more likely to regrow after they have been removed. People who exercise throughout their lives and who maintain a healthy weight have a lower rate of colorectal cancer. Some evidence suggests that taking aspirin and other NSAIDs or, better yet, natural inhibitors of prostaglandin may help (see the Tune-Up Tip).

Tune-Up Tip: When All Is NSAID and Done . . .

Evidence is mounting that aspirin and other pain-relieving drugs may prevent colorectal cancer. These drugs work by reducing production of prostaglandins, which can irritate cells or cause them to grow abnormally. It may be, too, that prostaglandins are involved in changing a harmless polyp into a potentially life-threatening tumor.

Rather than recommending aspirin, however, I encourage you to utilize turmeric or preparations containing the yellow pigment of turmeric, curcumin. This compound has been shown to exert even more impressive effects than aspirin in inhibiting colon cancer in animal studies. In addition to inhibiting prostaglandin formation, curcumin also exhibits potent antioxidant effects (in some experimental studies it was up to three hundred times more potent than vitamin E). In addition to eating more curries (turmeric is the major component of curries), you can take 100 to 200 mg of curcumin daily to reduce colon cancer risk.

Key Steps to Tuning Up Your Digestive System

- Eat in a relaxed setting.
- Take the time necessary to thoroughly chew (and enjoy) your meal.
- Identify problem areas, such as low output of hydrochloric acid or pancreatic enzymes, and take appropriate steps to rectify the situation.
- Maintain the right balance of bacterial flora by consuming a diet rich in plant foods for their dietary fiber. If necessary, take probiotics to promote the growth of beneficial bacteria (*Lactobacillus acidophilus*

and *Bifidobacterium bifidum,* five billion to ten billion organisms daily, or up to twenty billion if you are taking an antibiotic) until the problem resolves.

- Improve your stress response (see Lifestyle Tune-Up #2, following this chapter).

Lifestyle Tune-Up #2: Learn to Deal with Stress

Put simply, stress is anything that causes your body to react. That reaction is your body's effort to relieve the stress. In Chapter 1 I explained how the body works constantly to keep things running as steadily as possible. The term for this is *homeostasis*. Anything that throws your system out of homeostasis is a stressor. How seriously stress affects you depends on two main factors: the intensity of the stressor and the power of your body to respond.

The stomach and intestines are often hit hard by stress because the stress reaction diverts energy away from the digestive tract and toward the muscles. Under stress, the body prepares to fight or run. Digestion will just have to wait until the danger has passed. With the digestive system on hold due to stress, essential nutrients will not be absorbed. Without those nutrients, the supply of energy stored in the cells is not being replenished. Over time, as stress persists, the energy supply gets used up. As a result, we get tired, often to the point of exhaustion. At that point, disease organisms are more likely to penetrate our defenses and make us ill. The longer stress persists, the worse the problem gets. We humans are simply not designed to live under constant high stress.

In a sense, the numerous systems of the body are like a chain made of many links. Some of these links are stronger than others. Under stress, the weakest link is always the first to break. Which link is likely to snap depends on many factors. This is where the concept of biochemical individuality comes into play. Often the first signs of chronic stress are problems with digestion. However, for someone born with a tendency to develop heart disease, stress may be more likely to cause a heart attack or stroke. Constant high blood pressure can damage blood vessels, potentially causing them to rupture. The relentless onslaught of stress hormones can inflame tissues, leading to pain and soreness in the joints or to damage in the mucous membranes of the lungs. As a result, in some people, stress can lead to a range of debilitating conditions such as arthritis or asthma. In other individuals, the immune system may be the first to collapse, leaving the person vulnerable to chronic infections.

There are two main strategies for addressing the problem of stress in our lives. The first is to identify the causes of stress and take whatever steps possible to reduce the number of stressors or their severity. The other strategy is to tune up the body and provide it with all the resources it needs to fend off the damage resulting from stress. In other words, we can work to make all of the links of the chain stronger.

Conditions Linked to Stress

Angina	Headaches
Asthma	High blood pressure
Autoimmune disease	Irritable bowel syndrome
Cancer	Lowered immunity
Cardiovascular disease	Menstrual irregularities
Colds	Non-ulcer dyspepsia
Depression	Rheumatoid arthritis
Diabetes (type 2, non-insulin- dependent)	Ulcerative colitis
	Ulcers

Throughout our lives, each of us develops our own ways of coping with stress. Some of those strategies are healthier than others. For example, one person might relieve stress by taking long, relaxing walks or watching funny movies. Another might drink alcohol, use drugs, overeat, or have an inappropriate emotional outburst. If you want to be healthy (and happy), you must develop positive methods for managing stress.

One of the most important things you can do to battle stress is to learn how to breathe properly. I learned a lot about breathing by observing my daughter, Alexa, when she was just a baby. Like any doting father, I often stood over her crib and watched her as she slept. I was amazed to see how fully her chest rose and fell with each breath. One time I became aware of how tight my own chest felt just then. Not wanting to disturb Alexa, I had been holding my breath. As soon as I relaxed, I felt a wave of calmness and love wash over me. A baby's body is smart—it lets breathing happen as deeply and naturally as possible. Later in life, to our detriment, we begin to control breathing more consciously. Sometimes we forget how to do it right.

Proper breathing requires the use of the diaphragm, a dome-shaped muscle that separates the chest from the abdomen. When you breathe in, the diaphragm contracts and pulls downward, enlarging the chest. This helps you draw air into the lungs. When you breathe out, the diaphragm rises, helping you expel air. (The diaphragm also serves another function: It acts as a pump that promotes circulation of the lymph fluid. More about the lymphatic system appears in Chapter 5.) Using the diaphragm when you breathe directly activates the parasympathetic nerves. This, in turn, induces the relaxation response.

To improve your ability to breathe from the diaphragm, practice the following deep-breathing exercise for five minutes to ten minutes at least twice a day.

- Find a quiet, comfortable place to sit or lie down.
- Place your feet slightly apart. Place one hand on your abdomen near your navel. Place the other hand on your chest.
- Inhale through your nose and exhale through your mouth.
- Concentrate on your breathing. Notice which hand is rising and falling with each breath.
- Gently exhale most of the air in your lungs.
- Inhale while slowly counting to four. As you inhale, slightly extend your abdomen, causing it to rise about one inch. Make sure that you are not moving your chest or shoulders.
- As you breathe in, imagine the warmed air flowing in. Imagine this warmth flowing to all parts of your body.
- Pause for one second, then slowly exhale to a count of four. As you exhale, your abdomen should move inward.
- As the air flows out, imagine all your tension and stress leaving your body.
- Repeat the process for five to ten minutes or until you achieve a sense of deep relaxation.

Of course, there is more to dealing with stress than learning how to breathe, but it is the first step. I will give you other tips for dealing with stress in subsequent chapters.

Tuning Up Your Detoxification System

Without filters and an effective exhaust system to remove the gunk and combustion by-products from the engine, your car would quickly grind to a halt. In a similar way, your body works constantly to get rid of many dangerous substances. Some of these poisons are found in the environment, contained in things you eat, inhale, or touch. But others are the product of your body's own metabolic activity—the "exhaust" that results whenever chemical processes take place.

Substances that pose a threat to your body's cells are known as toxins. The job of detoxifying—neutralizing or eliminating toxins—is carried out partly by the intestines, the kidneys, and even the lungs and skin. But the lion's share of the work is handled by one of the most remarkable organs you have: the liver.

When either the liver or kidneys are not functioning properly, cellular waste and toxins accumulate in every body tissue. Imagine what your house would be like if you never took out the garbage. Gross, isn't it? If your liver or kidneys are not functioning properly, that's what happens to your body. Some of the sickest-looking people I have seen in my clinical practice have been patients with severe liver or kidney disease such as cirrhosis of the liver, hepatitis, liver cancer, and chronic renal failure.

You do not have to have liver or kidney disease to gain the enormous benefits of tuning up liver function. In fact, I will go so far as to say that if you are a relatively healthy person, this chapter is the most important one in the whole book. The recommendations I offer here can dramatically change your life.

The Liver

The liver is the second-largest organ in the body (your skin is the largest). It is also the largest gland (an organ that manufactures and secretes substances other tissues need). The liver performs over five hundred separate jobs. Here are some of its crucial functions:

- It produces glucose (blood sugar) from nutrients other than carbohydrates.
- It converts glucose to glycogen, the form of sugar that can be stored in your cells (including liver cells) for later use. When you are running low on energy, the liver converts glycogen back to glucose and ships it off to your cells via the bloodstream.
- Inside the liver, fatty acids, amino acids, vitamins, and minerals are converted into more usable forms.
- The liver makes important cellular structural components, including cell membrane compounds (phospholipids) and cholesterol. It is also the liver's job to manufacture the carrier proteins (lipoproteins) that transport these components throughout the body.
- To keep your body's supply of protein at the right level, the liver converts amino acids into glucose, proteins, or other types of amino acids, depending on what your body needs at any given moment.
- It breaks down excess amino acids to form a waste product called urea, which is then carried in the bloodstream to the kidneys and excreted in the urine.
- The liver produces many important blood proteins, including immune factors, proteins involved in blood clotting, and a crucial component of hemoglobin.
- Iron and vitamins A, D, and B_{12} are stored in liver cells. Old red blood cells are broken down in the liver and their components recycled to create new cells.

That's quite a list of tasks—and we haven't even discussed detoxification yet!

The liver takes care of poisonous substances in a complex series of steps. First it filters and removes toxins from the blood. Then it changes the chemical structure of those toxins to make them water soluble so that they can be excreted in the urine. (Many of the most dangerous toxins are fat soluble, which means that unless they are detoxified, they are more likely to lodge in your cells and remain there, causing trouble.) The liver also secretes bile, which collects the waste products and carries them away from the liver. As I discussed in Chapter 2, bile is also necessary for the proper digestion of fats.

How important is detoxification to your well-being? Extremely. Detoxification uses up over 80 percent of the amount of energy your body devotes to making new molecules. In other words, most of the molecules we synthesize every day are made for the sake of getting rid of *waste* molecules. You can see the connection between liver function and energy levels: If your liver is overloaded—as is the case for most Americans—you may be suffering from low energy levels, since even more of your body's energy is being devoted to detoxification. That leaves very little energy for other body processes. Supporting your liver by following the guidelines in this chapter will help your energy levels soar to new heights.

Because of its importance, the liver is high on the priority list for receiving oxygenated blood from the heart. Approximately one-fourth of the heart's output goes directly to the liver first, traveling through the hepatic artery. (The word *hepatic* means "pertaining to the liver.")

But blood also flows into the liver on its return journey to the heart. The portal vein brings nutrient-dense blood directly from the digestive system into the liver. The liver needs those nutrients to carry out its hundreds of functions. What's more, the liver also gets first crack at handling any toxic substances absorbed from your digestive system. Due to this two-level blood supply, nearly two quarts of blood pass through the liver every minute.

The liver is packed full of unique cells called hepatocytes, which are able to handle a greater variety of tasks than any other type of cell in the body. Hepatocytes are especially high in the tiny structures called mitochondria. These cellular "engines" produce the energy the liver needs to carry out its processes of synthesis and metabolism. Cells elsewhere in your body also contain mitochondria, but liver cells contain more of them—nearly two thousand per cell. In contrast, white blood cells (lymphocytes) contain only a half dozen or so.

Another sign that the liver is crucial to your well-being is its amazing efficiency. The liver could lose up to three-fourths of its cells (for example, due to disease or surgery) and still be able to function properly. But the liver doesn't take such damage lying down. It is the only internal organ in the body that is able to regenerate itself. This capacity to regenerate is not unlimited, however. Continuous or repeated damage—for example, due to chronic consumption of harmful drugs or alcohol—produces scar tissue that seriously interferes with the liver's ability to function. This condition is called cirrhosis.

Because it is responsible for so many different body functions, the liver must stay in peak condition. If your liver slows down, toxins can build up. When that happens, cells and organs throughout your body become susceptible to damage and disease.

To find out how well your detoxification system is doing, complete the following self-assessment.

DETOXIFICATION ASSESSMENT • PART A
Liver Function

Circle the number that best describes the intensity of your symptoms on the following scale:

0 = I do not experience this symptom
1 = Mild
2 = Moderate
3 = Severe

Yellow in white of eyes	0	1	2	3
Bad breath	0	1	2	3
Body odor	0	1	2	3
Fatigue	0	1	2	3
Strong-smelling urine	0	1	2	3
Sensitive to chemicals	0	1	2	3
Headaches	0	1	2	3
Tingling sensations in hands and feet	0	1	2	3
Mental confusion/cloudiness	0	1	2	3
Less than one bowel movement per day	0	1	2	3

Add the numbers circled and enter that subtotal here: _____

Circle the number of the answer that applies to you:
More than 20 pounds overweight   NO = 0   YES = 10

History of heavy alcohol use or chemotherapy	NO = 0	YES = 10
Blood test reveals elevated bilirubin or liver enzymes	NO = 0	YES = 10
Have or had hepatitis	NO = 0	YES = 10

Add the numbers circled and enter that subtotal here: _____

Add the two subtotals and enter that total here: _____

Scoring   *9 or more: High priority*
        5–8: Moderate priority
        1–4: Low priority

Interpreting Your Score

The symptoms addressed in this questionnaire are those that commonly result from the buildup of poisons or the failure of the organs to do their job. For example, one function of the liver is to metabolize hemoglobin, the red pigment left over when old blood cells die. The pigment is changed into a water-soluble form (bilirubin) and then excreted in the bile. However, if the liver is unable to keep up with the demand, bilirubin can build up in the skin or other organs, such as the whites of the eyes. This condition is called jaundice (from the Latin word for "yellow"). Similarly, dark-colored or strong-smelling urine may signal that the filtration system is not working effectively. The higher your score, the greater the need to address problems related to detoxification.

Heavy Metal Toxicity

Heavy metals include lead, mercury, cadmium, arsenic, nickel, and aluminum. Once they enter the body, these substances can collect inside cells, especially those of the brain, nerves, kidneys, and immune system. Like grit that gets inside the valves of your engine, the heavy metals can disrupt the ability of the cells to carry out their function. Worse, they can cause the cells to act in abnormal ways, for example, by causing the buildup of abnormal substances or making the cells reproduce in an out-of-control function, leading to cancer or other serious—potentially fatal—diseases.

Most of the heavy metals that enter the body result from environmental contamination. For example, industrial processes and fossil fuels spew thousands of tons of lead particles into the air each year. Some of the particles settle in soil, where they are absorbed by plants, or are washed into the water supply. Other sources of heavy metals include lead from pesticide sprays and the solder in tin cans; cadmium and lead from cigarette smoke; mercury from dental fillings and contaminated fish; and aluminum from antiperspirants, cooking utensils, food containers, and even some antacids.

Heavy-metal toxicity can cause a range of symptoms, depending on which cells and tissues are affected. Many of the symptoms, such as headache, fatigue, tremors, dizziness, lack of coordination, and impaired ability to think and concentrate, reflect damage to the central nervous system. There is a connection between heavy-metal poisoning and childhood learning disabilities, such as attention deficit disorder. Other possible symptoms include muscle aches, indigestion, constipation, anemia, and high blood pressure.

CASE HISTORY: Getting the Lead Out

Carl is a fifty-two-year-old man who works in the men's clothing department at a local store. He came to see me for help in getting his high blood pressure under control. He told me he was frustrated with the "medical world" and absolutely hated the drugs his doctors had prescribed. The side effects (dizziness, tingling sensations and numbness in his hands and feet— not to mention impotence) were driving him nuts. Worse, the treatment did not seem to be getting his blood pressure down. His typical reading was 150/105 (a normal reading is closer to 120/80).

Carl did not fit the mold of the usual high-blood-pressure patient. First of all, he was not overweight. He was an avid runner and ate a health-promoting diet. Except for his high blood pressure and some frequent headaches, he considered himself to be in excellent physical health.

The medical literature and my clinical experience have taught me that when I meet a patient like Carl, who doesn't fit the typical profile, I should suspect that the blood pressure problem may involve high body lead levels. Several studies have found that lead raises blood pressure by negatively affecting kidney function.

Because I know that people who live in large cities or areas with soft water typically have higher lead levels, I asked Carl where he lived. He replied that he had a nice old house right above a major freeway in downtown Seattle. He also told me that he ran twenty-plus miles a week, mostly on a busy road along the Seattle waterfront. His route was picturesque, but I was sure that he was sucking in too much pollution. I had the nurse collect a sample of Carl's hair so that we could send it out for a hair mineral analysis. Hair analysis is a very good screening test for heavy metal toxicity.

I was shocked by the results. Carl's lead levels were literally off the charts. Despite the high levels, Carl was unaffected by symptoms commonly seen in people with high chronic lead exposure, including depression and neurological complaints such as visual disturbances. (Note: MineralCheck is a hair analysis kit from BodyBalance, available in healthfood stores or by calling 1-888-891-3061 or visiting www.bodybalance.com.)

For some patients with high lead levels I will recommend intravenous chelation therapy. This process involves slowly infusing EDTA (ethylenediaminetetraacetic acid), an amino-acid-like molecule, into the bloodstream. EDTA chelates (binds with) minerals such as calcium, iron, copper, and lead and carries them to the kidneys, where they are excreted. EDTA chelation has been commonly used for lead poisoning, but it is also used for treating patients with atherosclerosis (hardening of the arteries).

In Carl's case, though, I thought oral (as opposed to IV) chelation might work to reduce his lead levels. I was optimistic because although Carl consumed a healthy diet, he did not take any nutritional supplements. I felt that we could "get the lead out" and lower blood pressure simply by flooding his body with calcium, magnesium, and zinc, as well as vitamin C, vitamin E, and the B vitamins. I prescribed the basic dietary recommendations given later in this chapter (pages 80–81) along with the following supplements:

- Doctor's Choice for Men, a high-potency multiple vitamin and mineral formula: two tablets three times daily (twice the normal dosage)
- Vitamin C: 1,000 mg three times daily
- A high-potency garlic preparation: one pill twice daily providing 8,000 mcg of allicin

I thought that, for the time being, Carl should continue to take his prescribed blood pressure medication (Atenolol, a beta-blocker). But I urged him to monitor his blood pressure carefully. The extra calcium and magnesium he would be putting into his system could cause his blood pressure to drop too low.

Carl's blood pressure slowly started coming down after about a month. By the end of two months he needed only half the dosage of Atenolol, and after three months he was totally off the drug. I think the garlic was also a big factor in Carl's case (see the Tune-Up Tip).

At his last visit, Carl's blood pressure had dropped to 110/70. He still runs, but I convinced him to change his route to one of Seattle's gorgeous parks overlooking Puget Sound. The view is still spectacular—but instead of lead, he's inhaling fresh sea breeze.

Tune-Up Tip: Garlic

Garlic and onions are rich sources of sulfur-containing compounds that are helpful in escorting heavy metals out of the body. Interestingly, patients with high blood pressure typically have low levels of sulfur-containing compounds in their blood. To lower cholesterol and/or blood pressure, fresh garlic or garlic products that clearly state the "allicin potential" or "allicin yield" should be used. To lower blood cholesterol and/or pressure, the recommended dosage of fresh garlic is roughly one or two cloves of garlic daily; uncooked garlic is best. An equivalent amount for a garlic product (preferably an odor-controlled one) would be an allicin potential or allicin yield of 4,000 mcg. For helping the body eliminate heavy metals, it does not matter as much if the garlic is fresh. Cooked garlic (as well as onions) is still rich in sulfur compounds. The bottom line here is that for removing heavy metals, try to include in your diet as much garlic as possible, in any form.

Toxic Chemicals

Toxic chemicals that affect the liver include:

- Certain chemicals such as food additives or colorings (especially tartrazine, a yellow coloring)
- Solvents such as cleaning products or formaldehyde
- Pesticides
- Herbicides
- Drugs (illicit, over-the-counter, and prescription)
- Alcohol
- Naturally occurring toxins in foods and herbs

Since all of these toxic chemicals are broken down by the liver, chronic exposure to these substances can damage liver function. Typically, symptoms of liver toxicity show up as problems involving the brain and nerves.

CASE HISTORY: Scene of the Crime

One of the most "toxic" people I have ever met was thirty-eight-year-old Beth. She suffered from headaches, odd neurological symptoms, occasional blurred vision, and severe bouts of depression and fatigue. She worked in a crime lab and loved her job. I was fascinated when she told me in detail about how she analyzed evidence. I soon realized, however, that her work was killing her—it was literally poisoning her.

The lab where she worked was poorly ventilated, so many of the toxic chemicals used to perform various tests, including chloroform, lingered in the air. Beth had seen other doctors, but none of them suspected that her chemical exposure was a significant cause of her illness. Fortunately for Beth, we were able to get her detoxification system back on track and she was able to keep the job she so enjoyed. She followed the same basic program that I outline in this chapter. Silymarin, a special extract of milk thistle (*Silybum marianum*), was a big part of her treatment.

I have seen this program work for other people in occupations where chemical exposure is a common problem: Sean, a cabinetmaker; Bill, an owner of a small copy and print shop; Gary, an auto mechanic; Dorothy, an office worker at a newspaper; and Kurt, a carpet layer. All of these patients had similar symptoms: fatigue, nausea, odd muscle aches or nerve pains. When I met each of them for the first time, I was struck by the impression that these people were just *beat*—something was wearing them down. And that is exactly what happens to people who are constantly exposed to toxic chemicals in the environment.

But when they take steps to support detoxification, the transformation can be amazing to see: The eyes become brighter, smiles are broader, there is more expression in the face, voice, and body, and there is a restored vibrancy of spirit.

I urge people with occupations that expose them to chemical toxins to take precautions to reduce their exposure—make sure ventilation is good and wear a protective mask, for example—and be sure to support their liver.

Tune-Up Tip: Silymarin

In cases of obvious chemical toxicity or impaired liver function, support your liver with silymarin, a flavonoid-rich extract of milk thistle (*Silybum marianum*). Silymarin enhances detoxification reactions and acts as a powerful antioxidant to protect the liver from toxic chemicals. Silymarin is even more potent than vitamins C and E in mopping up free radicals. Clinical studies in humans have shown silymarin to have positive effects in the treatment of virtually all types of liver disease, including cirrhosis, hepatitis, fatty liver, and inflammation of the bile ducts. The standard dosage for silymarin is 70 to 210 mg three times per day.

Balancing Your Detox System

To get the most out of your detox tune-up, it helps if you understand a little more about how the liver neutralizes harmful substances.

Detoxification is basically a two-step process involving a family of perhaps one hundred enzymes known as the cytochrome P450 enzymes. Generally, each enzyme is designed to metabolize certain types of chemicals, but there is also a lot of overlap among the P450 family. This "backup system" ensures that the liver is usually able to detoxify the body efficiently. This explains why some people can smoke without developing lung cancer and why certain individuals are more vulnerable to the effects of drinking. We also inhabit different environments: We eat different foods, are exposed to different chemicals, and have different metabolic and nutritional needs. For these reasons, the activity of different components of the cytochrome P450 system varies widely from person to person. Your health care professional can conduct tests to assess how well your liver enzymes function.

Phase I Detoxification

Detoxification enzymes work in different ways to neutralize chemicals. In one process, the enzyme simply breaks apart the toxic molecule into two or more harmless components. This is what happens when you metabolize caffeine, for example.

Another strategy is to change the molecule so that it can be dissolved in water. This makes it possible for the toxin to circulate in the bloodstream to the kidneys, where it can be excreted in urine. Or the toxin can attach itself to the bile and be excreted in feces.

The third method is to transform the molecule into another form so that other enzymes can then go to work on it.

Together, these three methods are known as Phase I detoxification. Symptoms that may indicate a dysfunctional Phase I system include:

- Sensitivity to or craving for alcohol—one or two drinks make you very drunk, or you have an uncontrollable urge to drink
- Caffeine intolerance—even a small amount keeps you awake at night (indicates underactive Phase I)
- Rapid metabolism of caffeine—ability to consume large amounts and still sleep (indicates overactive Phase I)
- Liver disease
- Parkinson's disease
- Illness resulting from exposure to perfumes or environmental chemicals

Phase II Detoxification

Toxins such as caffeine are completely neutralized during Phase I and do not need more processing. Many substances, however, require further action during the next step in the process, known as Phase II. Phase II works to detoxify substances not by breaking them down into smaller pieces, but by adding other molecules. In a way, this is like "handcuffing" the toxin so it can be escorted out of the body by the biological equivalent of security guards. The heavy metals are detoxified in this way.

The process of adding one molecule to another is called *conjugation*. Conjugation either neutralizes the toxin, so it will do no harm if it remains in the body, or changes the toxin to a water-soluble form, so it can be excreted.

THE STRANGE CASE OF ALCOHOL

It may seem strange, but during Phase I, many toxins are actually made more active—and thus potentially more damaging. For example, many molecules are oxidized, resulting in the production of large numbers of free radicals. If you don't have an adequate supply of antioxidants, such as beta-carotene and vitamins C and E, these free radicals can cause serious damage to your tissues.

Similarly, if your Phase II system is out of whack, these activated substances are not neutralized effectively and can cause even more harm. Alcohol is a prime example. Alcohol by itself is not that damaging to human cells. What causes the problem is acetaldehyde, a compound formed during Phase I detoxification. During Phase II, acetaldehyde is converted to a nontoxic compound, acetic acid. People who have an enhanced Phase I conversion of alcohol to acetaldehyde and a reduced Phase II conversion to acetic acid are more sensitive to the effects of alcohol. They are much more likely to become alcoholics as well as to suffer from the damaging effects of alcohol, including cirrhosis of the liver.

Some population groups, such as Native Americans and children of alcoholics, are inherently very susceptible to alcoholism, not because they are weak or immoral, but because of biology. They are born with genes that typically give them an overactive Phase I and an underactive Phase II detoxification of alcohol.

The Seven Pathways of Phase II Detoxification

There are seven main methods, or pathways, by which Phase II detoxification occurs.

Acetylation is the process of neutralizing toxins by attaching molecules of acetyl coenzyme A (acetyl CoA). It is through this pathway that certain antibiotics, such as the sulfa drugs used in the treatment of urinary infections, are eliminated from the body. You need good supplies of vitamins B_2 (riboflavin), B_5 (pantothenic acid), and C for this system to work properly.

Amino acid conjugation involves attaching an amino acid, most commonly glycine, to a toxin. People with chronic conditions such as hepatitis, alcoholic liver disorders, cancer, and other diseases, or those who are exposed to high levels of toxins for long periods of time, usually have a poorly functioning amino acid conjugation system. You need adequate protein intake for this system to work properly.

Glucuronidation is the pathway in which glucuronic acid is attached to toxins. This is the system through which you detoxify many commonly prescribed drugs, as well as aspirin, menthol, vanillin (synthetic vanilla), estrogen and other hormones, cigarette smoke, and food additives such as benzoates (preservatives). The glucuronidation pathway works pretty well in most people except those with a condition called Gilbert syndrome, which causes inadequate metabolism of bilirubin, a pigment left over from the breakdown of hemoglobin (see Case History on page 78).

Glutathione conjugation is the process by which a small protein called glutathione is attached to a fat-soluble toxin, converting it into a water-soluble form. If you want to rid your body of fat-soluble compounds—especially the heavy metals—you need to have a good supply of glutathione on hand (or rather, in your liver). To make glutathione, your body needs adequate levels of the amino acids methionine and cysteine. This is another reason for making sure you have sufficient protein in your diet. Glutathione also acts as an important antioxidant. This is crucial for good liver function, because liver cells contain so many of the energy factories (mitochondria) where free radicals are produced. The combination of detoxification and protection from free radicals makes glutathione one of your body's most important anticancer and antiaging agents.

Methylation is the pathway used to detoxify estrogen and other steroid hormones. A methyl group (a carbon atom plus three hydrogen atoms) is attached to the toxin, allowing it to then be more efficiently processed. Most of the methyl groups needed for this process come from a chemical called S-adenosylmethionine, or SAMe for short. SAMe, in turn, is made in the body from the amino acid methionine. For SAMe production to happen, your body needs certain key nutrients, including choline, vitamin B_{12}, and folic acid. Through methylation, SAMe neutralizes the female hormone estrogen, making methionine a useful substance for treating conditions involving excess estrogen such as premenstrual syndrome. It also prevents estrogen-induced cholestasis (blockage of bile flow from the gallbladder). SAMe is also available as a nutritional supplement.

Sulfation is the main pathway by which your body detoxifies environmental poisons, microbial products, and certain drugs and food additives. Similar to glutathione conjugation, sulfation involves attaching sulfur to toxins to make them water-soluble and easier to eliminate from the body. Stress hormones are neutralized through sulfation, so the more stress you experience, the harder your liver has to work to detoxify your system. What's more, when you increase activity in the sulfation pathway, you reduce activity in the glutathione pathway, increasing your risk of free-radical damage. If your sulfation pathway is on the blink, you may experience symptoms affecting the nervous system, such as "pins and needles" in the hands and feet. Diets low in the amino acids methionine and cysteine can reduce sulfation activity. So too can excess levels of molybdenum or vitamin B_6 (more than 100 mg per day).

Sulfoxidation is the process by which your body metabolizes the sulfur-containing molecules in drugs and foods. This pathway eliminates the sulfites commonly used as preservatives in such foods as potato salad, salad bar ingredients, dried fruits, and certain drugs, especially asthma medications. In most people, the enzyme known as sulfite oxidase converts sulfite to a safer form (sulfate), which then passes out of the body in the urine. But people whose sulfoxidation system isn't up to par become highly sensitive to sulfur-containing substances. For example, people with asthma are vulnerable to serious attacks when exposed to such substances.

Tune-Up Tip: Boost Glutathione Levels

Glutathione's combination of detoxification and free-radical protection makes it one of the most important cancer and aging fighters in our cells. The greater your exposure to toxins, the faster your body uses up its supply of glutathione. Without the protection of glutathione, your cells die at a faster rate, making you age more quickly and putting you at risk for toxin-induced diseases, including cancer. People who smoke, are chronically exposed to toxins, suffer from inflammatory conditions such as rheumatoid arthritis, or suffer from chronic conditions such as diabetes, AIDS, or cancer typically have lower levels of glutathione. It's a vicious cycle: Health problems deplete your supply of glutathione, and reduced levels of glutathione increase your risk of health problems.

Don't look to supplements containing glutathione to boost levels of glutathione in the body. While glutathione in food appears to be efficiently absorbed into the blood, the same does not appear to be true for glutathione supplements in humans. When healthy subjects were given a single dose of up to 3,000 mg of glutathione, researchers found there was no increase in blood glutathione levels. In contrast, blood glutathione levels rose nearly 50 percent in healthy individuals taking 500 mg of vitamin C. Vitamin C raises glutathione by helping the body manufacture it. In addition to vitamin C, other nutritional compounds that may help increase glutathione levels include N-acetylcysteine, alpha-lipoic acid, glutamine, methionine, and whey protein.

However, rather than looking to these higher-priced supplements to boost glutathione, I recommend supplementing your diet with at least 500 mg of vitamin C each day and focusing on food sources of glutathione, such as fresh fruits and vegetables, fish, and meat. Especially good sources of glutathione include asparagus, avocados, walnuts, and Brassica family foods such as cabbage, broccoli, and Brussels sprouts. You can also step up your body's production of glutathione by eating foods that contain a compound called limonene, such as citrus, dill weed, or caraway seeds.

CASE HISTORY: An Odd Case of Burning Feet

Richard, age forty, is a computer programmer. For some time he had suffered from fatigue, loss of appetite, dry and itchy skin, and odd burning sensations in his legs. Whenever he took a bath, he said, his legs "burned like fire." He consulted neurologists, who could find nothing wrong. Another doctor found that his serum bilirubin level was high. The diagnosis: Gilbert syndrome, which results from inadequate glucuronidation, one of the Phase II detoxification pathways. Previously considered rare, Gilbert syndrome now is thought to affect up to 5 percent of the general population. The doctor told him not to worry about it, that it was no big deal.

Well, Richard *did* worry. His symptoms persisted, and he was miserable. And he missed his long, relaxing soaks in the tub.

Unhappy with the care he'd been receiving, he came to see me. I agreed with the diagnosis—it was apparent from the slight yellowish tinge to Richard's skin and in the whites of his eyes—but I strongly disagreed with the do-nothing approach to treatment. I also suspected that his liver was unable to break down some kind of nerve toxin that was causing the unpleasant sensations in his legs. From my clinical experience, I knew that there are many steps that can be taken to support liver function, especially glucuronidation, to produce significant improvements in health.

My recommendations:

- Drink 8 ounces of water six times daily.
- Increase intake of citrus fruit (except grapefruit) and sulfur-rich foods (egg yolks, red peppers, garlic, onions, broccoli, Brussels sprouts, nuts, and seeds).
- Take a supplement containing lipotropic substances (see page 85).

After Richard had been following this program for six weeks, his bilirubin level had dropped by 75 percent, from 3.2 mg/dl down to 0.8 mg/dl. He had more energy, his skin was healthier-looking and no longer itched, and his odd burning sensations had disappeared. He was ecstatic because he was once again able to take a bath. I told Richard my theory that the treatment had helped his liver remove a nerve toxin. Richard didn't really care *why* he felt better, he was just happy that he did.

Your health care professional can conduct tests to identify which part(s) of your detox system may not be functioning properly. However, the pattern of symptoms you experience can usually provide a clue. Some symptoms that are directly tied to a specific dysfunction appear in Table 3-1.

Table 3-1: Symptoms of Dysfunctional Phase II Detoxification System

Symptom	System Most Likely Dysfunctional
Adverse reactions to sulfite food additives (such as in commercial potato salad or salad bars)	Sulfoxidation
Alzheimer's disease	Sulfoxidation
Asthma reactions after eating at a restaurant	Sulfoxidation
Chemical sensitivity	Glutathione conjugation
Eating asparagus results in a strong urine odor	Sulfoxidation
Garlic makes you sick	Sulfoxidation
Gilbert syndrome	Glucuronidation
Liver disease	General Phase II dysfunction
Prostate cancer	Sulfation
Rheumatoid arthritis	Sulfoxidation
Toxemia of pregnancy	Amino acid conjugation
Yellow discoloration of eyes and skin, not due to hepatitis	Glucuronidation

Tune-Up Tip: Detoxing Through Diet

- To promote Phase I detoxification, you need the right levels of the P450 enzymes. And like all enzymes, the P450s need adequate amounts of certain nutrients, especially copper, magnesium, zinc, and vitamin C.
- Boost your glutathione levels by following the guidelines given in the Tune-Up Tip on page 78.
- To ensure your amino acid conjugation is working well, be sure you are eating adequate amounts of protein-rich foods.
- To promote methylation, eat foods rich in folic acid, such as green leafy vegetables, and those that contain vitamin B_6, such as whole grains and legumes. Make sure you're getting enough vitamin B_{12}, which is found in animal products or dietary supplements.
- Enhance sulfation by consuming sulfur-containing foods, such as egg yolks, red peppers, garlic, onions, broccoli, and Brussels sprouts.
- To ensure effective acetylation, eat foods that are rich in the B vitamins, such as whole grains, and in vitamin C, such as peppers, cabbage, and citrus fruits (except grapefruit—see page 81).

- Glucuronidation depends on an enzyme with a tricky name, UDP-glucuronyl transferase (UDPGT). You can activate UDPGT by eating limonene-rich foods such as citrus fruits, dill, and caraway. Also be sure to consume sulfur-rich foods.
- For effective sulfoxidation, eat foods rich in molybdenum, such as legumes and whole grains. Molybdenum helps because it is needed for production of sulfite oxidase, the enzyme that "digests" sulfites.

From what you've read so far, it should be clear that detoxification is a complex process that depends on literally dozens of systems working in balance, in sync, and at the right level of intensity.

Not surprisingly, that doesn't always happen. Sometimes the Phase I process goes too rapidly or too slowly for the Phase II process to work smoothly. In a way, detox is like a car factory: If basic parts such as bolts or screws don't arrive in time, the workers can't assemble the final vehicle, no matter how many hubcaps and fenders they have in stock. People who have a very active Phase I system but a slow or inactive Phase II system may suffer severe toxic reactions to environmental poisons, because their bodies can't "handcuff" them and clear them out fast enough.

GRAPEFRUIT: NOT SUCH A GREAT FRUIT?

Citrus fruits are an important part of a good diet because they provide vitamin C and other essential nutrients. But grapefruit contains high levels of a flavonoid (plant compound) called naringin. This substance reduces the activity of a group of P450 enzymes known as CYP3A enzymes. These enzymes are the ones your body uses to break down certain drugs, such as calcium channel blockers (used in the treatment of high blood pressure), sedatives (for example, midazolam), and cyclosporin (an immune suppressant given to people who have received organ transplants). If the drugs are not metabolized, they remain in the body in higher concentrations. This increases the risk of unwanted toxic effects.

If you are taking a prescription medication, ask your doctor if you should avoid eating grapefruit or drinking grapefruit juice. Some drugs, such as Neoral (oral cyclosporin), already carry a warning.

For citrus lovers, there are plenty of other choices. Oranges, tangerines, and tangelos do not contain significant amounts of naringin but have lots of other important nutrients and flavonoids.

CASE HISTORY: Bringing Donna Back to Life

Three years ago, Donna was on top of the world. This attractive, vivacious redhead was attending a private college, where she loved her courses in literature and history. She'd met a great guy and they enjoyed a terrific relationship.

But then she came down with a bad bout of bronchitis, and since then she hadn't been feeling up to snuff. She had been prescribed an antibiotic, which many doctors now agree is often unnecessary for this condition. The drug caused an imbalance in her intestinal bacteria (dysbiosis). After taking the drug, she developed a severe vaginal yeast infection. Over time her health declined. Her once-healthy skin was now thin and pale, almost translucent. She had dark circles under her eyes. She moped about, feeling tired, apathetic, and depressed. Unable to complete her coursework, she had dropped out of college. Her boyfriend, upset by the changes in her personality, had broken up with her.

Donna made the rounds of conventional medical doctors and alternative health care providers. She received diagnoses ranging from chronic fatigue syndrome to multiple chemical sensitivities to fibromyalgia. She didn't care what label her doctors used for her illness; she just wanted to get better. Mysteriously, whatever drugs, supplements, and herbs she took only seemed to make things worse. Frustrated, she decided to consult me.

My instincts told me that something was wrong with her liver and detoxification system. I suspected an imbalance between Phase I and Phase II reactions. Such disturbances are common in patients who are thought to have chronic fatigue, allergies, or fibromyalgia. I ordered lab tests that analyzed Donna's detoxification profile. Before I received the results (which eventually confirmed my suspicions), I recommended that Donna eat a very limited diet and take three daily servings of a hypoallergenic meal replacement formula (UltraClear) that was developed by Jeffrey Bland, Ph.D., one of the world's leading authorities on clinical nutrition. The formula works to restore the balance between Phase I and Phase II detoxification. In Dr. Bland's practice, patients have reported a greater than 50 percent reduction in symptoms after just twenty days.

Since Donna was so thin (118 pounds on her five-foot-eight frame), I did not want to restrict her calories too severely. So I instructed her to eat plenty of pears, apples, berries of all types, carrots, lentils, celery, garlic, onions, turmeric, and cinnamon. I also recommended 4 to 6 ounces of fish every other day. These foods contain many of the nutrients needed to support active liver detoxification.

I had Donna follow this regimen for two weeks, after which she was significantly improved—not quite 100 percent, but better than she had felt in years. We then explored some of the other issues in her life that I suspected were interfering with her health. Chief among them was the deep loneliness she was feeling since losing her boyfriend. We spent more than one session talking about her broken heart. The very act of talking about it seemed to help heal the wounds.

Not long ago I called Donna just to check in, and was glad to hear her say that life is very good again. She was back at school and had a new boyfriend, her energy was high, and she had big plans for the future. She told me she was her old self again. When I commented that she sounded even better than her old self, she said, "You know, I think you're right."

Gallstones

In Chapter 2 I explained the role of bile in digestion. Bile also is crucial for detoxification, because it carries fat-soluble toxins with it into the digestive tract for elimination. For good detoxification, your liver must produce adequate supplies of bile, and the bile must flow properly to do its job. If the secretion of bile is blocked (a condition called cholestasis), toxins can build up.

There are several conditions that can lead to cholestasis (see Table 3-2). Damage to the liver can prevent bile from leaving the hepatocytes. Also, the ducts that collect and transport bile can become plugged.

Table 3-2: Causes of Cholestasis

Gallstones	Chemicals and drugs
Alcohol	Natural and synthetic steroid
Hereditary disorders such as	hormones
Gilbert syndrome	Anabolic steroids
Hyperthyroidism or excessive	Estrogens
thyroxine supplementation	Oral contraceptives
Viral hepatitis	Chlorothiazide
Pregnancy	Erythromycin

Gallstones—hard lumps of material that form in the gallbladder or the bile ducts—are the most common cause of blocked bile flow. Each year in the United States, doctors perform about half a million operations to remove gallbladders because of stones. There is a link between gallstones and the high-fat, low-fiber diet so common in this country. The stones, which can be as small as one-twentieth of an inch or as large as one inch, are usually made of cholesterol, but some contain bile pigments or other substances such as calcium carbonate (chalk). Stones form when the liver makes bile that contains either too much cholesterol or not enough of the detergent substances that keep cholesterol suspended in a kind of fatty soup. Symptoms of gallstones include fatigue, malaise, digestive disturbances, allergies and chemical sensitivities, and constipation. In some cases, liver function tests can detect abnormal enzyme levels, which can signify liver damage. However, in the early stages, many people with gallstones do not exhibit symptoms or liver abnormalities.

Another common cause of liver damage, and thus bile abnormalities, is excessive alcohol consumption. Even small quantities of alcohol—one or two drinks—can damage liver cells. As a result, fat accumulates in the liver, leading to further damage. Fat buildup reduces bile flow, leading to the buildup of toxins within the body.

Dealing with a Toxic World

The most effective therapy for promoting effective detoxification is a healthy dose of common sense. Avoid putting poisons in your body in the first place. Don't smoke; drink little or no alcohol; don't breathe polluted air; avoid caffeine; drink plenty of water that's been filtered; stay away from harmful chemicals, including solvents and pesticides; use medications only when absolutely necessary.

The most important dietary guidelines for supporting good liver function are also those that support good general health. Avoid saturated fats, refined sugar, and alcohol; drink at least 48 ounces of water each day; and consume plenty of fiber, especially soluble fiber, which promotes bile secretion.

As I indicated above, certain foods are particularly helpful because they contain the nutrients your body needs to produce and activate the dozens of enzymes involved in the various phases of detox. Such foods include:

- Garlic, legumes, onions, eggs, and other foods with a high sulfur content
- Good sources of soluble fiber, such as pears, oat bran, apples, and legumes
- Cabbage-family vegetables, especially broccoli, Brussels sprouts, and cabbage
- Artichokes, beets, carrots, dandelion greens, and many herbs and spices, such as turmeric, cinnamon, and licorice

Certain nutritional supplements help promote detoxification:

- A high-potency multiple vitamin and mineral supplement is a must. Make sure that it contains higher-than-RDA levels for all the B vitamins and at least 20 mg of zinc, 200 mcg of selenium, and 1 mg of copper, as these nutrients are critical to so many detoxification pathways.
- Take extra doses of vitamin C (500 to 1,500 mg daily) and vitamin E (400 to 800 IU) to neutralize the free radicals formed during detoxification reactions.
- Consider supplementing nutrients known as lipotropic agents. These substances accelerate the metabolism of fat, prevent its accumulation in the liver, and promote the flow of bile out of the liver. Such compounds are like decongestants for the liver. Among the key lipotropic agents are choline, betaine, and methionine. In my practice, I often recommend them for patients with such liver disorders as hepatitis, cirrhosis, and chemical-induced liver disease. Take a daily dose of 1,000 mg of choline and 1,000 mg of methionine or cysteine or both.
- Consider silymarin (see page 73).

Tune-Up Tip: Calcium D-Glucarate for Breast Cancer Patients

Detoxification is crucial in the fight against breast cancer. The main concern is making sure that estrogen is properly detoxified, as an excess of estrogen is linked to breast cancer. To reduce breast cancer risk, your body needs to neutralize and eliminate estrogen as well as synthetic compounds that mimic the action of estrogen in the body, such as certain pesticides, herbicides, and compounds in plastic.

One of the key ways in which the body gets rid of estrogen and estrogen mimickers is by the Phase II process of glucuronidation. The problem is that certain bacteria produce an enzyme, glucuronidase, that interrupts this process (by breaking the bond between estrogen and glucuronic acid). Not surprisingly, excess glucuronidase activity is associated with an increased cancer risk, particularly the risk of estrogen-dependent breast cancer. Enzyme activity is higher in people whose diet is high in fat and low in fiber. The level of glucuronidase activity may be the reason why certain dietary factors cause breast cancer and why other dietary factors are preventive.

You can reduce glucuronidase activity by establishing the proper bacterial flora. The strategy is to eat a diet rich in high-fiber plant foods and supplement the diet with the "friendly" bacteria *Lactobacillus acidophilus* and *Bifidobacterium bifidum* (see pages 52–53). Other foods that can dramatically reduce the activity of this enzyme are onions and garlic and foods high in glucaric acid, such as apples, Brussels sprouts, broccoli, cabbage, and lettuce.

Glucaric acid in a pill form, calcium D-glucarate, may turn out to be a vitally important strategy in the prevention of breast cancer, especially as a way to prevent its recurrence. Preliminary research is very encouraging. Currently, women with a history of breast cancer are prescribed the drug tamoxifen. This drug is associated with numerous side effects, and its overall effectiveness is still controversial. In contrast, calcium D-glucarate is completely safe and, if preliminary results hold true, is more effective than tamoxifen. Calcium D-glucarate is currently being investigated at some of the leading cancer research centers in America, including the M. D. Anderson Cancer Center in Houston, Texas. It is just entering the health food market as well (for more information, see Chapter 10). Meanwhile, if you are a woman at high risk for breast cancer, or if you have or have had breast cancer, I recommend taking at least 400 mg of calcium D-glucarate daily.

The Kidneys

Let's now focus on the liver's detoxification partner, the kidneys. These paired organs are located in the lower back just above the waist, on either side of the spinal column. The kidneys are responsible for filtering the blood and excreting waste products and excess water in the form of urine. The kidneys empty urine into the ureters, tubes that carry the urine from the kidney to the bladder.

In addition to eliminating waste products, the kidneys regulate the body's acid-alkaline balance (pH) and fluid volume. They also secrete several important hormones, such as erythropoietin, which stimulates production of red blood cells in the bone marrow, and they convert vitamin D into its most active form.

DETOXIFICATION ASSESSMENT • PART B
Kidney Function

Circle the number that best describes the intensity of your symptoms on the following scale:

>   *0 = I do not experience this symptom*
>   *1 = Mild*
>   *2 = Moderate*
>   *3 = Severe*

Fluid retention in arms and legs	0	1	2	3
Dry, itchy skin	0	1	2	3
Infrequent urge to urinate	0	1	2	3
Consumption of less than 48 ounces of water daily	0	1	2	3
Cloudy urine	0	1	2	3
Strong-smelling urine	0	1	2	3
Fatigue	0	1	2	3
Metallic taste in the mouth	0	1	2	3
Dark circles under the eyes	0	1	2	3
High blood pressure (>140/90)	0	1	2	3

Add the numbers circled and enter that total here: _____

Scoring   *8 or more: High priority*
     3–7: Moderate priority
     1–2: Low priority

Interpreting Your Score

The questionnaire reflects the need to focus on supporting kidneys that display mild to moderate dysfunction. Even a score of 8 or more (high priority) does not necessarily mean that you are experiencing a kidney "disease." The questionnaire can point out several symptoms that indicate dehydration, such as dry and itchy skin, strong or cloudy urine, or rarely feeling the need to urinate. Fatigue with a metallic taste in the mouth may indicate uremia, the situation when components of urine back up into the blood. Fluid retention, high blood pressure, and dark circles under the eyes also may indicate the kidneys are not doing a good enough job regulating fluid volume in the body. In fact, although we think of high blood pressure as being a cardiovascular disease, it is really a disorder of the kidneys.

Following the guidelines for enhancing liver function go a long way in supporting proper kidney function. When the liver does not properly detoxify, it leaves the kidneys vulnerable to damage. My key recommendation for tuning up your kidneys is one that you probably have heard a thousand times: Drink at least six to eight glasses of water each day. Don't wait till you're thirsty; schedule regular water breaks throughout the day instead. Drink a glass of water at least every two hours throughout the day and you will reach your goal.

SIXTY PERCENT OF THE BODY IS WATER

Water is essential for life. The average person has a total body water content of about 10 gallons. We need to drink at least 48 ounces of water per day to replace the water that is lost through urination, sweat, and expired through our lungs. If we don't, we are likely to become dehydrated.

Even mild dehydration results in impaired physiological and performance responses. Many nutrients dissolve in water so they can be absorbed more easily in your digestive tract. Similarly, many metabolic processes need to take place in water. Water is a component of blood and thus is important for transporting chemicals and nutrients to cells and tissues. Each of your cells is constantly bathed in a watery fluid. Water also carries waste materials from cells to the kidneys so they can be filtered out and eliminated. Water absorbs and transports heat. For example, heat produced by muscle cells during exercise is carried by water in the blood to the surface, helping your body maintain the right temperature balance. The skin cells also release water as perspiration, which helps keep you cool.

Recent research indicates that low fluid consumption in general and low water consumption in particular increases the risk of kidney stones; cancers of the breast, colon, and urinary tract; childhood and adolescent obesity; and heart disease (e.g., mitral valve prolapse).

Several factors are thought to increase the likelihood of chronic mild dehydration, including a poor thirst mechanism, dissatisfaction with the taste of water, common consumption of the natural diuretics caffeine and alcohol, regular exercise increasing water lost through sweat, and living in a hot, dry climate. Surprisingly, if you drink two cups of water and two cups of coffee, cola, or beer, you may end up with a net water intake of zero. Be aware of your "water budget." If you drink coffee or other dehydrating beverages, compensate by drinking an additional glass of water.

Avoid Alcohol or Use It Only in Moderation

Keeping alcohol intake moderate is critical to proper liver and kidney function. Alcoholic beverages have been part of human culture for thousands of years. (Beer has even been found in the tombs of Egyptian pyramids.) Alcohol is used for all kinds of social gatherings, celebrations, and rituals. Millions of people drink moderately several times a week and experience no ill effects. But others are more vulnerable to the problems alcohol can cause. Your response to alcohol is in part a matter of biochemical individuality.

Alcohol is a drug. As is true of other drugs, the impact of alcohol depends to a significant degree on the dose. Its main ingredient, ethanol, acts as a stimulant at low doses, but at higher doses it acts as a depressant—even as an anesthetic. Continued drinking of alcohol creates tolerance: The more you drink, the more you need to consume to achieve the same effect.

Alcohol passes quickly from the stomach into the bloodstream, where it travels to the brain. As a depressant, it decreases activity in the central nervous system, reducing anxiety, tension, and inhibitions. That's why alcohol is so often used as a "social lubricant," and why many events begin with a cocktail party. Drinking makes many people feel more relaxed and confident, more at ease in social settings. However, with continued drinking or drinking at high levels, alcohol slows reactions, impairs concentration, and interferes with judgment.

At low doses alcohol causes the blood vessels to widen, causing increased blood flow and sensations of warmth. As a blood thinner, alcohol may help reduce the risk of clotting and heart attacks. However, with high doses, you can actually lose body heat. Having a drink can trigger the flow of gastric juices. This stimulates appetite and can improve digestion, which again is one reason people have a drink before a meal. But continued drinking at high levels can cause inflammation and weakening of the stomach lining, increasing the risk of gastric ulcers.

As any beer drinker can tell you, drinking increases urine flow. Obviously, drinking large amounts of fluid means your body must increase the output of urine to maintain its balance. But alcohol also acts to inhibit production of antidiuretic hormone (ADH). Without instructions from this hormone, your kidneys speed up the process of filtering water out of the blood. For this reason, alcohol causes you to lose more fluid than you take in, increasing the risk of dehydration. The hangover from excessive drinking is largely the result of lack of body water.

Molecules of alcohol are broken down by liver enzymes. However, if you drink too much, you can overwhelm this detoxification system. Damage to liver cells can cause the development of a kind of scar tissue, resulting in cirrhosis, which severely—even fatally—impairs liver function. Also, some people have bodies that simply do not produce adequate levels of the enzymes needed to break down alcohol. These people are particularly vulnerable to alcoholism.

There are many other physiological problems associated with excess alcohol intake. Just a few examples: Alcohol doubles the risk of cancer of the mouth and throat. (Smoking and drinking combined increases the risk fifteenfold.) Alcohol kills brain cells, leading to nerve, muscle, and cognitive impairment. Immune system cells decline in number and activity with alcohol intake, increasing the risks of infection.

I do not tell my patients that they must never drink. In fact, I will often point out that population studies are showing that moderate alcohol consumption, particularly of red wine, is associated with some protection against heart disease. I myself enjoy a glass of good red wine with meals. However, to gain the health benefits from alcohol you must drink only in moderation. Limit alcoholic drinks to one a day—two at most. Keep in mind that 12 ounces of beer, 5 ounces of wine, and 1½ ounces of distilled beverages all contain the same dose of alcohol. If you drink, I suggest you select fermented beverages (beer and wine), whose alcohol is produced by the natural fermentation of fruits and grains, rather than distilled beverages such as vodka, gin, and whiskey.

Whole-Body Detoxification

Fasting

For centuries, many people have used fasting—the act of abstaining from all food and drink (except water) for a specified period of time—as a means of cleaning out the body. Fasts are part of many religious traditions. For example, Native Americans would fast during the vision quest, a days-long ritual involving the search for deep spiritual insight. Jews fast on Yom Kippur, the most solemn of holidays, as a sign of repentance. Fasts are also used for therapeutic reasons, to increase the elimination of wastes and enhance the healing processes.

Fasting can be used as a form of detoxification. In fact, I like to recommend that a person fast once a year as part of an annual internal "spring cleaning." However, there are some important safety guidelines you should follow if you choose to fast.

Keep in mind that many toxins are fat-soluble and are stored in fat cells. Examples include heavy metals such as mercury and pesticides such as DDT. If you abstain from food, your body will get its energy by burning its reserves of fat. But when the cells burn fat, they also release the poisons they've been storing. As toxin levels in the blood increase, so does the risk of serious damage to tissues, especially the brain and nerves. Thus, instead of eliminating toxins, fasting can sometimes release them to wreak their deadly havoc.

Another concern is that if you fast, you aren't getting the nutrients you need to keep the detoxification system running. Your liver needs a steady supply of proteins, vitamins, and minerals to produce the substances that make detox happen, such as enzymes and bile. Without raw materials, liver cells—and their thousands of little factories—simply shut down. A fast can cause blood sugar levels to plummet, so people with diabetes are at risk of lapsing into a coma.

What's more, unless you eat fruits, vegetables, legumes, and whole grains, you may not get enough fiber. Fiber helps the feces absorb water. Water lubricates the stool so you can pass it more easily and quickly. But by absorbing water, your stool also picks up the toxins the water contains. And remember that the whole goal of the Phase II detox system is to make toxins water soluble. Having adequate fiber makes all that Phase II effort pay off.

Fiber also picks up the poison payload carried by molecules of bile. Almost all of the bile you produce each day—perhaps 99 percent—is reabsorbed by the intestine and recycled to the liver. The bile goes back to work, but it leaves behind the crud it picked up along its journey. Like a biological trash hauler, fiber grabs the once-toxic molecule and carries it out of the body. Although fiber provides almost no nutritional value, it is vital for keeping our passageways clean.

For these and other reasons, fasting should be done only with care and caution. Talk to your medical doctor before you begin. You need to know if you have any medical condition, such as diabetes, that may worsen due to fasting.

If your doctor approves, you can probably fast for up to three days at home. Longer fasts usually require medical supervision in a hospital or clinic.

During the fast, drink only fresh fruit and vegetable juices (ideally prepared from organic produce) for the next three days. You will need a juice extractor to prepare the juice yourself. In my opinion, the Juiceman models from Salton are the best because of their good performance and ease of use. Any department store or store that sells small kitchen appliances should have juicers for sale. I think they are a good investment, especially if you have kids. While it is often difficult to get kids to eat their fruits and vegetables, you can make some delicious, highly nutritious fresh juices that they will absolutely love.

During the three-day juice fast, drink four 8- to 12-ounce glasses of fresh juice throughout the day. In addition to the fresh juice, an equal amount of pure water should also be consumed. More is okay if you feel thirsty. Juice reduces the side effects often associated with a water fast, such as light-headedness, fatigue, and headaches. Stay away from coffee and soft drinks. Herbal teas (unsweetened) are fine, especially green tea, rose hip tea, dandelion tea, and licorice tea. You need fluids, but fresh juice, especially vegetable juice, gives you the nutrients you need—vitamins, flavonoids, antioxidants—for good detox activity.

If you do not want to invest in a juice extractor, let me offer an alternative. There are a number of "green drinks" on the market that can be used instead. These products contain dehydrated barley, wheat grass, or algae sources such as chorella or spirulina that are then rehydrated by mixing with water. Some of the more popular brands are Green Magma, Kyo-Green, Greens +, and ProGreens. Although I think it is best to make these green drinks mixed with water, you can use a little apple juice if desired. Use the appropriate amount for two servings and drink four of these double servings throughout the day.

Plan to rest during your fast. Schedule it for a time when activity levels and stress will be low. Don't exercise during the fast, although light stretching and short walks are fine. I encourage napping. Resting improves detoxification, because less metabolic activity means that the body produces fewer toxins that have to be eliminated. Practice good breathing and relaxation techniques. (See Lifestyle Tune-Up #2, following Chapter 2.)

Because a fast slows down your metabolism, you may find that your body temperature drops a little, as will your blood pressure, pulse, and breathing rate. You may sleep less. This is all normal, but to make sure things don't slow down *too* much, always keep yourself warm.

For your final meal before the fast, eat only fresh fruits and vegetables. To break the fast, reintroduce solid foods gradually, in limited portions and at room temperature. Eat slowly, chew thoroughly.

For added nutritional support during a fast:

- Take a high-potency multiple vitamin and mineral formula.
- Take extra doses of the lipotropic (fat-metabolizing) agents: 1,000 mg of choline and 1,000 mg of methionine or cysteine or both daily.
- Take at least 500 mg of vitamin C and 200 IU of vitamin E three times per day.
- Take 1 to 2 tbsp of a fiber supplement before bed. The best fiber sources are those that contain soluble fiber, such as powdered psyllium seed husks, guar gum, or oat bran.
- If you are particularly overloaded with toxins, take silymarin, 70 to 210 mg three times per day.

Gentle Heating

Your body removes many toxins by shipping them out through the pores in the skin. Exposure to heat causes your pores to open. Heat also makes you sweat, because your body sends moisture where it is needed to cool the skin. Since Phase II detoxification makes toxins water soluble, sweating can help purify your insides.

Saunas and hot-water foot baths are healthy and pleasant ways to promote whole-body (systemic) detoxification. A prolonged low-temperature sauna (less than 110 degrees F) for up to an hour once or twice a week is a great way to aid detoxification. It will do you more good than a few minutes in a very hot sauna. Take the slow and steady approach. Pregnant women, children, and adults with heart disease or seizures should not take saunas. Nor should you sauna after intense exercise or after drinking alcohol. Check with your doctor before taking a prolonged sauna.

Since not everyone has access to a sauna, or the time for an hour-long session, here's an alternative. Soak your feet in about six inches of hot water, as hot as you can handle comfortably (it does not have to be unbearable). Soak your feet for at least twenty minutes, adding hot water as necessary. This technique should get your pores open and help you work up a light sweat. You can take a full bath or shower when you are finished. It is not as effective as the prolonged sauna, but you can do it more often—as many as two to four times a week—to make up the difference.

Key Steps to Tuning Up Your Detoxification System

- Decrease the toxic load by avoiding exposure to harmful chemicals and by eating fiber-rich foods.
- Take additional antioxidants to neutralize free radicals: vitamin C, 500 to 1,500 mg per day; vitamin E, 400 to 800 IU per day.
- Improve liver function by eating garlic and onions, and foods from the Brassica family (cabbage, broccoli, Brussels sprouts, etc.); if needed, take lipotropic formulas or silymarin.
- Improve kidney function by drinking at least six to eight glasses of water each day.
- Avoid alcohol or consume it only in moderation.
- Do a three-day juice fast every spring (consult your physician first).
- Use an extended sauna or hot-water foot baths frequently.

Lifestyle Tune-Up #3: Boost Your Intake of Antioxidants

The terms *antioxidants* and *free radicals* are becoming familiar to most health-minded individuals. Loosely defined, a free radical is a highly reactive oxygen molecule that can destroy body tissues, especially cell membranes. Like tiny ornery BBs, these particles shoot through the cell's membranes, tearing gaping holes and putting the cell at risk.

All atoms contain small particles called electrons. Normally electrons come in pairs. When you burn oxygen, though, one of the electrons can sometimes get stripped away. The atom—now a free radical—becomes unstable and goes on a frantic search to find another electron to complete the set. It will grab on to any electron it can find. In the process, though, it can destroy the molecule it has robbed. This process is known as oxidation, and it is similar to what happens when an apple turns brown or a car gets rusty.

Free radicals assault us from all directions. Some of these come from our environment, in pollutants such as chemicals or cigarette smoke. But they are also the result of our own metabolic activity. Our cells need to burn oxygen to produce their endless supply of life-giving chemicals. In the process, though, they produce free radicals. Approximately 15 percent of the oxygen we breathe combines with fats and other substances to produce free radicals.

Because free radicals destroy cells, damage by free radicals is what makes us age. Free radicals are partly responsible for many diseases, including the two biggest killers of Americans, heart disease and cancer.

Antioxidants, in contrast, are compounds that protect against free-radical damage. They work by "calming down" the free radical, lending it one of its own electrons and thus putting an end to its rampage. By mopping up free radicals, antioxidants prevent degenerative diseases. They slow down the aging process, enhance immune function, reduce inflammation, and fight allergies.

A diet rich in antioxidants has shown protective or therapeutic effects against:

- Heart disease and strokes
- Cancer
- Cataracts and age-related macular degeneration
- Cognitive impairment and Alzheimer's disease
- Age-related immune dysfunction
- Diabetes
- Virtually every chronic degenerative disease

The best-known antioxidant nutrients are beta-carotene, selenium, and vitamins C and E. Supplementation with these nutrients is important in boosting antioxidant levels, but it is even more important to consume a diet rich in plant foods, especially fruits and vegetables.

One of the most exciting recent developments in nutrition and natural medicine is our growing understanding of various plant compounds known as phytochemicals (*phyto-* means "plant"). Neither vitamins nor minerals, these substances are abundant in many leaves, seeds, beans, fruits, and vegetables. They produce a wide range of natural effects in the body. By increasing our intake of certain phytochemicals, we can improve body function and help prevent a number of debilitating illnesses, especially cancer.

Table 3-3: Examples of Anticancer Phytochemicals

Phytochemical	Actions	Sources
Carotenes	Antioxidants; enhance immune functions	Dark-colored vegetables such as carrots, squash, spinach, kale, tomatoes, sweet potatoes; fruits such as cantaloupe, apricots, and citrus fruit
Coumarins	Antitumor properties; enhance immune functions; stimulate antioxidant mechanisms	Carrots, celery, fennel, beets, citrus fruits

Phytochemical	Actions	Sources
Dithiolthiones, glucosinolates, and thiocyanates	Block cancer-causing compounds from damaging cells	Cabbage-family vegetables—broccoli, Brussels sprouts, kale, etc.
Flavonoids	Antioxidants; direct antitumor effects; immune-enhancing properties	Fruits, particularly darker fruits such as berries, cherries, and citrus fruits; also vegetables, including tomatoes, peppers, and greens
Isoflavonoids	Block estrogen receptors	Soy and other legumes
Lignans	Antioxidants; modulate hormone receptors	Flaxseed and flaxseed oil; whole grains, nuts, and seeds
Limonoids	Enhance detoxification; block carcinogens	Citrus fruits
Polyphenols	Antioxidants; block carcinogen formation; modulate hormone receptors	Green tea, chocolate, red wine
Sterols	Block production of carcinogens; modulate hormone receptors	Soy, nuts, seeds

One important group of phytochemicals are *pigments*. As the term suggests, pigments give foods their color. Color contributes to food's "eye appeal." Equally important for survival, color helps us recognize when a food has spoiled. But pigments do more than just make food look pretty (or rotten). They are powerful chemicals that contribute to your body's metabolic activity.

The best-known pigments, and the ones found most widely in foods, are the carotenes. These are the red and yellow pigments found in vegetables such as carrots, peppers, sweet potatoes, and tomatoes, and in fruits such as apricots, watermelons, and cherries. Carotenes are also found in green leafy vegetables, such as spinach, and in legumes, grains, and seeds.

Carotenes are one family in a larger clan of plant chemicals called the carotenoids. Scientists have identified over six hundred types of carotenoids. During metabolism, some carotenes—perhaps as many as fifty—are converted into vitamin A. Beta-carotene is perhaps the most biologically active. That means the body converts most of it into vitamin A. But additional carotenes are also necessary for a complete diet, because they produce other healthy effects in the body. I'll have more to say about the vitamins a little later.

Another important group of phytochemicals are the *flavonoids*. As a class of compounds, flavonoids have been referred to as "nature's biological response modifiers" because of their anti-inflammatory, antiallergenic, antiviral, and anticancer properties. In addition, flavonoids act as powerful antioxidants, providing remarkable protection against oxidative and free-radical damage. These substances work primarily as antioxidants to protect your cells. Good dietary sources of flavonoids include citrus fruits, berries, onions, parsley, legumes, green tea, and red wine. A large number of the beneficial effects of many herbal medicines, such as *Ginkgo biloba* extract, are due to their flavonoid components. So far, researchers have discovered over four thousand flavonoids.

TYPES OF FLAVONOIDS

- The PCOs (short for proanthocyanidin oligomers) are the blue or purple pigments found in grapes, blueberries, and other foods. They can also be extracted from pine bark. These substances work as antioxidants and help prevent destruction of collagen, an important protein for healthy skin and connective tissue. Extracts of grape seeds and pine bark are popular supplements that provide PCOs. They are also referred to as oligomeric proanthocyanidins [OPC].
- Quercetin is found in many foods. One of the best dietary sources is onions. Besides serving as an antioxidant, quercetin helps reduce the effects of inflammation and promotes activity of hormones such as insulin. Quercetin is a popular flavonoid supplement often used in the treatment of allergies. The usual dosage is 100 to 200 mg before meals.
- Citrus bioflavonoids are found in fruits such as oranges, limes, lemons, and grapefruit. Besides providing antioxidant activity, they also appear to improve blood circulation and increase the ability of key nutrients to leave the tiny blood vessels (capillaries) and reach cells more efficiently. Citrus bioflavonoids are especially important

in protecting against colon cancer. They are often included in vitamin C supplements because they enhance the activity of vitamin C.
- Polyphenols are complex flavonoids found in such foods as green
tea, red wine, and even chocolate. These substances are potent antioxidants that offer significant protection against heart disease and
various cancers, especially in the gastrointestinal tract. They work
by blocking the formation of cancer-causing chemicals such as
nitrosamines.

Based on extensive data, it appears that a combination of antioxidants will provide greater antioxidant protection than any single nutritional antioxidant. Therefore, in addition to consuming a diet rich
in plant foods, especially fruits and vegetables, I recommend using a
combination of antioxidant nutrients rather than high dosages of any
single antioxidant. Mixtures of antioxidant nutrients appear to work
together harmoniously to produce the phenomenon of synergy. In
other words, 1 + 1 = 3.

The two primary antioxidants in the human body are vitamin C
and vitamin E. Vitamin C is an "aqueous phase" antioxidant. This
means that it is found in body and cell compartments composed of
water. In contrast, vitamin E is a "lipid phase" antioxidant because it
is found in lipid (fat) soluble body compartments such as cell membranes and fatty molecules. If you are taking a high-potency multiple
vitamin and mineral formula, many of the supportive antioxidant nutrients such as selenium, zinc, and beta-carotene are provided for.
Therefore, your primary concern may be simply to ensure beneficial
levels of vitamin C and vitamin E. Here are my daily supplementation
guidelines for these key nutritional antioxidants for supporting general health. Be sure to note how much your multiple vitamin and
mineral formula is providing.

Vitamin E (d-alpha-tocopherol)   400 to 800 IU
Vitamin C (ascorbic acid)   500 to 1,500 mg

NATURAL VITAMIN E IS BEST
Vitamin E is available in many different forms. Natural forms of vitamin E
are designated d-, as in d-alpha-tocopherol, while synthetic forms are dl-,
as in dl-alpha-tocopherol. The letters *d* and *l* reflect mirror images of the
vitamin E molecule (just as your right hand [d] and left hand [l] are mirror

images of each other). In the human body, only the d form is recognized. Although the l form has antioxidant activity, it may actually inhibit the d form from entering cell membranes. Therefore, my recommendation is to avoid synthetic vitamin E.

Natural forms	Synthetic forms
d-alpha-tocopherol	dl-alpha-tocopherol
d-alpha-tocopheryl acetate	dl-alpha-tocopheryl acetate
d-alpha-tocopheryl succinate	dl-alpha-tocopheryl succinate

I recommend choosing a flavonoid-rich extract to provide extra antioxidant protection. The antioxidant activity of flavonoids is generally more potent and effective against a broader range of oxidants than traditional antioxidant nutrients such as vitamins C and E, selenium, and zinc. We can use certain flavonoid-rich extracts as tissue-specific antioxidants because of their ability to be concentrated in specific body tissues. For example, I recommend *Ginkgo biloba* extract to most of my patients over the age of fifty because of its ability to act as an antioxidant in the brain and in the vascular lining throughout the body. Use the table below to identify which flavonoid-rich extract is most appropriate for you and take it according to the recommended dosage.

Flavonoid-Rich Extract	Daily Dosage for Antioxidant Support	Indication
Grape seed extract (95% proanthocyanidin oligomers)	50 to 100 mg	Systemic antioxidant, specific. Best choice for most people under the age of 50. Also specific for the lungs, diabetes, varicose veins, and protection against heart disease.

Flavonoid-Rich Extract	Daily Dosage for Antioxidant Support	Indication
Green tea extract (60–70% total polyphenols)	150 to 300 mg	Systemic antioxidant. Best choice for protection against cancer. Also protects against heart disease.
Ginkgo biloba extract (24% ginkgo flavonglycosides)	120 to 240 mg	Best choice for most people over the age of 50. Protects brain and vascular lining.
Milk thistle extract (70% silymarin)	100 to 300 mg	Best choice if the liver or skin needs additional antioxidant protection.
Bilberry extract (25% anthocyanidins)	80 to 160 mg	Best choice to protect the eyes.
Hawthorn extract (10% procyanidins)	100 to 300 mg	Best choice in heart disease or high blood pressure.

CHAPTER 4

Tuning Up Your Metabolism

Why is it that some people can eat all the food they want and still stay thin while others seem to gain weight if they merely look at a cookie? The answer can be summed up in one word: metabolism.

The term *metabolism* refers to all the chemical processes that take place in your body. Strictly speaking, everything I talk about in this book—digestion, detoxification, activity in the immune system, and so on—is all part of your metabolism. In this chapter, though, I'll focus mainly on the ways your body produces and uses energy.

Each of us has a different rate of metabolism. Whatever your starting point, tuning up your metabolism will help you use energy more efficiently (this means you spend less energy to achieve the same level of function). A metabolic tune-up provides many benefits. You'll feel better, have more pep, control your weight, and sleep more soundly.

Your Metabolic Rate

There are two basic types of metabolism. The first breaks molecules into smaller parts (catabolism). The second builds them into larger units (anabolism). Catabolism creates and releases energy, while anabolism uses up energy.

Before you can use energy, your body has to create and release it. A key player in this transaction is a molecule called adenosine triphosphate, or

ATP for short. In simple terms, your cells take in the nutrients that have been digested by your intestinal tract. Inside the cells, the nutrients (especially glucose, the simplest form of sugar) are reassembled into molecules of ATP. In the process, energy is temporarily stored in the bonds between the atoms of this molecule. When energy is needed, enzymes step in and break the bonds, releasing the stored energy. The ability of your cells to make ATP is essential for life, because ATP provides energy that all body cells need. Without ATP, the body's chemical factory shuts down, cells can't import nutrients or make proteins, and muscle cells lose their ability to contract and move. In short, life grinds to a halt.

At all times you are burning energy to keep your heart beating, your lungs pumping air, your brain working, and your tissues in good repair. You also use up energy maintaining proper body temperature. The rate at which these basic functions use energy when you are awake but not moving is known as the basal metabolic rate, or BMR. The BMR is sometimes referred to as the "energy cost of living."

WHAT IS YOUR BMR?

To calculate your approximate basal metabolism rate, determine your weight in kilograms. Divide the number of pounds you weigh by 2.2. If you are a man, the result is your hourly BMR.

Example: John weighs 176 pounds (80 kilograms). His BMR is 80, which means he burns up 80 calories an hour, or 1,920 calories per day, just staying alive.

If you are a woman, you need to take an additional step. Multiply your weight in kilograms by 0.9. The result is your hourly BMR.

Example: Mary weighs 121 pounds, or 55 kilograms. Her BMR is about 50 (55 × 0.9), which means she needs to consume at least 1,200 calories per day to fuel her basic body functions.

Any type of movement—getting up out of a chair, typing on a keyboard, scratching your nose—increases your energy expenditure. The more effort required, the faster the rate at which you use up energy (see Table 4-1). Even a few seconds of very intense activity can significantly increase your metabolic output. One reason for this increase is that skeletal muscles make up nearly half of your body's mass, and so they consume a proportionate amount of energy. When you exercise vigorously, even for only a few minutes, your metabolic rate increases to fifteen to twenty times normal. The rate remains high for several hours afterward.

Exercise raises your metabolic rate, not just during your workout but for several hours afterward. The impact on your metabolism depends on how intensely you exercise. A light workout might help you burn another 5 or 10 calories after the session ends, while a moderate workout will use up another 12 to 35 calories. In contrast, strenuous exercise can increase postexercise energy burning by up to 180 calories.

Table 4-1: Typical Energy Expenditure (kilocalories per hour)

Activity	Man (150 pounds)	Woman (120 pounds)
Sleeping	65	50
Sitting quietly	75	60
Walking	350	300
Cycling	450	350
Gardening	550	450
Jogging	600	450
Swimming	700	550
Running	900	700

WHAT ARE CALORIES?
Calories are units of heat energy (*calor* means "heat" in Latin). One calorie is the amount of energy it takes to raise the temperature of a gram of water (about three-hundredths of an ounce) by one degree centigrade. That's not much energy. In fact, the calories listed on food labels are actually kilocalories, or units of 1,000 calories. For simplicity's sake, I will use the term *calorie* here to reflect kilocalories.

Factors Affecting BMR

Your BMR depends on many factors: the quantity and quality of food you eat (certain foods require more energy to digest than others, and eating more food slows metabolism), adequate supplies of water and oxygen, and the amount of heat your body produces. Genes play a major part in determining the BMR. Remember the concept of biochemical individuality: Each of us has a different energy requirement. Some people burn more calories to maintain body temperature and weight; others burn fewer calories to get the same result. Other important factors are:

- *The body's general size and shape.* As the ratio of body surface area to body volume increases, so does the rate of heat loss. The metabolism must work harder to make up for the lost heat. For this reason, a person who weighs 150 pounds and is five feet tall will have a lower BMR than one who weighs the same but is six feet tall.
- *The proportion of muscle (lean) tissue compared with fat tissue.* Even at rest, muscles use up energy at a faster pace just to stay alive. The more muscle you have, the higher your energy needs.
- *Gender.* As a rule, women have proportionately more body fat and less lean tissue than men. Because of this, their BMR is 5 to 10 percent lower.
- *Age.* As we get older, our muscle mass tends to decrease. This is partly due to natural body changes over time, but it is also the result of a decline in activity. Many older people put on weight because they do not decrease their calorie intake to compensate for their slowing metabolism.
- *Stress.* Physical or emotional stress activates the body's energy-producing system, known as the "fight-or-flight response," causing the BMR to soar. The longer stress continues, the more rapidly your body uses up its energy supply. This, in turn, leads to deep fatigue and leaves you vulnerable to infections and other illnesses.
- *Growth rate.* We need extra energy during growth periods, which is one reason why babies feed so often and why teenagers seem to be ravenously hungry all the time. During pregnancy and while breast-feeding, a mother's energy requirement increases by perhaps 50 percent, because she is sharing her body's energy supply with her developing baby.
- *Environmental temperature.* Your body works hard to maintain a steady temperature. To keep cool, people who live and work in tropical climates use about 20 percent more energy during the day than people in a temperate climate. Likewise, people in cold climates burn more energy to keep warm.
- *Certain drugs, especially stimulants such as caffeine, nicotine, or amphetamines.* Many people find that they gain weight after they quit smoking, due partly to the slowing down of their metabolism and partly to the fact that they eat more to relieve the oral cravings that cigarettes formerly satisfied.
- *Illness.* If you develop an infection, your body's metabolism gears up to fight off the invading microbe. The immune system deploys an army of immune cells that seek out and destroy the disease-causing bugs. Your brain boosts your temperature, which makes your body an uncomfortable place for the microbe to be. The fever that makes you so

miserable is actually a metabolic strategy to make you well. For each degree your body temperature rises, your BMR increases by 10 to 15 percent. Overall, an illness can increase your resting energy expenditure by up to 40 percent. Recovery from surgery pushes the rate higher by a whopping 50 percent.

Weight Control

Your ability to maintain a desired body weight is the result of a simple equation: the difference between the number of calories consumed and the number of calories spent. If you take in, say, 2,000 calories a day and burn 2,100 calories, you will eventually lose weight. But if you eat more than you burn, you gain weight, because your body stores unused nutrients (fats, sugars, and carbohydrates) in your cells. If your energy requirement suddenly increases—during exercise, for example—your body will first use up the most easily available source of calories: blood sugar. Once that supply is gone, your cells will release their stores of fats and use those to produce energy. That's why exercise is so valuable in maintaining a healthy weight. Muscle activity, including increased heart and breathing rates, uses up calories that are just sitting around taking up space.

The types of foods in your diet play a big role in determining your calorie intake. Carbohydrates and proteins supply about 4 calories per gram. But fat packs 9 calories into each gram. Ounce for ounce, fatty foods give you more than twice as many calories as other foods.

WHY MOST DIETS DON'T WORK

If you've been struggling to lose weight on a low-calorie diet, I have an important tip for you: Eat more. Yes, in order to lose weight, you must feed your metabolism. The key is to choose high-fiber, low-calorie foods instead of high-calorie foods loaded with fats and sugars. These healthy foods can help you achieve long-term results. What are high-fiber, low-calorie foods? Vegetables, legumes (beans), most fruits, and whole grains.

The very act of eating and digestion requires a significant amount of energy. Eating breakfast, for example, can boost your resting metabolism rate by 10 percent or more. On the other hand, dieting or fasting will cause your total energy expenditure to fall. The biggest mistake people make when trying to lose weight is trying to starve themselves thin. This creates a phenomenon that too many Americans know firsthand—the yo-yo effect. They lose weight only to put it right back on and then some. When the body is not fed properly, it feels that it is starving. The result is that metabolism slows down and less fat is burned. This is a natural response that our bodies have developed to help us survive famine and starvation.

Diets do not work if the focus is on restricting food intake rather than on enhancing metabolism. If you need to get your weight under control, then your first step should be tuning up your metabolism.

Tune-Up Tip: Successful Exercise

Regular physical exercise is an absolute must for a healthy metabolism. Exercise is also an effective strategy for weight control because it causes a favorable shift in body composition, increasing muscle mass and decreasing body fat; the greater your muscle mass, the greater your fat-burning capacity. When you diet to lose weight, most of the reduction comes from loss of water. In addition, dieting lowers your basal metabolic rate (BMR)—in other words, your body slows down to compensate for the reduced caloric intake, thus keeping your weight basically the same. Exercise has been shown to compensate for a reduced BMR due to calorie restriction, and it helps your body lower your "set point," the weight to which your body naturally returns. Here are seven tips to help you develop an effective exercise program.

1. *Recognize the importance of physical exercise.* Make regular exercise a top priority in your life.
2. *Before starting, consult your physician.* This is especially important if you are over forty years of age. Suddenly launching into vigorous exercise when you're not used to it can cause dangerous strain on your heart. Regardless of your age, before exercising see a physician if you are a smoker or if you have known heart disease, high blood pressure, or irregular heartbeat. Consult a doctor if you become breathless with moderate exertion or if you experience pain or pressure in your chest, arm, teeth, jaw, or neck during exercise.
3. *Make it fun.* If you like what you're doing, you have a better chance of sticking with it. Find a workout buddy and plan to exercise together. For example, you and your neighbors might enjoy taking brisk walks early in the morning or in the evening.
4. *Give yourself time to exercise.* To do you the most good, exercise must cause an increase in your heart rate and must be sustained for a minimum of twenty minutes. Evidence suggests that exercising in this way three times a week is usually enough to provide you with benefits. (More

frequent exercise of longer duration is even better.) Aerobic exercise—movement that increases utilization of oxygen—includes walking briskly, jogging, bicycling, cross-country skiing, swimming, aerobic dance, and racquet sports. Strength-training (anaerobic) exercise, such as lifting weights, is just as critical to long-term weight control as aerobic exercise because it is able to build muscle mass.

5. *Monitor exercise intensity.* This is determined by measuring your heart rate (beats per minute). To check your pulse, put your index and middle fingers on the opposite wrist or on your neck just below the jaw. Count the number of beats in twenty seconds and multiply by three. This is your resting heart rate per minute. Your goal should be to increase your heart rate to within the appropriate training rate range for the duration of aerobic exercise (say twenty minutes). The training rate depends on your age. To determine your rate range, subtract your age from 185 to get the top of the range, and subtract another twenty to determine the bottom range. Thus a forty-year-old would have a target training heart rate of 125 to 145 beats per minute. Do not exceed the higher figure in this range.

6. *Exercise regularly.* You need to commit to your exercise plan. Exercise at least three times a week throughout the year. Some people find it easier to exercise every day, so that it becomes a habit. With strength-training exercise, however, most experts recommend taking a day off to allow your body to recover.

7. *Stay motivated.* If you are goal-oriented, set realistic targets for your exercise—more laps, more lifts—and keep track of how you're doing. Reward yourself when you reach the goal. Vary your routine to avoid boredom. Read exercise books or magazines for tips on getting the most out of your program and learning other exercise strategies.

————— Stoking Your Fat-Burning Furnace —————

When you increase your metabolic rate, you stoke your internal furnace to burn fat more quickly. As a result, pounds melt away. In addition to regular exercise, one of the best natural methods to increase your fat-burning machinery is to use a thermogenic formula. *Thermogenesis* means "heat production."

A certain amount of the food we consume is converted immediately to heat. This process, known as diet-induced thermogenesis, is the method by which the body "wastes" calories. There is evidence that rate of diet-induced thermogenesis is the key factor in determining whether an individual is likely to be overweight. In lean individuals, a meal may stimulate up to a 40 percent increase in heat production. In contrast, overweight individuals often display only a 10 percent or less increase in heat production following a meal. The food energy is stored as fat instead of being converted to heat.

Factors that decrease thermogenesis in overweight people include loss of sensitivity to the hormone insulin and impaired sympathetic nervous system activity. Insulin sensitivity is a bit of a Catch-22—obesity decreases insulin sensitivity, and a decrease in insulin sensitivity promotes obesity. Tuning up insulin sensitivity is an important goal in weight loss and is discussed on pages 117–119.

The sympathetic nervous system controls many body functions, including metabolism. Many overweight individuals may have a slow metabolism due to lack of stimulation by the sympathetic nervous system. Several natural plant-derived stimulants, described below, can activate the sympathetic nervous system, thereby increasing the metabolic rate and thermogenesis. The result: weight loss.

Free Foods

Most vegetables are fantastic diet foods, as they are very high in nutritional value but low in calories. In fact I consider some to be "free foods" for people counting calories. They can be eaten in any amount because the calories they contain are offset by the number of calories your body burns in the process of digestion. If you are trying to lose weight, these foods can help keep you feeling satisfied between meals.

Alfalfa sprouts	Endive
Bell peppers	Escarole
Bok choy	Lettuce
Cabbage	Parsley
Chicory	Radishes
Celery	Spinach
Chinese cabbage	Turnips
Cucumber	Watercress

THE LOW-CARB DIET CRAZE

Fad diets come and go. In the 1970s high-protein, low-carbohydrate plans like the Scarsdale Diet and Dr. Atkins' Diet Revolution were in. Twenty years later these diets have resurfaced as The Zone, The Carbohydrate Addict's Dietary Program, Sugar Busters, and Dr. Atkins' New Diet Revolution. Can you really lose weight by feasting on beef, eggs, bacon, and other high-protein, high-fat foods? And should you?

The bottom line for any diet to be able to promote weight loss is that it must provide fewer calories than you burn. Most people in the United States eat way too much sugar and refined carbohydrates, so when they knock these foods out of their diet they lose weight. That is the real key to the success of these programs.

The concern that I have with these programs is that they focus too heavily on consuming calories from animal foods. I worry that people chowing down on all these high-protein, high-fat animal foods may be successful in their short-term goal of weight loss but may be increasing their risk of cancer, heart disease, and other degenerative diseases. Most Americans already derive well over 50 percent of their calories from animal foods.

What is a healthy diet? First take a look at what your body is designed for. Is your body designed to eat plant foods, animal foods, or both? Based on detailed anatomical and historical evidence, it is clear that humans evolved as "hunter-gatherers." That is, humans appear to be omnivores capable of surviving on both gathered (plant) and hunted (animal) foods. However, while the human gastrointestinal tract is capable of digesting both animal and plant foods, there are indications that it can accommodate plant foods much more easily than the harder-to-digest animal foods. Specifically, the makeup of our teeth, the manner in which our jaws swing, and the long length of the human intestinal tract all point to our bodies being built to consume primarily plant foods. Nonhuman primates eat mainly fruits and vegetables but may also eat small animals, lizards, and eggs if given the opportunity. Based upon all of this evidence, it appears that humans are designed to eat a diet that includes around 2 percent of their calories as animal foods.

In addition to anatomical evidence, there is a tremendous amount of data showing that a diet high in animal foods is a major factor in the development of heart disease, cancer, strokes, arthritis, and many other chronic degenerative diseases. It is now the recommendation of many health and medical organizations that the human diet should focus primarily on plant-based foods—vegetables, fruits, grains, legumes, nuts, seeds, and so on. Personally, I am in this camp as well. That being the case, I am philosophically opposed to many of the principles of these low-carbohydrate diets. However, there is one key notion in the low-carb diets that I agree with wholeheartedly: If you want to lose weight, cut out refined sugars and reduce your intake of bread, pasta, and other starches. But I recommend that instead of loading up on high-protein, high-fat foods, you should concentrate on consuming nonstarchy vegetables, fish, and low-fat meat choices, including poultry. I believe these dietary changes not only will help people lose weight, but will make them healthier as well.

Herbal Thermogenic Formulas

Herbal thermogenic formulas, designed to enhance thermogenesis, have become quite popular weight-loss aids. Some well-known brands are Metabolife, Metabolift, Escalation, Thermogenics +, Ultra Diet Pep, and Thermogenic Power. Their active ingredients are ephedrine, derived from an herb called ephedra (also known as ma huang), and natural sources of caffeine, such as the kola nut or the herb guarana. Ephedrine and caffeine act by stimulating the nervous system, which in turn ratchets up your metabolism and the production of heat.

Use of herbal thermogenic formulas is somewhat controversial. In my opinion, these products can be quite useful as part of a well-designed overall weight-reduction program. I became quite a proponent of thermogenic formulas when I witnessed a 280-pound woman transform herself into a 130-pound woman in a little over one year as a result of taking an herbal thermogenic formula.

The bottom line is that for people prone to obesity, thermogenic formulas address the underlying metabolic problems. In many instances they may help reset the internal fat-burning thermostat. Once that has occurred, the emphasis then shifts to weight loss through more conventional means: diet and exercise. If you choose to take an herbal thermogenic formula, do so with caution.

THERMOGENIC FORMULAS: PROCEED WITH CAUTION If you choose an herbal thermogenic product for weight loss, use common sense and take only recommended dosages. Do not exceed these amounts; with products of this type, more is not necessarily better. Products standardized for their stimulant levels offer considerable benefits over herbal products that do not specify their ephedrine or caffeine content. I recommend products that provide a daily dose of 30 mg ephedrine and 100 mg caffeine. Higher doses are more likely to cause nervousness, irritability, insomnia, and increased blood pressure and/or heart rate.

The FDA advisory review panel on nonprescription drugs recommended that ephedrine not be taken by patients who have heart disease, high blood pressure, thyroid disease, diabetes, or difficulty in urination due to enlargement of the prostate. In addition, ephedrine should not be used to treat patients who are taking medicines to lower blood pressure (antihypertensives) or antidepressants.

Tune-Up Tip: Spice It Up to Burn It Off

Several studies have shown that increasing the intake of red (cayenne) pepper *(Capsicum frutescens)* may be an effective method to increase BMR, diet-induced thermogenesis, and the burning of fat for energy (lipid oxidation). In the most recent study, after ingesting a standardized dinner on the previous evening, the subjects ate one of the following for breakfast: a high-fat meal, a high-fat meal with 10 g red pepper, a high-carbohydrate meal, or a high-carbohydrate meal with 10 g red pepper. Diet-induced thermogenesis was significantly enhanced by the addition of red pepper to either meal, but especially the high-fat meal. Similar results have been noted with garlic and ginger in animal studies. The bottom line from this study and others is that adding red pepper (as well as garlic and ginger) to your diet is a safe, natural way to enhance the burning of fat.

5-HTP

Another new approach to weight loss involves use of a special form of the amino acid tryptophan, known as 5-hydroxytryptophan, or 5-HTP. 5-HTP is the middle step in the process by which the body transforms tryptophan into the important brain chemical serotonin. Commercially available 5-HTP is isolated from a natural source—a seed from an African plant *(Griffonia simplicifolia)*.

Serotonin is involved in many body processes, including mood regulation. Antidepressants such as Prozac work by keeping serotonin flowing between brain cells. With more serotonin available, the cells stay charged up and running smoothly. Because your brain eventually changes serotonin into melatonin, you also need serotonin for proper sleep. (Certain foods, such as milk and turkey, contain tryptophan, which means they help your body make serotonin. That's why you fall asleep after a Thanksgiving meal of turkey and eggnog!)

A massive amount of evidence suggests that low serotonin levels are a common consequence of modern living. High levels of cortisol, a hormone produced by the adrenal glands in response to stress, and loss of sensitivity to insulin, which can be caused by eating too many foods high in simple sugars, are two of the biggest culprits, because they impair conversion of tryptophan to 5-HTP. In short, the lifestyle and dietary practices of many people living in this stress-filled era result in lowered levels of serotonin within the brain. Consequently many people are overweight, crave sugar and other carbohydrates, experience bouts of depression, get frequent headaches, and have vague muscle aches and pain. All of these conditions have been helped by raising brain serotonin levels with 5-HTP.

Serotonin also plays a role in controlling our eating behavior. Normally, when we eat, the body senses when it has taken in enough food. The digestive tract signals the brain, which throws a switch that basically tells the body to stop eating. Research suggests that serotonin helps make sure that switch is working properly, so that when you've eaten enough, you'll push yourself away from the table.

The trouble is, you can't just take a pill containing serotonin. The molecules would break down in the stomach before they reached the brain. Besides, the brain has a powerful filtering system to keep out certain substances. Serotonin is one of them. Rather than importing serotonin, the brain prefers to make its own supply from 5-HTP.

I have recommended 5-HTP as a weight control strategy to hundreds of people who have gone on to tell me they are very pleased with the results. The substance helps reduce their appetite. But even though they eat less food, they still felt satisfied after a meal. As a bonus, it appears that 5-HTP not only reduces calorie intake, but increases metabolism (specifically, it raises the BMR). Studies in Italy found that overweight women who took 5-HTP lost an average of just under 12 pounds in twelve weeks. If this rate of weight loss was maintained—easier said than done!—it would translate to a loss of roughly 50 pounds a year.

While the studies in Italy used 5-HTP at a dosage of 300 mg three times per day, lower dosages are proving to be as effective for many people. One of my patients, a thirty-eight-year-old mother of three, lost 17 pounds and went down three dress sizes within three months simply by taking 50 mg three times per day twenty minutes before meals. Another lost 26 pounds in six months by taking 100 to 200 mg of 5-HTP three times per day. Taking the lowest dosage of 5-HTP will be easier on your pocketbook.

GUIDELINES FOR USING 5-HTP

Weight Control

- Start with 100 mg three times a day taken twenty minutes before meals.
- If results are unsatisfactory after four weeks of use at 100 mg, take 200 mg three times a day for a month.
- If results are again unsatisfactory after another four weeks, increase the dosage to 300 mg three times for one additional month. If there is no positive result, 5-HTP is not likely to be of benefit. Never exceed the maximum total daily dose of 900 mg (300 mg three times daily).
- If you experience nausea, take 5-HTP with a little food or with ginger capsules (take two 500 mg capsules) or ginger tea. If significant nausea persists, reduce dosage to 50 mg for two weeks before increasing back to 100 mg.

Depression

- Start with 50 mg three times a day taken twenty minutes before meals. After two weeks, if needed, increase the dose to 100 mg three times per day. If results are unsatisfactory after four weeks, increase to a maximum dose of 150 mg three or four times per day.

Sleep

- 100 mg half an hour before bedtime. If results are unsatisfactory after three days, gradually increase to 200 mg, then after two weeks to 300 mg (if needed), in a single dose.

Blood Sugar Control

Your body's endocrine system works hard to maintain the level of blood sugar (glucose) within a narrow range. If something happens to disrupt these mechanisms, your health is at risk. The consequences include hypoglycemia (low blood sugar) or diabetes (high blood sugar). For your tune-up to succeed, you need to get control over blood sugar levels.

ASSESSING BLOOD SUGAR CONTROL

Circle the number that best describes the intensity of your symptoms on the following scale:

0 = I do not experience this symptom
1 = Mild
2 = Moderate
3 = Severe

Part A: Hypoglycemia

Dizziness when standing suddenly	0	1	2	3
Loss of vision when standing suddenly	0	1	2	3
Craving for sweets	0	1	2	3
Headaches relieved by consuming sweets or alcohol	0	1	2	3
Feelings of shakiness two to three hours after a meal	0	1	2	3
Irritability after missing a meal	0	1	2	3
Waking up in the middle of night craving sweets	0	1	2	3
Tiredness or weakness if a meal is missed	0	1	2	3
Heart palpitations after eating sweets	0	1	2	3
Need to drink coffee to get started	0	1	2	3
Impatience, moodiness, nervousness	0	1	2	3
Tiredness 1 to 3 hours after eating	0	1	2	3
Poor memory	0	1	2	3
Poor concentration	0	1	2	3
Forgetfulness	0	1	2	3
Eating produces feelings of calm	0	1	2	3

Add the numbers circled and enter that total here: _____

Scoring   *12 or more: High priority*
            6–11: Moderate priority
            1–5: Low priority

Part B: Hyperglycemia

Night sweats	0	1	2	3
Increased thirst	0	1	2	3
Lowered resistance to infection	0	1	2	3
Fatigue	0	1	2	3
Boils or leg sores	0	1	2	3
Lesions and cuts take a long time to heal	0	1	2	3
Overweight	0	1	2	3
Exercise provides a pickup	0	1	2	3
Failing eyesight	0	1	2	3
Craving for sweets, but eating sweets does not relieve symptoms	0	1	2	3

Add the numbers circled and enter that subtotal here: _____

Circle the number of the answer that applies to you:

Family history of diabetes	NO = 0	YES = 10
Personal history of diabetes	NO = 0	YES = 10

Add the numbers circled and enter that subtotal here: _____
Add the two subtotals and enter that number here: _____

Scoring   *12 or more: High priority*
6–11: Moderate priority
1–5: Low priority

Interpreting Your Score

The questionnaires above are excellent screening tools for identifying problems with blood sugar control. Part A deals with hypoglycemia while Part B is suggestive of diabetes. Both of these conditions are best diagnosed by your physician. This recommendation is especially important if you scored high on Part B. A score of 12 or more on either section means that you will definitely need to follow closely the recommendations for tuning up blood sugar control. If your score is between 6 and 11, it indicates that you need to devote some attention to improving blood sugar control while a score of 5 or less indicates that you may only need to follow the most basic recommendations to improve or maintain proper blood sugar control.

—————————— **Avoid Simple Sugars** ——————————

Eating foods that are high in simple sugars can hinder your efforts to keep your blood sugar under control, especially if you are prone to hypoglycemia or have diabetes. Simple sugars are digested and absorbed too quickly, causing a rapid rise in blood sugar levels. In response to high blood sugar, your pancreas pours out insulin, which causes cells to take up the sugar, thus rapidly lowering the amount in the blood. But your metabolic control system reads those plummeting sugar levels as a sign that your energy supplies are dwindling and that your life may be in danger. Consequently, your adrenal glands step up their production of adrenaline, which works to raise the blood glucose level again. Over time, the adrenal glands become exhausted by the repeated stress, and they can no longer function properly. Eventually the body becomes insensitive to insulin. Left untreated, this situation can lead to adult-onset diabetes (also known as type 2 or non-insulin-dependent diabetes) or Syndrome X.

SYNDROME X

A term increasingly used today to describe a collection of metabolic abnormalities (including glucose or insulin disturbances, high blood cholesterol and triglyceride levels, high blood pressure, and upper-body obesity) that results from elevated insulin levels, which in turn are the product of excessive intake of highly refined carbohydrates.

The human body simply was not designed to handle the amount of refined sugar, salt, and saturated fats that many people in the United States consume. Syndrome X is the label that modern medicine has given to a condition caused primarily by poor dietary and lifestyle choices. Medical researchers spend millions of dollars to develop drugs to address these problems, when it would cost far less and be more effective to prevent them by teaching people how to choose a healthier diet and lifestyle.

For most people, watching their diet is the only step needed to help regulate blood sugar levels. The best strategy is to eliminate all highly refined carbohydrates from your diet. Examples include white sugar, white bread and pastries, pasta made from white flour, and processed breakfast cereals. In the process of manufacture, these foods are stripped of most of their important nutrients.

Boost your intake of complex carbohydrates, including starchy vegetables such as yams and potatoes, legumes, and whole grains. The body breaks down the carbohydrates in these foods more gradually, leading to better blood sugar control. A growing amount of evidence suggests that complex carbohydrates should form a major part of your diet.

Tune-Up Tip: Watch for Hidden Sugar

Read food labels carefully for clues about the amount of sugar the product contains. Words ending in -ose indicate a sugar. Examples include *sucrose, glucose, maltose, lactose,* and *fructose.*

Other "hidden" sugar sources include corn syrup and white grape juice concentrate. More than half of the carbohydrates consumed in this country come from sugars added to foods as sweetening agents.

I became interested in nutrition in the 1970s, at the time hypoglycemia was a popular self-diagnosis. There were a number of popular books (such as *Sugar Blues* by William Duffy, *Hope for Hypoglycemia* by Broda Barnes, and *Sweet and Dangerous* by John Yudkin) attributing every symptom on the hypoglycemia questionnaire (as well as many more) to hypoglycemia. In these books, the dangers of too much sugar in the diet were clearly spelled out. Yet since those books were published the per capita of sugar consumption has risen. The average American now consumes over 100 pounds of sugar and at least 40 pounds of other sweeteners each year. This sugar addiction plays a major role in the high prevalence of poor health and chronic disease in the United States.

A deficiency in the trace mineral chromium can contribute to problems with sugar control. Your body needs chromium to maintain normal glucose levels, use insulin effectively, and keep blood lipid levels down. Some people with diabetes have been able to reduce their need for extra insulin by up to 50 percent after a few months of supplementation with 200 to 400 mcg of chromium per day. I recommend supplements containing chromium in the form of either chromium picolinate or chromium polynicotinate. Both forms are well absorbed by the body.

CASE HISTORY: Chromium Control for Sugar Cravings

Stacey, age thirty-four, came to see me with a long list of complaints, including symptoms of irritable bowel syndrome, migraine headaches, fatigue, depression, and sugar cravings. Stacey's diet largely consisted of high-sugar foods—pastries and coffee (with sugar) for breakfast, candy bars as snacks throughout the day. She never skipped dessert. She knew that too much sugar was probably a factor in her health problems, but she felt powerless to resist her urges. Taking 400 mcg of chromium picolinate did the trick. It reduced her sugar cravings, and as a result, she saw improvement in all of her other related problems. Her case reminded me of an important lesson in natural approaches to healing: Always start with the simple things first.

EXTRA SUPPORT FOR PEOPLE WITH DIABETES

If you have diabetes, I recommend a number of dietary and lifestyle strategies designed to promote a healthy metabolism.

- Consume a diet rich in whole, unprocessed foods: whole grains, legumes, vegetables, nuts, and seeds.
- Eliminate intake of alcohol, caffeine, and sugar.
- Get regular exercise.
- Take supplements:
  High-potency multiple vitamin and mineral formula (including 200–500 mcg of chromium)
  Vitamin C: 500–1000 mg three times a day
  Vitamin E: 400–800 IU daily
  Flaxseed oil: 1 tbsp per day
  Gamma-linolenic acid (GLA), an essential fatty acid, available in extracts of evening primrose, borage, or black currant oil: 240–480 mcg per day
  Magnesium: 250 mg two or three times daily
  Garlic preparation containing 4,000 mcg of allicin potential per day
  Gymnema sylvestre extract (standardized to contain 24% gymnemic acid): 400 mg per day

---

Your Metabolic Control System

Your body's metabolism is primarily controlled by hormones and their effects on nerves and tissues. Hormones are chemicals that are produced by glands and released into the bloodstream, where they travel to produce effects on other tissues. All together, the thyroid and parathyroid glands, adrenal glands, pineal gland, hypothalamus, pituitary gland, pancreas, and sex glands (ovaries in women, testicles in men) make up the endocrine system. The word *endocrine* comes from Greek words meaning "secreting internally."

—— The Hypothalamus and the Pituitary Gland ——

Much of the activity in the endocrine system is under the control of two closely connected control centers in the brain, the hypothalamus and the pituitary gland. This connection is actually a bridge between the nervous system (hypothalamus) and the glandular system (pituitary). In response to stress, these two control centers work together to speed up the heartbeat and breathing rate, widen the pupils of the eyes (the better to see danger), and increase blood flow to the muscles. They also work together to control body temperature, causing you to shiver if you're cold (to generate heat from the muscle activity) or sweat if you're hot (to cool the skin). It is primarily the hypothalamus and pituitary that are in charge of regulating hunger and thirst, and they also play a major role in regulating sleep, sexual behavior, and mood.

The pituitary is sometimes called the "master gland" because it governs the secretion and activity of other endocrine glands via its vital hormones, but much of this activity is actually controlled by the hypothalamus. Here are a few of the control hormones secreted by the pituitary:

- Adrenocorticotropic hormone (ACTH), which activates the adrenal cortex to release steroids
- Growth hormone, which causes cells to divide and produce proteins
- Thyroid-stimulating hormone (TSH), which signals the thyroid to get busy
- Prolactin, which causes milk production in the female breast
- Sex hormones that control the function of male and female sex organs
- Melanocyte-stimulating hormone (MSH), which activates pigment cells and controls skin color
- Antidiuretic hormone (ADH), which controls the rate at which the kidneys produce urine
- Oxytocin, which stimulates uterine contractions during birth

Primary disorders of the pituitary and hypothalamus are rare. Most of the time disturbances of the hypothalamus and pituitary are the result of stress or problems with the endocrine glands. By tuning up the individual components of the system, you will be indirectly reducing the stress on these important control centers.

The Thyroid and Parathyroid Glands

The thyroid gland is located in the front of the neck below the voice box. It is just about the same size and shape—and is in the same location—as a small bow tie. The parathyroid glands are pea-sized glands (there are usually four of them) attached to the back edges of the thyroid gland (*para-* means "beside" or "near").

The thyroid secretes two hormones that are crucial for regulating metabolism: triiodothyronine (T_3) and thyroxine (T_4). The numbers refer to the numbers of iodine atoms each molecule of hormone contains. T_4 is the major player, because it affects virtually every cell in the body.

One of T_4's most important roles is to stimulate the enzymes that digest glucose. T_4 controls BMR, oxygen consumption, and heat production. It triggers the release of digestive juices, is involved in metabolism of fats and proteins, and helps the liver produce cholesterol, needed for transporting fat around the body. T_4 regulates tissue growth and is crucial for development and function of the nerves, bones, and reproductive organs. Finally, it keeps the skin moist and promotes normal secretion by skin cells. Quite a lot of jobs for one hormone to handle!

The thyroid also secretes a hormone called calcitonin, whose function is to lower the level of calcium in the blood. When calcium levels rise, the thyroid releases more calcitonin, which causes the bones to absorb calcium. When calcium levels fall too low, the parathyroid glands go to work. Parathyroid hormone causes the bones to release calcium, the intestines to absorb more calcium from food, and the kidneys to release less calcium in the urine. As a result, calcium levels rise again.

You need to have the right balance of these hormones. Too little thyroid hormone causes the BMR to plummet, leading to low body temperature, reduced heart rate, low blood pressure, intolerance to cold, decreased appetite, and weight gain. Low levels affect the brain and nervous system, causing such symptoms as depression, unusual sensations in the arms and legs, and lack of concentration. Because the digestive system slows down, constipation may result. The skin becomes pale, thick, and dry. The hair develops a coarser texture and thins out, while the nails become hard and thick. In some cases, people who lack sufficient thyroid hormone become infertile.

Too much thyroid hormone can be equally troublesome, but in opposite ways. The metabolic rate kicks into high gear, resulting in high body temperature, inability to tolerate heat, increased appetite, weight loss, and muscle weakness and atrophy. Rapid heartbeat and high blood pressure are common, posing a risk of heart failure. Effects on the brain and nerves include irritability, restlessness, insomnia, and bulging eyes. An overstimulated digestive system can lead to diarrhea and loss of appetite. The skin becomes flushed, thin, and moist, and the nails become soft and thin. Men often lose their ability to get an erection.

It's rare that the parathyroid glands produce too much hormone. When they do, the result is loss of calcium from the bones, leading to risk of fractures. Excess calcium also reduces nerve activity and can lead to kidney stones. In contrast, deficiency of parathyroid hormone causes nerve damage, leading to twitching, convulsions, and possibly paralysis.

ASSESSING THYROID FUNCTION

Circle the number that best describes the intensity of your symptoms on the following scale:

0 = I do not experience this symptom
1 = Mild
2 = Moderate
3 = Severe

Thick skin and fingernails	0	1	2	3
Dry skin	0	1	2	3
Sensitivity to the cold	0	1	2	3
Cold hands and feet	0	1	2	3
Excessive menstrual bleeding	0	1	2	3
Chronic fatigue	0	1	2	3
Trouble waking up in the morning	0	1	2	3
Depression, apathy	0	1	2	3
Low sex drive	0	1	2	3
Puttylike, wrinkled skin	0	1	2	3
Irritability and mood swings caused by sugar	0	1	2	3
Premenstrual tension	0	1	2	3
Constipation	0	1	2	3
Thinning or loss of outside portion of eyebrow	0	1	2	3
Easy weight gain	0	1	2	3

Anemia unaffected by iron	o	I	2	3
Slow reflexes	o	I	2	3

Add the numbers circled and enter that subtotal here: _____

Circle the number of the answer that applies to you:

Axillary (armpit) temperature below 97.6°F	NO = o	YES = IO
Infertility	NO = o	YES = IO

Add the numbers circled and enter that subtotal here: _____
Add the two subtotals and enter that total here: _____

Scoring   *9 or more: **High priority***
*5–8: **Moderate priority***
*1–4: **Low priority***

Interpreting Your Score

The questionnaire above is an excellent screening tool for identifying problems with thyroid function. A score of 9 or more on either section means that you will definitely need to follow closely the recommendations for tuning up the thyroid. If your score is between 5 and 8, it is less of a concern, but I would still strongly recommend making tuning up your thyroid gland a top priority. A score of 4 or less indicates that there are probably other things going on that are impacting your thyroid gland. For example, if your adrenal gland is a bit underactive, it can lead to some of the same sort of symptoms as low thyroid. Remember the body is a system: improving the functioning of one component affects the functioning of all the other components.

Thyroid Tune-Up

A low level of thyroid hormone is a common problem, affecting perhaps one out of five women and a smaller percentage of men. If your thyroid activity is reduced, your body may not respond as well as it should to nutritional or supplemental strategies. For that reason, a crucial step in tuning up your metabolism is to make sure your thyroid is working properly.

Your doctor can conduct blood tests that measure thyroid hormone levels. The test assesses the quantity of T_4 and T_3 and determines how well your body's cells respond to the hormones. It also measures quantities of thyroid-stimulating hormone (TSH), a chemical released by the pituitary gland. High levels of TSH indicate that the pituitary is in over-drive, frantically trying to signal the thyroid to step up its hormone output. However, in milder cases of thyroid hormone insufficiency, the blood test may show that hormone levels are within "normal" ranges, even if the person is experiencing symptoms. In my practice, I usually suggest that patients take thyroid hormone supplements if the TSH value is greater than 2.0 or if there are low levels of either T_4 or T_3. This recommendation is especially valid for patients suffering from depression—usually the first sign of low thyroid function.

Before rushing off to your doctor for a blood test, however, I suggest that you first determine your basal body temperature. Your body temperature reflects your metabolic rate, a rate that in turn is largely determined by thyroid hormone activity. When your thyroid is out of whack, your temperature often falls. Many experts agree that the basal body temperature is the most sensitive functional test of thyroid function. The test is simple: All you need is a thermometer.

TAKING YOUR BASAL BODY TEMPERATURE

1. **Plan to take the test first thing in the morning after you wake up, because it's important to measure temperature after you have had adequate rest.**

2. **Before going to sleep, shake down the thermometer to below the 95-degree mark and place it by your bed.**

3. **Immediately upon waking, place the thermometer in your armpit for a full ten minutes if using a conventional thermometer (newer digital thermometers can give almost immediate results). Hold your elbow close to your side to keep the thermometer in place.**

4. **Move as little as possible. Lying and resting with your eyes closed is best. Do not get up until the full ten minutes have passed.**

5. **After ten minutes, read and record the temperature and date.**

6. **Repeat the test for least three mornings (preferably at the same time of day). Give the information to your physician.**

Note: Women of childbearing age must perform the test on the second, third, and fourth days of menstruation, as hormonal fluctuations related to ovulation cause the basal body temperature to rise and fall in a predictable pattern during the monthly cycle. Men and postmenopausal women can perform the test at any time.

The underarm temperature is more reflective of basal body temperature than a temperature taken using the under-the-tongue method, and it should be lower than the normal oral temperature of 98.6 degrees Fahrenheit. The typical basal range is between 97.6 and 98.2 degrees. Lower than that may indicate a problem with hypothyroidism. If your basal body temperature is below 97.2 degrees, I recommend seeing your doctor for the blood test, paying close attention to the TSH level. If the temperature is between 97.2 and 97.6 degrees, try alternative methods to raise thyroid function (discussed below). I urge anyone with hypothyroidism, even a mild case, to take the appropriate steps to correct the problem. An underlying state of low thyroid function means that virtually every cell of your body is underperforming. Conversely, restoring proper thyroid hormone levels can dramatically increase the metabolism within your cells.

The medical treatment of most cases of low thyroid hormone levels involves the use of either desiccated thyroid (the dried form of natural thyroid from pigs) or synthetic versions of T_4 (for example, Synthroid). As a naturopathic physician, I think pharmaceutical grade (USP) desiccated thyroid is the better choice. This product contains all the thyroid hormones and so provides a better balance than a single-hormone synthetic product.

Tune-Up Tip: Thyroid Extracts

Thyroid extracts are available in health food stores. The FDA requires that these products not contain any T_4. However, it is nearly impossible to remove all of the hormone from the gland. For this reason, thyroid extracts you buy in health food stores are like milder forms of desiccated natural thyroid because they contain at least some T_4. If your problem is mild (e.g., your basal body temperature is between 97.2 and 97.6 degrees), these preparations may provide all the thyroid support you need. Follow the dosage recommendation on the product label.

Supporting Thyroid Function

In addition to thyroid extract, health food stores sell nutritional formulas that support thyroid function. These supplements often contain iodine, tyrosine, zinc, and specific vitamins.

The thyroid gland needs iodine to make its hormones. In fact, iodine's only role in your body is in making thyroid hormones. Too little iodine can cause enlargement of the thyroid, a condition known as goiter. Most table salt today is iodized, which means iodine has been added. However, too much salt (specifically, the sodium that salt contains) poses its own risks to health. The RDA for iodine is pretty low—just 150 mcg. Yet the average daily intake of iodine in the United States is estimated to be more than 600 mcg per day. So most people don't have to worry about getting enough iodine. In fact, too much iodine can actually interfere with the thyroid's ability to produce hormones. I have seen patients who suffer from symptoms of low thyroid because they eat too much salt or take too many kelp tablets. (Kelp is a popular iodine supplement.)

Remember, the key to metabolic harmony is *balance*. I recommend that you limit your intake of iodine from all sources to no more than 600 mcg per day. Read the labels on your multivitamin supplement and on any thyroid preparations you are taking. Keep your intake of iodized salt to a bare minimum. Make sure that your total amount of iodine intake is within the recommended range—not too low or too high.

Tune-Up Tip: Go Easy on Goitrogens

Some foods, especially when eaten raw, contain substances that interfere with your body's ability to absorb and use iodine. Because these foods can contribute to the risk of goiter, they are classified as goitrogens. Examples include turnips, cabbage, mustard, cassava root, soybeans, peanuts, pine nuts, and millet. Because these foods contain many other valuable nutrients, I recommend that you avoid them only if low thyroid hormone levels are a problem for you. Cooking usually inactivates goitrogens, so don't be concerned about these items in your diet if you serve them cooked.

Another key ingredient in thyroid hormones (and in the neurotransmitters epinephrine and norepinephrine) is the amino acid tyrosine. If you consume adequate protein, your body should have all the tyrosine it needs. However, if extra tyrosine is needed, supplements are available, and tyrosine is often included in nutritional formulas designed to enhance thyroid function.

A deficiency in the mineral zinc or in any of the vitamins A, B_2, B_3, B_6, C, and E could cause or contribute to hypothyroidism. This is of special concern for people over the age of sixty-five. Eating a balanced diet and taking a multiple vitamin and mineral supplement will ensure that you get adequate levels.

Exercise is another important factor for a properly functioning thyroid. By speeding up your metabolism, exercise stimulates the thyroid gland to secrete hormones. Exercise also makes your other tissues more sensitive to the effects of thyroid hormones. Many of the general health benefits resulting from exercise are in fact directly due to its impact on thyroid function. Exercise is especially important if you are overweight and following a reduced-calorie diet, because exercise counteracts the drop in metabolic rate that occurs when you diet.

CASE STUDY: More than a Weight-Loss Problem

Danielle, age thirty-seven, is the manager of a local flower shop. At five feet seven inches tall, she weighs 155 pounds—about 20 more than is healthy for her height and age.

She came to see me because of her depression. "I feel like crying all the time," she said. She also complained of fatigue and frustration over the fact that, no matter what she tried, she couldn't lose those excess pounds. When I saw her, I noticed that the back of her arms and elbows were extremely dry. Tellingly, she was missing the outer third of her eyebrows. I commented that her skin looked red and irritated. "I itch like mad," she said. The problem— an allergic reaction called hives—had started about six months before. "Maybe it's some new plant in the shop," she mused. She had been taking frequent doses of antihistamines to keep the hives under control. Her other symptoms had started four years earlier, after the birth of her second child.

Normally, when a patient presents with severe hives, I suspect allergies to foods or to food additives. I suggested Danielle undergo the standard food allergy study. I also felt that hypothyroidism was a likely diagnosis, especially when I saw that she had scored high on almost every question on the thyroid survey. Her dry skin and thinning eyebrows were other clues to hypothyroidism.

I ordered blood tests to measure her thyroid hormone levels (among other things) and to evaluate for food allergies. The results clearly showed she was suffering from hypothyroidism—her TSH was significantly higher than normal. I also told her to take her basal body temperature on the second, third, and fourth days of her upcoming period. When she reported that her first basal body temperature reading was 96.2 degrees F, the diagnosis was confirmed. I had her start with 1 grain (65 mg) of USP thyroid daily.

Two weeks later Danielle came back to the office so we could discuss the results of her food allergy tests. To my surprise, she told me that her hives had cleared up. There are reports in the medical literature of patients whose allergic skin conditions clear up during thyroid hormone therapy, but I had not expected such treatment would help her. Happily, I was wrong. Still, Danielle's food allergy test results indicated a significant allergy to milk, wheat, and peanuts. I instructed her to avoid these foods entirely.

After six weeks, during a routine recheck, Danielle's thyroid hormone levels were perfect and her basal body temperature was up to 97.2 degrees F. Her hives vanished, her energy levels soared, her mood was brighter, and her crying spells had disappeared.

When I saw Danielle three months later, she was noticeably thinner. She had finally gotten rid of those extra pounds. I lowered her thyroid to 0.5 grain per day based upon her blood work. I will continue to monitor the dosage based upon half-yearly blood tests.

The Adrenal Glands

These two little glands play the major role in our ability to handle stress. They also contribute to our sex drive and ability to fight off allergies, inflammation, and infections. It is important to understand these glands so that you can appreciate how vital it is that they receive the right support.

Each pyramid-shaped adrenal gland sits on top of a kidney. (The prefix *ad-* means "near," and *renal* comes from the Latin word for "kidney".) There are two main layers in the adrenal glands. The outer layer, or cortex, produces more than two dozen steroid hormones, known as *corticosteroids*.

Aldosterone, one of these hormones, is a key player in regulating electrolytes such as potassium and sodium, which in turn regulate the flow of electricity in your nerves and cells. Aldosterone lowers the rate at which you excrete sodium from the body and helps the body retain water. Because water is an important component of blood, aldosterone also plays a role in maintaining blood pressure. Too much of the hormone can lead to high blood pressure and swelling. Generally, when sodium levels are too high, potassium levels fall. Thus excess aldosterone can lead to loss of potassium, causing nerve damage, muscle weakness, and possibly paralysis.

Cortisol (also known as hydrocortisone) and similar adrenal hormones play a major role in your response to stress. Cortisol keeps your blood sugar levels constant by triggering formation of glucose from fats and proteins. It also maintains blood volume by regulating the amount of water in cells. Cortisol blocks inflammation by preventing release of inflammatory chemicals from cells.

Normally, your body releases high amounts of cortisol early in the morning but only low levels at night. If you are under stress, though, your adrenals will release cortisol whenever it is needed. Constant stress means constant hormone secretion, and here is where we see the negative side of this finely tuned response. Excessive levels of cortisol and other glucocorticoids, usually the result of the use of steroid drugs or severe stress, can lead to symptoms such as depression, fatigue, insomnia, high blood sugar, loss of muscle and bone, poor wound healing, and impaired immune function.

Table 4-2: Conditions Linked to Elevated Cortisol Levels

Atherosclerosis	Immune system depression
Chronic fatigue syndrome	Insomnia
Cushing's syndrome	Menstrual abnormalities
Depression	Obesity
Fibromyalgia	Osteoporosis
High blood pressure	Rapid aging
Hypoglycemia	Stress
Hypothyroidism	

The androgen DHEA, another hormone produced by the adrenals, is a source molecule that your body converts to major sex hormones, including estrogen, progesterone, and testosterone.

The most familiar adrenal hormone, adrenaline, is produced in the inner core of the gland, known as the medulla. Adrenaline (also called epinephrine) and the related hormone noradrenaline (norepinephrine) provide a short-term full-body alert in response to danger. These chemicals, classified as catecholamines, control nerve activity. Epinephrine stimulates the heart, widens air passages to permit deeper breathing, and controls certain metabolic activities, while norepinephrine causes blood vessels to constrict and thus plays more of a role in regulating blood pressure. They also speed up the production of glucose in the liver. Excess levels of catecholamines increase metabolic rate, causing high blood sugar levels, rapid heartbeat, high blood pressure, nervousness, insomnia, and sweating.

As you have probably noticed, symptoms of too much adrenaline are very similar to the symptoms of drinking too much coffee. That is because caffeine increases the output of adrenaline as well as prevents its breakdown. So the net result of consuming caffeine can be a substantial increase in adrenaline levels. Too much caffeine is a major problem for many people with anxiety, depression, and insomnia.

Both physical stress and psychological stress impact your adrenal glands. Under prolonged stress, the adrenals may initially increase the output of hormones such as cortisol, but in time they will actually shrink in size and lose their ability to function, leading to total exhaustion. I tend to see more people with overactive adrenals than exhausted ones.

The general state of adrenal health and function can be assessed by measuring the level of cortisol in the saliva at different times throughout the day. This test is often performed as part of the adrenal stress index (see box). Your tune-up will help you maintain the proper level of cortisol and other adrenal hormones. Lifestyle Tune-Up #2, following Chapter 2, describes a deep breathing exercise you can perform to help relieve stress.

THE ADRENAL STRESS INDEX

The adrenal stress index measures cortisol and DHEA levels in the saliva. (Salivary levels of these hormones correlate with the free-circulating, biologically active forms of these hormones.) Prolonged stress raises cortisol and depresses DHEA levels. Elevated cortisol and low DHEA are associated with accelerated aging, poor mental function and memory, fatigue, depression, osteoporosis, and heart disease.

The adrenal stress index is a popular diagnostic tool among alternative medical practitioners. When a person's system is not reacting to stress properly, there also will be an altered circadian rhythm of these hormones. Normally cortisol levels are highest in the morning and lowest at night. But in people experiencing too much stress, not enough sleep, or depression, the level of cortisol will be much higher at night.

"StressCheck," an adrenal stress index test kit from BodyBalance, is available in health food stores and pharmacies, or by calling 1-888-891-3061 or visiting www.bodybalance.com. If you wish to monitor your adrenal tune-up, do a test at the very beginning of your tune-up and then follow it up two months after you have instituted therapy.

Tuning Up the Adrenal Glands

Potassium

The most important dietary recommendation for adrenal health is to restore your potassium-sodium balance. Most Americans consume half as much potassium (which scientists abbreviate K) as they do sodium (abbreviated Na), leading to a K:Na ratio of 1:2. Ideally, however, we should get at least *five times* as much potassium as sodium (a ratio of 5:1). In other words, most people today are getting only one-tenth of the potassium they need.

Reduce sodium in your diet by avoiding the intake of salt. Eat at least five servings of fruit and vegetables per day, because most of these foods have a K:Na ratio of at least 100:1 (see Table 4-3). As you probably know, bananas are the princes of potassium because they have over four hundred times as much of this nutrient as they do sodium.

Table 4-3: Potassium-to-Sodium Ratio in Fruits and Vegetables

Fruit	K:Na Ratio
Apples	90:1
Asparagus	165:1
Bananas	440:1
Carrots	136:1
Potatoes	110:1
Oranges	260:1
Strawberries	125:1

Other nutrients especially important in supporting adrenal function are vitamins B$_5$, B$_6$, and C, zinc, and magnesium. The easiest way to get these nutrients is by eating a good diet and taking a high-potency multivitamin and mineral supplement.

Ginseng

There are two main kinds of ginseng: Chinese or Korean (*Panax ginseng*) and Siberian (*Eleutherococcus senticosus*). For thousands of years, people have taken ginseng to restore vitality, increase feelings of energy, boost mental and physical performance, enhance resistance to stress, and reduce anxiety. It appears to accomplish these goals primarily by tuning up the adrenal gland and reestablishing proper cortisol levels.

Chinese ginseng tends to be the more potent of the two. Consider using Chinese ginseng if you have been under a great deal of stress, if you are recovering from an illness, or have been taking corticosteroid drugs (such as prednisone) for a long time. However, if your stress is mild or moderate and your adrenal function seems less affected, Siberian ginseng may be a better choice.

There are many types and grades of ginseng and ginseng extracts. The quality of the product depends on the source, the age, and parts of the root used, as well as the method of preparation. Unfortunately, most ginseng available in the United States is of poor quality, derived from the lowest-grade root, diluted with excipients, blended with adulterating substances, or low in active ingredients.

When shopping, choose only products that have been standardized for ginsenoside content. For adrenal support, the dosage for products such as Ginsana, which contains 5 percent ginsenosides, would be 100 mg one to three times daily. For milder support, use fluid extracts of Siberian ginseng at a dosage of 1 to 2 tsp one to three times daily, or the dry powdered extract at a dosage of 100 mg one to three times daily.

In my practice, I've noticed that patients have varying degrees of response to ginseng. I recommend that you start by taking lower doses and gradually increase the daily amount. If you overdo it, you may notice such side effects as anxiety, irritability, nervousness, insomnia, hypertension, breast pain, and menstrual changes. Should these problems develop, reduce your intake or discontinue using ginseng entirely.

Tune-Up Tip: Supplement to Support the Adrenals

Your adrenals will function better if they have access to all the vitamins and minerals they need, especially vitamins B_5, B_6, and C, magnesium, and zinc. Here are the key supplement strategies for stress (total daily dose):

Vitamin B_5	100–500 mg
Vitamin B_6	50–100 mg
Vitamin C	500–1,500 mg
Magnesium	250–500 mg
Zinc	20–30 mg
Ginseng extract	100–200 mg

Kava

Because stress activates so many hormones and neurotransmitters, many people under stress feel agitated and anxious, and they experience difficulty sleeping. They may experience anxiety attacks, during which the metabolic rate speeds up. This causes rapid heartbeat, chest pains, difficulty breathing, sweating, dry mouth, dizziness, and digestive disturbances.

If this describes you, I recommend you try another herbal product, known as kava. Kava extracts are widely used in Europe to treat anxiety and panic attacks without side effects (however, see box). The active ingredients in kava are a group of compounds known as kavalactones. The dose of kava depends on its concentration of kavalactones, which in the natural plant can vary from 3 percent to 20 percent. For this reason, choose a kava product that specifies kavalactone content. To relieve anxiety, I recommend a dose that provides 45 to 70 mg of kavalactones three times daily.

WARNING Although no side effects have been reported using standardized kava extracts at recommended levels, kava may increase the effect of prescription sleeping pills and may worsen Parkinson's disease. Until this issue is resolved through more studies, kava extract should not be used by people taking prescription sleeping pills or by Parkinson's disease patients.

CASE STUDY: Getting the Stress Out

Patty, thirty-nine, was a Web site manager for an Internet company. She complained of stress, anxiety, and insomnia. When she did sleep, she didn't remember her dreams.

In taking her medical history, I identified many possible contributing factors. First was her diet, which did not support health at all. Like many people living in Seattle, Patty had a great affection for Starbucks coffee. She was regularly drinking four tall lattès a day; when she wasn't sipping java, she was guzzling Diet Pepsi (another major source of caffeine). Instead of breakfast, she opted for a double latte. Her first "food" of the day was usually a candy bar from the vending machine during her first coffee break. Lunch was often her only significant meal. For dinner, she usually had a bowl of popcorn washed down with (you guessed it) a Diet Pepsi.

To make matters even worse, stress was a major factor in Patty's life. She was going through a divorce, changing jobs, and looking for a new apartment. She told me she felt like she was "going nuts." She had tried benzodiazepines (Valium-like drugs) as well as Ambien, an insomnia drug, but did not like the way they made her feel. She also reacted quite poorly to the antidepressant Prozac. "I just can't take it anymore," she said, adding that I was her "last resort."

After taking her medical history, I asked Patty what changes in her diet and lifestyle she thought she needed to make to support her body and mind. In my experience, most patients pretty much know what they need to do to improve their health. Patty was no different. She admitted she needed to eat more nutritiously, cut down on the caffeine intake, and start exercising more regularly.

I told Patty that maybe the anxiety she was feeling arose from excitement over the endless possibilities that were now available to her (plus, of course, her excess caffeine intake). If we took away the caffeine, perhaps everything else would fall into place. We spent most of the hour-long office visit discussing what an exciting time it was in her life. If you think about it, the physical feeling of excitement is very close to the feeling of anxiety (imagine a roller-coaster ride). Perhaps the biggest difference is the label we put on it. I asked Patty such questions as "What are the things in life that you are most excited about?" and "Why does this make you feel excited?" It was amazing to watch the transformation occurring before me. Her anxiety and fear were being replaced with excitement and hope. I could tell that Patty was going to be okay, but we needed to improve her physiology so that her natural positive mental attitude could shine. Here was her prescription:

- Switch to decaffeinated coffee.
- Quit eating those candy bars and drinking those diet soft drinks!
- Eat breakfast, even if it was simply an apple or banana on her drive to work.
- Consume a salad (no dressing) at lunch. Continue with her other healthy lunch choices.
- Don't fill up on popcorn at dinner. Plan ahead and plan meals at least a day in advance.
- Join a health club.
- Take the following supplements:
  - Doctor's Choice for Women (a high-potency multiple vitamin and mineral formula): one tablet three times daily.
  - KavaTone: one capsule three times daily. Each capsule of this product provides 200 mg of an extract standardized to contain 30 percent kavalactones and 100 mg of an oat straw extract.
  - 5-HTP: 100 to 300 mg at bedtime (see page 112).

A repeat office visit four weeks later was phenomenal. Her whole life had been transformed. Patty told me that the first week was hard, as she did experience some caffeine withdrawal (she took acetaminophen to help with headaches). But after that first week she noticed that her energy levels were higher. She felt "the weight of the world" was finally off her shoulders. At the same time, she had found a great place to live, her divorce had been finalized, she had several men pursuing her at the health club she joined, she was sleeping normally again, and she was dreaming again for the first time in years. We eventually weaned her off the kava, but she continued to use the 5-HTP because she liked the way it helped her get a good night's sleep.

DEALING WITH STRESS

Throughout our lives, each of us develops our own ways of coping with stress. Some of those strategies are healthier than others. For example, one person might relieve stress by taking long, relaxing walks or watching funny movies. Another might drink alcohol or use drugs. If your coping strategy appears on the following list, you will definitely need to develop better methods for managing stress.

- Dependence on chemicals
  - Drugs (legal and illegal)
  - Alcohol
  - Tobacco
- Overeating
- Watching too much television
- Emotional outbursts
- Feelings of helplessness
- Overspending
- Excessive or reckless behavior (promiscuous sex, thrill-seeking, etc.)

DHEA

Recently there has been a lot of interest in the use of DHEA as a strategy for tuning up the metabolism and supporting adrenal function. After age twenty-five or so, your DHEA levels decline significantly. Proponents claim that taking DHEA supplements boosts energy and well-being, increases sexual appetite and performance, and offsets age-related changes in sexuality and mental function. In short, many people regard DHEA as a kind of hormonal fountain of youth.

I believe that DHEA may offer significant benefits to certain people, but only when used appropriately. In my practice, the only time I recommend use of DHEA by people under forty years of age is if the patient is a woman with an autoimmune disease such as lupus, rheumatoid arthritis, or multiple sclerosis. If you fall into this category, have your doctor evaluate your DHEA levels. The dosage of DHEA I suggest for patients with these autoimmune diseases is 50 to 100 mg daily. The most common side effect from this regimen is acne.

I do not recommend use of DHEA by other women who have not gone through menopause, because many women naturally experience an increase in DHEA levels as they approach the "change of life." Too much DHEA can cause masculinizing side effects, such as growth of facial hair as well as menstrual abnormalities. For most premenopausal women, there simply is no reason to take DHEA. For women after menopause, I usually recommend conservative doses, no higher than 5 to 15 mg daily. However, for older women with lupus, higher dosages may be helpful. In a series of clinical studies conducted at Stanford University in women with lupus, dosages were as high as 200 mg daily. Again, if you have an autoimmune disease such as lupus, I suggest talking to your doctor about DHEA.

Most men who ask me about DHEA complain about low energy and low sex drive. They are hoping for treatment that will increase their sense of well-being and help them feel younger. Before suggesting the use of DHEA, I measure the blood levels of DHEA and testosterone. If these are abnormally low, I recommend that men between the ages of forty and fifty take between 15 and 25 mg of DHEA per day. Older men usually need somewhat higher doses, 25 to 50 mg per day. People over age seventy may need even larger doses to compensate for the continuing decline of their own natural supply of DHEA.

If you are taking DHEA and you are not under the care of a physician, I strongly urge you to contact either BodyBalance, 1-888-891-3061 or www.bodybalance.com, or Aeron LifeCycles, 1-510-729-0375 or www.aeron.com. These labs offer test kits directly to consumers that measure salivary DHEA levels. The BodyBalance test kits are also available in health food stores. You can use the results to make sure that you are not taking too much. I have heard stories of younger men taking DHEA in very high doses—2,000 mg a day or more—in an effort to build up their muscles. This practice is unsafe, dangerous, and very stupid.

Tune-Up Tip: Use 7-KETO for Weight Loss

7-KETO (3-acetyl-7-oxo-dehydroepiandrosterone) is a naturally occurring metabolite of DHEA. The development of 7-KETO as a dietary supplement is the result of research conducted under the direction of Henry Lardy, Ph.D., at the Enzyme Institute at the University of Wisconsin. They were looking for the biologically active components of DHEA that are not converted into testosterone and estrogen. 7-KETO emerged as the answer to their quest, as it was shown to be more potent than DHEA in all experiments.

In addition to a safety trial in humans, 7-KETO has been shown to promote weight loss in a double-blind trial that also required each participant to exercise three times per week for forty-five minutes per session and eat a 1,800-calorie diet. Each subject was given either a placebo or 100 mg of 7-KETO twice daily. The results of the study indicated a statistically significant decrease in body weight and body fat in the 7-KETO group at four and eight weeks. At the end of the eight-week trial, there was a 2.88 kg (6.34 pound) weight loss and a 1.8 percent drop in body fat percentage in the 7-KETO group. In comparison, in the placebo group there was a 0.97 kg (2.13 pound) weight loss and a 0.57 percent drop in body fat at eight weeks. The weight-loss effect of 7-KETO was attributed to its producing a statistically significant increase in T_3 thyroid hormone activity, although it did not raise it out of the normal range. T_3 plays a major role in determining a person's metabolic rate.

Although there are no long-term studies with 7-KETO, researchers believe the weight loss is likely to be permanent because 7-KETO appears to affect a person's "set point." Every person's weight has a "set point," a weight that our body's natural feedback mechanisms work to maintain. This set point can be a weight that is higher than is healthy. Unless the set point changes, our bodies will automatically adjust metabolism and appetite in an attempt to return to this weight when the diet program stops. This is likely one of the reasons so many people have trouble keeping off the weight they've lost. 7-KETO is thought to produce permanent weight loss because it is able to influence the set point down to a lower weight.

CASE STUDY: Boosting Fred's Libido

Fred, a fifty-two-year-old successful entrepreneur, came to me complaining of reduced libido and sexual performance. His soon-to-be wife was twenty-eight years old, and he was feeling a "bit old." He came to me to get my opinion on the testosterone patch. This patch is used by some physicians to treat "male menopause" much as estrogen patches are used to treat female menopause.

I told Fred that we could probably raise his testosterone levels indirectly by using DHEA, but there were risks involved. While higher levels of DHEA appear to offer protection against aging and heart disease, they may contribute to an increased risk for prostate cancer by raising testosterone levels too high.

I began Fred at the conservative dosage of 25 mg per day for three months. In follow-up visits, we found that the DHEA level did increase testosterone, but levels were still at the low end of normal for his age. We upped the dosage to 50 mg per day for the next three months, at which point I remeasured his hormone levels. When I called to tell Fred the results—that he now had the testosterone levels of a twenty-five-year-old—he laughed and said that his wife had been telling him that for the past two months. We have continued to monitor Fred's DHEA and testosterone levels and now have him on a dosage of 25 mg one day and 50 mg the next.

The Pineal Gland

The pineal gland is a tiny clump of tissue deep within the brain shaped (as the Latin root of its name suggests) like a pine cone. Its exact function is still a bit of a mystery. Apparently its main job is to secrete a hormone called melatonin. Because melatonin levels rise to their highest at night, the hormone may help regulate the sleep cycle. Your body seems to use light as its signal for regulating melatonin production. As soon as your eyes start receiving light—for example, when you wake up in the morning— your pineal gland shuts off the melatonin supply. Many scientists believe that the pineal gland and melatonin regulate your body's internal clock. If so, the pineal helps coordinate various functions and cycles such as body temperature, sleep, and appetite throughout the course of a day. Such cycles are called *circadian* rhythms; the word comes from the Latin terms meaning "about" (*circa-*) and "a day" (*diem*). The biological timekeeper is melatonin. Specifically, melatonin controls periods of sleepiness and wakefulness and plays a role in regulating mood. Some evidence suggests that melatonin may act as an antioxidant and as a cancer-preventing agent.

THE EFFECTS OF SLEEP LOSS ON CORTISOL LEVELS

Our society seems to attach high value to sleeping as little as possible and to extending the waking period. Also wreaking havoc on sleep cycles is shift work at around-the-clock operations—including hospitals. Sleep deprivation is a major problem in America.

Researchers are attempting to discover a physiological marker of sleep loss and stress. One of the best appears to be measuring cortisol levels at various times during the day. One recent study showed that even partial sleep loss of only four hours resulted in loss of cortisol regulation by the body.

Chronic sleep loss may set the stage for poor stress response and symptoms of cortisol excess, including depression, fatigue, and loss of blood sugar control. A vicious cycle ensues: High cortisol levels mean that your body converts less tryptophan into serotonin. Since serotonin is an important initiator of sleep and is also converted to melatonin, insomnia and poor sleep quality are generally associated with elevated cortisol levels. Low serotonin levels can also lead to craving of carbohydrates, depression, migraine headaches, and other problems. The amino acid 5-hydroxytryptophan (5-HTP) can be quite helpful to break the vicious cycle of high cortisol levels. The dosage recommendation in this application is 50 to 100 mg at bedtime.

Many people take melatonin to promote sleep. It can help, but only if melatonin levels are already low. A dosage of 3 mg at bedtime is usually sufficient for this purpose, although there is some evidence that much lower doses, 0.1 to 0.3 mg, may be just as effective. There is some concern that taking melatonin in excessive doses (8 mg or more) or at the wrong time of day may artificially reset your biological rhythms or lead to depression. If you stick to the recommended dosage, the risk of adverse reactions is low.

While low nighttime melatonin can lead to insomnia, higher daytime levels can lead to excessive daytime sleepiness. The levels of melatonin can be assessed in the saliva at various times during the day and night to accurately diagnose faulty melatonin secretion. You can contact Body-Balance (see page 130) to get a melatonin assessment kit (SleepCheck). Or, you can simply give vitamin B_{12} therapy a try.

Several studies have shown that vitamin B_{12} in the form of methylcobalamin (dosage 1.5 to 3 mg upon awakening) is an effective treatment to improve sleep in shift workers as well as in people with excessive daytime sleepiness, restless nights, and frequent nighttime awakenings. The subjects taking methylcobalamin experienced improved sleep quality, increased daytime alertness and concentration, and in some cases they also reported improved mood. Much of the benefit appears to be a result of methylcobalamin's influence on melatonin secretion. The substance causes a significant decrease in daytime melatonin levels while increasing nighttime levels.

Vitamin B_{12} is available in several forms. Methylcobalamin is active immediately upon absorption. Another form, cyanocobalamin, must be converted to methylcobalamin by the body, and is not active in many situations.

Key Steps to Tuning Up Your Metabolism

- Realize your metabolic rate depends on such factors as genetic inheritance, age, body weight, diet, exercise, and stress levels.
- To lose weight, avoid severe calorie restriction. Focus on nutrient-dense but low-calorie vegetables, especially the "free foods."
- Thyroid function is crucial for metabolism. Check your basal body temperature and make sure that it is between 97.6 and 98.2 degrees Fahrenheit.
- Avoid eating foods that are high in simple sugars. They can hinder your efforts to keep your blood sugar under control, especially if you are prone to hypoglycemia or have diabetes.

- Read food labels carefully and watch out for "hidden" sugar.
- Maintain a balance of potassium and sodium intake of at least 5:1. Eat fruits rich in potassium, such as bananas and oranges.
- Get enough sleep each night, exercise regularly, and be sure to practice deep breathing exercises at least for five minutes twice daily.

Lifestyle Tune-Up #4: Take a High-Potency Multiple Vitamin and Mineral Formula

There are thirteen vitamins and twenty-two minerals that you need to ingest in proper amounts for your tissues and organs to do their jobs. Required only in small amounts, vitamins and minerals are crucial for the manufacture as well as the activity of enzymes and other important proteins. Certain vitamins serve as a kind of cellular repair crew, repairing damage to delicate cell membranes. You need minerals to construct new cells and maintain the integrity of tissues, including bones, muscles, and blood. Without these substances, many body processes would grind to a halt. Significant lack of any one of them can lead to metabolic malfunction, accelerated aging, and disease.

There are two groups of vitamins. Those that dissolve in fat (fat-soluble) are vitamins A, D, E, and K. Those that dissolve in water (water-soluble) are vitamins C, the B vitamins, biotin, and folic acid.

Fat-soluble vitamins can be stored in fat cells. For that reason your body is able to keep a supply of these vitamins handy for release when needed. The downside is that you can also store too much of some of them, which can lead to toxic side effects. In contrast, the water-soluble vitamins are stored in only small amounts. Normally any quantity of these vitamins that your body does not use is excreted in the urine. Thus it's harder to build up toxic amounts of water-soluble vitamins, but by the same token it's easier to develop deficiencies of them.

Minerals are inorganic elements. They are classified as being either major or minor (trace), depending on the required dose. Major minerals require an intake of more than 100 mg per day. Minor minerals are no less important to your health, but you need them in smaller amounts.

Nutritional Supplementation Is Essential

While a health-promoting diet is an essential component of good health and an efficient metabolism, so too is proper nutritional supplementation. While some experts say that you can theoretically meet all of your nutritional needs through diet alone, the reality is that most Americans do not. Beyond this argument is the difference in how some experts view "optimal" nutrition. Does optimal nutrition mean simply no obvious signs of nutrient deficiency? Or is optimal nutrition the level of nutrition that will allow a person to function at the highest degree possible with vitality, energy, and enthusiasm for living? What it comes down to, then, is an argument of philosophy.

The World Health Organization defines health as "a state of complete physical, mental, and social well-being, not merely the absence of disease or infirmity." This definition of health provides a positive view of health that goes well beyond the absence of sickness. It is the goal of optimal health that drives people to take nutritional supplements.

Guidelines for Selecting a Multiple Vitamin and Mineral Formula

I believe that everyone needs to take a high-potency multiple vitamin and mineral supplement. By "high-potency," I mean that the supplement provides high levels of all the essential vitamins and minerals. The recommended daily allowances (RDA) that appear on food labels are based on government calculations of the amounts needed to prevent deficiency. Generally, the RDA levels are too low to provide optimum levels for optimum health. That's why throughout this book some of my recommendations for daily intake may be tens, even hundreds, of times higher than the RDA.

When taking a multiple vitamin and mineral formula, you may experience higher energy levels, improved brain function, fewer colds or infections, and other health benefits, or you may feel nothing. But even if you feel no different, it doesn't mean that the higher levels of nutrients you are ingesting are not being used by your body. For example, there is evidence that people taking nutritional supplements may have a lowered risk for heart disease, certain cancers, and cataracts. You may not feel the benefits immediately, but you will definitely realize them in the long term.

The following recommendations provide an optimal intake range to guide you in selecting a high-potency formula.

Vitamin	Range for Adults
Vitamin A (retinol)[a]	2,500–5,000 IU
Vitamin A (from beta-carotene)	5,000–25,000 IU
Vitamin B_1 (thiamin)	10–100 mg
Vitamin B_2 (riboflavin)	10–50 mg
Vitamin B_3 (niacin)	10–100 mg
Vitamin B_5 (pantothenic acid)	25–100 mg
Vitamin B_6 (pyridoxine)	25–100 mg
Vitamin B_{12} (cobalamin)	100–400 mcg
Vitamin C (ascorbic acid)[b]	100–1,000 mg
Vitamin D[c]	100–400 IU
Vitamin E (d-alpha tocopherol)[d]	100–800 IU
Vitamin K (phytonadione)	60–300 mcg
Niacinamide	10–30 mg
Biotin	100–300 mcg
Folic acid	400–800 mcg
Choline	10–100 mg
Inositol	10–100 mg

Notes:

[a]Women of childbearing age who may become pregnant should not take more than 2,500 IU of retinol daily due to the possible risk of birth defects.

[b]It may be easier to take vitamin C separately.

[c]Elderly people in nursing homes living in northern latitudes should supplement at the high range.

[d]It may be more cost effective to take vitamin E separately rather than as a component of a multiple vitamin.

Mineral	Range for Adults
Boron	1–6 mg
Calcium[e]	250–1,500 mg
Chromium[f]	200–400 mcg
Copper	1–2 mg
Iodine	50–150 mcg
Iron[g]	15–30 mg
Magnesium[h]	250–500 mg
Manganese	10–15 mg

Notes:

[e]Women at risk of or suffering from osteoporosis may need to take a separate calcium supplement to achieve higher doses.

[f]For diabetes and weight loss, doses of 600 mcg can be used.

[g]Men and postmenopausal women rarely need supplemental iron.

[h]When magnesium therapy is indicated, take a separate magnesium supplement.

Mineral	Range for Adults
Molybdenum	10–25 mcg
Potassium	200–500 mg
Selenium	100–200 mcg
Silica	1–25 mg
Vanadium	50–100 mcg
Zinc	15–45 mg

To find a multiple vitamin and mineral formula that meet these criteria, read labels carefully. Be aware that you will not find a formula that can provide all of these nutrients at these levels in one single pill—it would simply be too large. Usually it will require at least three to six tablets to meet these levels. While many "one-a-day" supplements provide good levels of vitamins, they tend to be insufficient in the levels of minerals. Your body needs the minerals as much as the vitamins—remember, the two work hand in hand.

CHAPTER 5

Tuning Up Your Immune System

The tragedy of the emergence of acquired immunodeficiency syndrome (AIDS) has dramatized to us all just how vital the immune system is to good health. When working properly, the immune system has a remarkable arsenal of weapons with an enormous capacity to fight off microorganisms that can infect us and do us harm. At all times, day and night, we are constantly exposed to various "bugs"—bacteria, viruses, fungi, and other microscopic invaders. They are in the food we eat and the air we breathe. They're in everything we touch or smell. Despite this onslaught, most of us are usually not sick—because of the strength of the immune system. With a strong immune system, we're safe from attack by all but the most virulent microorganisms. Even if infection does gain a foothold, it's usually just a matter of time before the immune system mounts an effective counterattack.

The workings of the immune system involve some of the body's most complex mechanisms. After all, its job is to protect every one of the body's trillions of cells against literally millions of invaders—including some the body may not yet have met. As clearly illustrated since the beginning of the AIDS outbreak in the 1980s, without a strong immune system, ordinary infections can fester into life-threatening catastrophes.

It is also the immune system's job to be on constant surveillance for cancer cells. When found, the scout cells send out powerful chemical messages that call troops of white blood cells to the area to bombard and destroy the cancerous cells. Low immune function sets the stage not only for constant struggles with infections, but also for cancer.

While many people may be aware of the consequences of low immune function (hypoimmunity), what they may not know is that for many people the immune system is a double-edged sword—it protects them, on one hand, but on the other, it can literally destroy them. What I am referring to is hyperimmunity, a state in which the immune system is out of control; this occurs with allergies (especially asthma) and conditions such as rheumatoid arthritis, lupus, and multiple sclerosis, where the immune system starts attacking the body.

The principles involved in tuning up your immune system are basically the same whether you are suffering from hypo- or hyperimmunity. The first goal is to make sure that you provide the immune system with all the vital ammunition (nutrition). Next is following a healthy lifestyle. These two simple steps can go a long way in supporting the central control mechanisms that keep the immune system in proper balance. The bottom line is that by tuning up your immune system, you'll not only increase your resistance to colds, flu, and other infections, but also protect yourself against cancer and other potentially deadly diseases.

A Quick Tour of the Amazing Immune System

Let me take you on a quick tour of this astonishing system. Your skin is the first line of protection against invasion. Good thing, too, because at all times there are trillions of bacteria milling about on the surface of your skin. Other potential invaders, such as yeasts, like to live in areas that offer warm, moist folds, such as the groin or between the toes. Skin that is dry or cracked creates openings that allow these invaders to enter your body. Moist, supple, and healthy skin not only feels and looks better, it helps you fend off infection.

Of course, your body already has a number of openings through which invaders can attack, including the mouth, nostrils, and genital openings. The linings of these passageways are protected by membranes that secrete a thick fluid called mucus. *Mucous membranes* are also found in many of your organs, including your airways, lungs, genitals, and digestive tract. The fluid they produce serves as a barrier that traps microbes and prevents them from damaging the underlying layers of cells. During a cold or the flu, your body steps up its secretion of mucus as a way of reinforcing the barrier. That's why you cough, sneeze, and blow your nose—

your body is attempting to expel the troublemakers before they do any more harm.

The skin and mucous membranes are remarkably effective barriers. But as you know, disease-causing organisms are wily and resourceful enemies. If they sneak past these first-line barriers, your immune system has additional troops to deploy: specialized cells that are trained to recognize and destroy invaders. The organs that produce these immune cells, or that play a role in their activity, include the bones, thymus, lymph nodes, spleen, and tonsils.

Your *bones* contain spongy matter called marrow, in which the red cells and most white blood cells are formed. (Red blood cells don't play a role in immunity; they're too busy ferrying molecules of oxygen and carbon dioxide around the body.) As I'll explain below, there are several kinds of white blood cells, each of which has a different part to play in mounting an immune response.

The *thymus* has two soft pinkish gray lobes lying just below the thyroid gland and above the heart in the upper chest area. To a great extent, the health of the thymus determines the health of the immune system. Without a healthy and well-functioning thymus, your immune system cannot function effectively. Inside the thymus, immature white blood cells mature to form T lymphocytes (the *T* stands for "thymus-dependent"). People with low thymus function are prone to frequent or chronic infections, allergies, migraine headaches, and rheumatoid arthritis. The thymus gland also produces hormones that regulate many immune functions. A low level of these hormones can reduce your immune response and leave you more vulnerable to disease. Common causes of low thymus hormone levels include advancing age, presence of a debilitating disease such as cancer or AIDS, and stress. Chronic viral or yeast infections or the presence of cancer are signs that your thymus gland desperately needs support.

Tune-Up Tip: Support Your Thymus

Your thymus reached its largest size shortly after you were born. Normally the thymus shrinks with age. However, high levels of free radicals—resulting from poor nutrition, disease, stress, or exposure to environmental toxins—can destroy thymus tissue and cause it to shrink faster than normal. Lowered immune function can result. To slow the rate of thymus shrinkage, it is important to eat a diet rich in antioxidant nutrients and to supplement your diet with extra antioxidants such as beta-carotene, vitamins C and E, selenium, and zinc.

The white blood cells travel through the *lymphatic system,* a network of vessels that collect the fluid found in the spaces between cells. This fluid, called *lymph,* contains primarily waste products that result from activity inside your cells. As lymph fluid travels, it passes through the *lymph nodes,* which filter the lymph to remove impurities. Inside the nodes, white blood cells called *macrophages* (the word means "big eaters") engulf and destroy the particles. During an infection, the nodes work overtime to collect and destroy infectious agents. That's why the nodes often swell during an illness. (Many people call these "swollen glands," but, strictly speaking, the lymph nodes aren't glands because they don't secrete chemicals.) Lymph fluid flows in one direction, so that the fluid leaving the node is always cleaner than the fluid that enters it.

The lymphatic vessels generally run alongside the blood vessels. At a point just below the neck, major lymph ducts drain into two major veins. In this way, lymph fluid, now filtered of its impurities, is put back into circulation as part of the liquid portion of blood.

Tune-Up Tip: Keeping Lymph Moving

There is no real "pump" that forces lymph to circulate through your body, the way the heart pumps blood. Instead, lymph circulation depends on breathing and movement by your body. Muscular contractions pump lymph out of the arms and legs into larger lymphatic vessels in the chest and abdomen. But the main mechanism of lymph circulation is breathing. Inhaling expands the diaphragm, which puts pressure on the large lymphatic vessels in the abdomen and chest. In turn, this eventually forces lymph to empty into the heart, so it can then be distributed through the blood circulation. This is another reason why exercise and breathing exercises are so important for your tune-up: Body movement and deep breathing with the diaphragm speed up the rate at which the lymph nodes filter out impurities.

The *spleen,* located in the upper left portion of the abdomen behind the lower ribs, plays several roles in the immune system. It produces some white blood cells, destroys and removes bacteria, and cleans up debris from worn-out cells such as old red blood cells. The spleen also serves as a reservoir of red blood, which it can release in case of emergency such as injury. The spleen produces several compounds that enhance immune system activity, and it is particularly important in fighting off bacterial infections.

The *tonsils* are a pair of oval masses of tissue located at the back of the throat. The tissue contains small cul-de-sacs, called crypts, that trap bacteria and particles entering from your nose and mouth. Immune cells living in the tonsils then destroy the invaders. Tonsils often become infected and swollen as a result of this activity, especially during childhood. But there's a payoff: The immune cells are able to "remember" which invaders they meet, which helps your body fend off attacks later in life. Forty or fifty years ago doctors were quick to recommend removing a kid's tonsils if they got infected frequently. We now realize that such tissue serves a purpose and that usually the tonsils should be left in place to carry out their natural immune function.

White Blood Cells

The infantry of the immune system are the white blood cells. Amazingly, every minute of your life, your body is making about *twelve million* new white blood cells to replace an equal number that have just worn out. At the same time, each living immune cell is busy making its own special mix of chemical messengers or antibodies. As you can imagine, your body devotes a tremendous amount of its resources to keeping your immune system running. By providing your body with the nutrients and energy it needs to keep up with this challenging task, you go a long way toward tuning up your immune system.

Lymphocytes are a type of white blood cell that act as the "special forces" of the immune system, a combination of the Green Berets and Navy SEALs. Their strategy is to use special destructive chemicals, search-and-destroy tactics, and highly sophisticated communication techniques. About 80 percent of your lymphocytes are T cells that mature in the thymus gland. T cells are responsible for an important immune response known as *cell-mediated immunity*. *Killer T cells* directly destroy invaders by attaching to them and causing them to break apart. *Helper T cells* release chemicals that act as messengers, recruiting other types of immune cells to the scene of attack and stimulating them to do their job. *Suppressor T cells* arrive on the scene once the mission is complete and issue orders to the troops to pull back.

The mix of T cell types is a sign of how efficiently your immune system is working. Too many suppressor cells and not enough helper cells—a situation often found in people with AIDS—means the system can't mount an effective defense against infection. In contrast, having too many helper cells and not enough suppressor cells causes the immune response to go into overdrive. This can lead to allergies or autoimmune disorders such as rheumatoid arthritis or lupus.

White blood cells that mature in the bone marrow are called *B lymphocytes*. B cells account for about 10 percent of your lymphocytes. They are responsible for the immune response called *humoral immunity*. Like alert sentries, B cells recognize the specific types of foreign particles present, including bacteria, yeast, and viruses. These foreign particles are referred to as *antigens*. In response to an antigen, B cells produce an *antibody*. Antibodies (also known as immunoglobulins) are special protein molecules that attach to antigens. If the antigen is on the surface of an invading organism, the antibody will bind to it and lead to its destruction. Each antibody must be tailor-made to fit the specific invader, so it takes a few days for B lymphocytes to crank out enough of them to be effective. In contrast, the cell-mediated response by T cells is immediate.

Cell-Mediated (T Cell) Immunity Protects Against:	Humoral (B Cell) Immunity Protects Against:
Most viruses (e.g., herpes simplex)	Some viruses (e.g., measles)
Most mycoplasmas (e.g., tuberculosis)	Most bacteria (e.g., strep and staph)
Most yeasts (e.g., candida)	Most parasites (e.g., giardia)

Helper T cells and B lymphocytes have relatively long lives—and, as noted, they have good memories. The next time an invader pops up uninvited, the cells remember how they mounted the previous attack. The T cells send messages to the B cells, ordering them to produce the same type of antibodies that worked before. Basically, this memory effect translates to lifelong immunity and is the same mechanism by which vaccines work. Vaccines produce a simulated infection by introducing the antigen without a viable organism. The body mounts an attack just as if it were infected. However, unlike actual infections, many vaccines do not produce lifelong immunity and require booster shots to continue to be effective. Also, some organisms, such as the flu viruses, outsmart the body's defenses by mutating.

HYPOIMMUNITY ASSESSMENT

Circle the number that best describes the intensity of your symptoms on the following scale:

    0 = I do not experience this symptom
    1 = Mild
    2 = Moderate
    3 = Severe

Inflamed or bleeding gums	0	1	2	3
Runny nose	0	1	2	3
Tendency to get boils or sties	0	1	2	3
Fatigue	0	1	2	3
Throat infections	0	1	2	3
Cold sores, fever blisters	0	1	2	3
Poor wound healing	0	1	2	3
Swollen lymph nodes	0	1	2	3
Slow recovery from colds or flu (lasts more than 4 days)	0	1	2	3
Tendency to catch colds or flu easily (more than two colds per year)	0	1	2	3

Add the numbers circled and enter that subtotal here: _____

Circle the number of the answer that applies to you:

Suffering from chronic infection	NO = 0	YES = 10
History of cancer	NO = 0	YES = 10

Add the numbers circled and enter that subtotal here: _____
Add the two subtotals and enter that total here: _____

Scoring   *12 or more: High priority*
           6–11: Moderate priority
           1–5: Low priority

Interpreting Your Score

If you suffer from recurrent infections, you probably already know the importance of tuning up your immune system. Be sure to take the hyperimmunity assessment on page 164 as well; sometimes a person can be suffering from hyperimmunity and signs of low immune function at the same time. The reason is that chronic allergies or the use of drugs such as prednisone can suppress the body's ability to fight infections.

Your Immune System Tune-Up

Now let's discuss the practical steps you can take to improve immune system function. The first goal is to take a look at your lifestyle to see if there are any factors that may be interfering with your body's ability to fend off illness. Among the most likely culprits:

- Chronic or severe stress
- Too much simple sugar in the diet
- Dysbiosis—overgrowth of unfriendly organisms, especially yeast (candida), in the bowel
- Excessive consumption of alcohol
- Exposure to environmental toxins
- Cigarette smoke
- Obesity
- Lack of exercise
- Food allergies

Once you've identified any harmful influences, of course, the next step is to do what you can to correct them.

Stress and Immunity

For most people, the biggest factor in an immune system disturbance is stress. When a person comes to see me complaining of chronic infections or a flare-up of their allergies, most often we can pinpoint stress as the underlying factor. Stress suppresses immunity by stimulating the *sympathetic nervous system*. This is a part of the autonomic nervous system that is responsible for the fight-or-flight response. When you are stressed out, your adrenal glands pump out more adrenaline and corticosteroids. These hormones inhibit white blood cell formation and function and cause the thymus gland to shrink.

Good immune function requires that the other part of the autonomic nervous system, the *parasympathetic nervous system,* be in control. This system automatically assumes control during periods of rest, relaxation, visualization, meditation, and sleep. But staying relaxed and calm during our waking hours can balance out the negative effects exerted by the sympathetic nervous system. During the deepest levels of sleep, potent immune-enhancing compounds are released, and many immune functions are greatly increased. At least seven hours of sleep per day is essential for helping the immune system function at its peak.

If you want a properly functioning immune system, it is absolutely vital that you reduce the amount of stress in your life as well as learn to control it better. Because stress exerts an influence on so many body systems, I provide a wide variety of stress busters in Lifestyle Tune-Up #2 (following Chapter 2).

The basic strategy for stress reduction is to find positive, relaxing ways of releasing excess tension and help your autonomic nervous system function under parasympathetic control. Stress reduction does not mean that you have to give up a high-energy lifestyle that you really enjoy. Find a routine that works for you. Doing so will not only help your immune system but also improve your relationships and free up energy and focus, so you can actually accomplish more—without sacrificing your health.

Tune-Up Tip: Creative Solutions to Stress

My patient Linda bought a personal CD player with headphones so she can listen to her beloved classical music whenever the opportunity arises.

Another patient, Sean, took lessons in yoga at the local YMCA. It not only helped his immune system, but helped him bring his rapid heartbeat under control.

Bill bought a relaxation video at the local Blockbuster—he tells me it features great music and scenes of nature, including underwater shots of whales and dolphins complete with their characteristic mating calls and other greetings.

Nutrition and Immunity

A deficiency of virtually any single nutrient can significantly impair immunity. Throughout the world, nutrient deficiency is by far the most common cause of poor immune function. This fact is by no means limited to people whose diets are restricted by poverty. In America, many people are overfed but undernourished. They choose foods that have a lot of calories but little real nutritional value. Every week I see people in my practice who are suffering from poor immune function. They benefit tremendously by following these simple guidelines:

- *Eat a diet that is rich in a variety of vegetables (especially the green leafy ones), fresh fruits, whole grains, beans, nuts, and seeds.* These plant foods are rich in essential nutrients and immune-boosting chemicals.
- *Cut out the sweet stuff.* Sugar makes your white blood cells sluggish. Studies show that eating 100 g of sugar (about 3.5 ounces) reduces the effectiveness of a type of white blood cell known as a neutrophil, which engulfs and destroys bacteria, by as much as 40 percent within two hours after ingestion. Since neutrophils account for about 60 to 70 percent of your white blood cells, interfering with them can seriously impair your immune function.
- *Decrease the intake of saturated fats and cholesterol.* A diet high in saturated fat suppresses immunity. Many of my patients initially presenting with high levels of cholesterol and triglycerides also report more frequent colds and flu. When cholesterol and triglyceride levels are normalized, proper immune function is restored.
- *Eat sufficient but not excessive amounts of protein.* Adequate protein intake is critical in the making of white blood cells, antibodies, and chemical messengers such as interferon. You also need protein to make antioxidant enzymes such as glutathione, which is found in abundance in white blood cells. Elevated glutathione levels are associated with better immune function. Patients with low immune function can benefit from eating more protein from fish, lean poultry, and lean cuts of meats. I have seen many vegetarians who are suffering from low immunity solely as a result of not consuming enough protein. In these patients, I recommend either soy protein isolate if they eat absolutely no animal products, or whey protein if they eat dairy. An additional 40 to 50 g per day for one month will boost protein stores back to normal. After the month is up, I would still recommend 20 g of either choice daily.
- *Take a high-potency vitamin and mineral supplement.* Doing so will increase your intake of the key nutrients for immune function, discussed below. Not long ago, a study of adults found that those who took a multiple vitamin and mineral supplement had a 50 percent decrease in the number of days of illness due to infection compared with

the group that took a placebo (dummy pill). Those taking the supplement also showed improvement on eight out of twelve objective measures of immune function. Pretty good results for such little effort!

The Magnificent Seven Nutrients in Immune Support

1. *Vitamin A* is necessary for maintaining the cells of the skin and the mucous membranes that act as the first lines of defense against infection. In addition, vitamin A is necessary for proper white blood cell function, and it enhances many of your immune system's activities, including thymus function, tumor-fighting activity, and antibody response. Vitamin A is especially important for fighting off viruses. For example, it has been found that children with lower vitamin A levels are much more prone to measles and viral respiratory tract infections. It also reverses immune suppression resulting from such conditions as high levels of stress hormones (glucocorticoids), severe burns, or surgery.

2. *Carotenes* are important in protecting your thymus gland because of their antioxidant effects. Studies back in the 1940s showed that the higher a child's carotene intake, the fewer the number of school days missed due to infections. More recent research has documented that carotenes enhance many aspects of immune function. Carotenes are found in green leafy vegetables, carrots, and other colorful vegetables.

3. *B vitamins*, especially B_1, B_6, and B_{12}, are required for making disease-fighting antibodies. In addition, B vitamins are essential to normal cell division. Therefore, low levels of B vitamins prevent your body from manufacturing new white blood cells. What's more, the lymphoid tissues (such as the thymus and spleen) shrink if they don't get enough B vitamins.

4. *Vitamin C* literally turns on white blood cells to attack intruders and also boosts interferon levels, antibody levels and response, and secretion of hormones from the thymus. Vitamin C acts directly against viruses, which is one reason it is used to fight off colds. When you have an infection or are under stress, your need for vitamin C increases.

5. *Vitamin E* supports immunity by encouraging the proliferation of white blood cells and improving antibody formation. Vitamin E supplementation has been shown to boost the immune response, especially in elderly subjects. Be careful, though: Too much vitamin E (doses over 800 IU per day) may actually inhibit immune response in healthy individuals. We can put this effect to good use by giving patients high doses of vitamin E for the treatment of autoimmune diseases such as rheumatoid arthritis, lupus, and multiple sclerosis.

6. *Zinc* is directly involved with immune function on many levels. Like vitamin C, zinc can act against certain viruses, such as those that cause the common cold (see box). When zinc levels are low, the number of T cells plummets, thymus hormone levels fall, enzyme production and activity declines, and certain white cell functions shut down. What's more, zinc is crucial for proper absorption of nutrients by the intestinal tract.

7. *Selenium* is involved in important antioxidant mechanisms that protect the thymus gland. People who are low in selenium have reduced levels of cellular and humoral immunity and lower antibody levels. It appears that selenium works, in part, by enhancing the ability of white blood cells to produce interleukin-2, a chemical that stimulates white blood cells to proliferate and attack foreign cells. One study found that people who took supplements of 200 mcg per day showed nearly a doubling in the activity of white blood cells, including their ability to kill tumor cells. The typical American diet does not contain enough selenium. I believe that supplementation is necessary for most people who want to enjoy its immune-boosting effects.

COLD FACTS ABOUT ZINC

A double-blind clinical trial found that lozenges containing zinc significantly reduced the average duration of the common cold. The lozenges used in the study contained 23 mg of elemental zinc, dissolved in the mouth every waking hour after an initial double dose. After seven days, 86 percent of the patients were symptom-free, compared to only 46 percent of those treated with placebo. Apparently zinc works in two ways: by reducing the ability of viruses to reproduce, and by boosting other aspects of immune function. This study led to an explosion of interest in the use of zinc as a strategy for reducing the severity of colds.

Not all studies on zinc have produced positive results. It appears that to be effective, zinc lozenges must be free of sorbitol, mannitol, and citric acid. These compounds bind with the zinc and reduce its effectiveness. The best lozenges are those that utilize the amino acid glycine as a sweetener. Use lozenges that supply 15 to 25 mg of elemental zinc. If you feel a cold coming on, take a double dose, then take one tablet every two hours. Let the tablet dissolve in your mouth. Continue for up to seven days.

Remember not to overdo it. Too much zinc can have the undesired effect of lowering immune function. For treatment of colds, I recommend that you take a total dose of no more than 150 mg a day for no more than a week.

Table 5-1: Nutrient Dosing Strategies for Immune Support

Vitamin A*
  Maintenance dose: 20,000 IU
    per day
  During infection: up to 50,000
    IU per day for no more than
    one month
Beta-carotene
  Maintenance dose: 25,000 IU
    per day
  During infection: up to 180,000
    IU per day
Vitamin C
  Maintenance dose: 500 to 1,000
    mg per day
  During infection: up to 5,000 mg
    per day in divided dosages

Vitamin E**
  Maintenance dose: 200 to
    400 IU
  During infection: 200 IU or less
Zinc
  Maintenance dose: 25 mg
    per day
  During infection: 75–150 mg per
    day (maximum 150 mg) for
    no more than one week
Selenium
  Maintenance dose: 200 mcg
    per day
  During infection: 400 mcg
    per day

*If you are now or may become pregnant, do not take vitamin A; in high doses, vitamin A can cause birth defects.

**At higher dosages (more than 800 IU), vitamin E may actually inhibit some immune functions important in fighting an acute infection.

Immune Support from Herbs

Eating a good diet and taking extra doses of vitamins and minerals, especially antioxidants, are important steps for boosting immunity. Herbs can provide extra immune support. As a rule, such herbal products should be used only for short periods of time (up to two months), for example, to stimulate the immune system during an acute infection, to help cure a chronic infection, or just to bring your system back up to normal.

Echinacea

The most widely used herb for enhancing the immune system by far is *echinacea*. Many Native American peoples used the herb, especially the root, as a remedy for more illnesses than any other plant. Echinacea (pronounced eck-uh-NAY-sha) was used externally for healing wounds, burns, abscesses, and insect bites. Taken internally, it was effective against infections and joint pain, and as an antidote to snake bites. Today, people take echinacea as a treatment for many types of infectious diseases, including flu and infections of the upper respiratory tract, urinary tract, or genitals. One of the most popular uses of echinacea is in treating the common cold.

APPLICATIONS OF ECHINACEA, BASED ON CLINICAL RESEARCH
Therapy and prevention of viral respiratory tract infections
Treatment of temporary immunodeficiency and increased susceptibility to infections
    Children in day care or nurseries
    Adults experiencing undue stress
    Sport-induced immunodeficiency
Adjuvant therapy to enhance the effectiveness of antibiotics in bacterial infections
Chemotherapy- and radiation-induced immunosuppression
Herpes simplex infections

Tune-Up Tip: Stopping a Cold—Cold

The common cold is caused by a variety of viruses that infect the oral and nasal passages and the sinuses. The symptoms of a cold are well known: low-grade fever, headaches, nasal congestion, sore throat, a general blah feeling (more technically known as malaise).

If you are an adult and you get more than one or two colds a year, or if your cold lasts more than four or five days, you probably have a weakened immune system. Kids have a tendency to get more colds because of increased exposure to cold viruses, but any more than three or four per year is excessive.

As is true of all health concerns, prevention is the smartest strategy. By boosting your immunity, you'll have a better chance of keeping colds from developing in the first place.

When you do get a cold, follow these recommendations.

Be sure to:
- Rest
- Drink plenty of liquids (water, diluted vegetable juices, soups, or herb teas), 8 ounces every hour

- Avoid sugar (including natural sugars such as honey, orange juice and other fruit juices, and fructose), because sugar depresses the immune system
- Eat a healthy, balanced diet

And take:
- High-potency multivitamin-multimineral supplement
- Vitamin C: 500 mg every hour that you are awake with a glass of water (if excessive gas or diarrhea is produced, reduce dosage to 500 mg every two hours)
- Thymus extract: 750 mg of the crude polypeptide fraction once or twice daily (see page 160)
- Echinacea: Dosages of *one* of the following preparations, three times daily:
  - Dried root (or as tea): 1–2 g
  - Freeze-dried plant: 325–650 mg
  - Juice of aerial portion of *Echinacea purpurea* stabilized in 22% ethanol: 2–3 ml (½ to ¾ tsp)
  - Tincture (1:5): 3–4 ml (¾ to 1 tsp)
  - Fluid extract (1:1): 1–2 ml (¼ to ½ tsp)
  - Solid (dry powdered) extract (6.5:1 or 3.5% echinacosides): 150 to 300 mg
  - Esberitox: three tablets three times daily

Echinacea products are available in many different forms: crude plant (ground, powdered, or freeze-dried); alcohol-based or aqueous tinctures; and others. You may become quite confused trying to figure out what is the best product to use. Although there are many effective echinacea products on the market, three products really stand out. The two products backed with the most scientific research are EchinaGuard (Nature's Way) and Esberitox (Enzymatic Therapy). EchinaGuard contains the fresh-pressed juice of *Echinacea purpurea* leaves and flowers while Esberitox contains standardized extracts of the roots from two species of echinacea (*E. purpurea* and *E. pallida*), as well as special extracts of *Thuja occidentalis* and *Baptisia tinctoria*—two other herbal medicines valued for their immune-enhancing activity. The third outstanding product is Echinamide (Natural Factors), which is extracted from echinacea grown under strict organic conditions. The standardization process for Echinamide includes a detailed chemical analysis prior to harvesting to assure a high level of the key active components in the extract. The Echinamide family of products includes liquids, softgel capsules, lozenges, throat sprays, and cough syrups.

Astragalus

Astragalus root is a traditional Chinese medicine commonly used for viral infections. Research in animals has shown that astragalus stimulates virtually all aspects of immune function, especially cell-mediated immunity. Like thymus extracts (see below), astragalus appears particularly useful in cases where the immune system has been damaged by chemicals or radiation (for example, in patients undergoing chemotherapy or radiation). Clinical studies in China have shown that astragalus protects against the common cold and that it reduces the duration and severity of symptoms should a cold develop. Take 100 to 150 mg of astragalus extract three times daily.

Oral Thymus Extracts

Perhaps the most effective method for reestablishing a healthy immune system is to support and promote the function of the thymus. As noted previously, you can prevent premature shrinkage of the thymus gland by ensuring adequate dietary intake of antioxidant nutrients, including beta-carotene, vitamins C and E, and the minerals selenium and zinc. Supplementation has been shown to increase thymus function and to enhance immunity provided by T cells.

Substantial scientific evidence supports the use of calf thymus tissue concentrates to boost thyroid activity and provide broad-spectrum immune enhancement. Different products are available that contain varying doses of thymus extract. I recommend products that have been concentrated and standardized for their polypeptide content, rather than products that contain crude preparations. Based on current clinical research, the daily dose should be equivalent to 120 mg of pure polypeptides with molecular weights less than 10,000 or approximately 500 to 750 mg of crude polypeptide fraction (these data will appear on the label). There have not been any reports of harmful side effects in clinical trials. I have recommended use of thymus extracts to many patients over the years with no complaints of side effects or adverse events. Quite the contrary—they report a lower incidence of colds, flu, and other diseases and are less affected by chronic infections and fatigue. Some people with low immune function seem to require thymus extract much the same way a person with low thyroid levels requires thyroid hormone. In other words, they will need to take it indefinitely. Most people, however, can simply take thymus extracts whenever they need to give their immune system a boost.

CONDITIONS IMPROVED BY ORAL THYMUS EXTRACTS
- Allergies, including asthma, hay fever, and food allergies
- Recurrent respiratory infections (especially in children)
- Immune function in cancer patients receiving chemotherapy, radiation, or both
- Viral hepatitis (acute or chronic)
- Susceptibility to infections by people infected by the human immunodeficiency virus (HIV)
- Acute and chronic viral infections
- Low or high ratios of helper to suppressor T cells
- Impaired cell-mediated immunity

CASE HISTORY: Fighting Back Against Herpes

The first time I saw Jamie was in 1989. She looked beat—tired, sallow skin, bags under her eyes. She could barely drag herself into my office. But what was most alarming was the fact that about a third of the left side of her face had erupted in fever blisters. It was the worst case of cold sores I'd ever seen in my years of practice. Such sores result from infection by a type I herpes simplex virus. To make matters worse, she also suffered from genital herpes.

Her history of viral infection went back at least nine years. During her second year of college, she had contracted infectious mononucleosis (mono). This debilitating disease is caused by infection with Epstein-Barr virus (EBV). Most people are infected with EBV, but only some develop symptoms. Experts suspect that EBV is also the cause of at least some cases of chronic fatigue syndrome (CFS). Back then, before CFS was recognized as a true illness, it was often called chronic Epstein-Barr virus (EBV) infection or "yuppie flu." Since her bout with mono, Jamie said, she had never felt quite as good as she had before she got the disease, although she had been enjoying relatively high energy levels for several years.

Six months before coming to see me, however, she started feeling lousy—

as she put it, "It's been worse than it ever was during the mono." Then the cold sores erupted. A normally attractive twenty-eight-year-old, Jamie was understandably upset and embarrassed. In addition to the recurrent cold sores and genital infection, she had been battling severe fatigue and depression. Her family physician was so convinced that she was suffering from AIDS that she sent Jamie to the University of Washington Immunology Clinic for a complete workup. Fortunately she did not have AIDS, but blood tests showed she did have severe immune deficiency.

It was easy to identify key stressors in Jamie's life. Her workload was intense. As an executive at a high-pressure company, she typically put in work-weeks of sixty or seventy hours. She also had an even more extensive travel schedule than I did, logging over 150,000 miles a year. She was getting married in two months and was in the process of buying a new home with her husband-to-be.

My immediate prescription was a vacation, but Jamie would have none of that kind of talk. She wanted me to fix her but did not want to adjust her lifestyle at all. She loved what she was doing and did not want to give it up. She just wanted to get her old self back. "That's fine," I told her, "but the problem is that your current self has an immune system that's shot."

Since Jamie did not want to make any significant changes to her lifestyle, we would need to be very aggressive in our therapy. In addition to suggesting that she follow the dietary recommendations described elsewhere in this chapter for tuning up immunity, I told her to follow a diet that avoids arginine-rich foods while promoting lysine-rich foods. Herpes viruses need a lot of arginine, an amino acid, to replicate; in fact, the very presence of arginine appears to stimulate replication. In contrast, lysine, another amino acid, appears to block the effects of arginine and thus has antiviral activity. Foods high in arginine are chocolate, peanuts, seeds, and nuts such as almonds. Foods high in lysine include most vegetables, legumes, fish, turkey, and chicken.

I also recommended the following supplements:

- High-potency multiple vitamin and mineral formula
- Vitamin C: 1,000 mg three times per day
- Lysine: 1,000 mg three times per day
- Thymus extract: two tablets twice daily, providing a total of 1,500 mg of thymus polypeptide fraction

For topical relief, I suggested Herpilyn from Enzymatic Therapy. Herpilyn contains a special extract of lemon balm (*Melissa officinalis*) that reduces the healing time and pain associated with cold sores and genital herpes.

Our primary goal was for Jamie to be free of fever blisters and genital sores on her wedding day. We not only accomplished this goal, but in the past six years Jamie has stayed free from herpes outbreaks.

Exercise and Immune Function

Regular exercise has been shown to lead to improved immune status. However, there is an important distinction that needs to be made. Although relatively strenuous exercise is required to benefit the cardiovascular system, light to moderate exercise may be best for the immune system. In particular, studies have shown that immune function is significantly increased by the practice of tai chi exercises. Tai chi is a martial art technique that features flowing movements from one posture to the next. The tai chi movements are quite dancelike, and interestingly, the same sort of improvement in immune function was noted with ballet. The research thus far suggests that light to moderate exercise stimulates the immune system, while intensive exercise (such as training for the Olympics) can have the opposite effect. Excessive exercise (leading to painful exhaustion two or more times a week) actually depresses the immune system for several hours after exertion, thus increasing the risk of infection during that time. One reason is that by stepping up metabolic activity, exercise results in a more rapid production of free radicals. If you exercise—and you should—be sure to take adequate doses of antioxidants, as detailed throughout this book.

You should also consider supplementing your diet with glutamine (3 to 5 g daily) or a glutamine-rich whey protein concentrate (20 to 30 g daily). Double-blind studies have shown that glutamine supplementation boosts immune function and fights infection in endurance athletes and critically ill patients.

HYPERIMMUNITY ASSESSMENT

Circle the number that best describes the intensity of your symptoms on the following scale:

>   *0 = I do not experience this symptom*
>   *1 = Mild*
>   *2 = Moderate*
>   *3 = Severe*

Entire body is painful to touch	0	1	2	3
Swollen joints	0	1	2	3
Food sensitivity or allergy	0	1	2	3
Certain foods make you sick, depressed, jittery	0	1	2	3
Chronic pain or inflammation	0	1	2	3
Painful stomach and/or intestine	0	1	2	3
Hay fever symptoms (eyes itch, nasal discharge)	0	1	2	3
Puffiness or dark circles under eyes	0	1	2	3
Chronic sinusitis/rhinitis	0	1	2	3

Add the numbers circled and enter that subtotal here: _____

Circle the number of the answer that applies to you:

Current use of cortisone, prednisone, or antihistamines	NO = 0	YES = 10
Eczema	NO = 0	YES = 10
Asthma/bronchitis	NO = 0	YES = 10
Autoimmune disease (rheumatoid arthritis, lupus, etc.)	NO = 0	YES = 10

Add the numbers circled and enter that subtotal here: _____
Add the two subtotals and enter that total here: _____

Scoring   *12 or more: High priority*
             6–11: Moderate priority
             1–5: Low priority

Interpreting Your Score

If you are suffering from asthma, rheumatoid arthritis, or some other clear-cut condition linked to an overactive immune system, you will definitely need to make tuning up your immune system a top priority. As noted in the hypoimmunity assessment, a person can be suffering from hyperimmunity and signs of low immune function at the same time. The reason is that chronic allergies or the use of drugs such as prednisone can suppress the body's ability to fight infections.

All of the recommendations previously given in regard to boosting your immune system apply here as well, with one exception: If you are not suffering from low immune function but definitely have signs of hyperimmunity, I would recommend boosting your vitamin E intake to 800 to 1,200 IU daily. All of the other nutritional and herbal guidelines apply, because they are really helping your immune system regain control; although they amplify normal immune reactions, there is no evidence that they push a hyperactive response even higher. I want to stress that for people suffering from allergies, autoimmune disease, or any other sign of hyperimmunity, the importance of eating an allergen-free diet that is also free of animal foods must not be underestimated. (The exception is fish, because of their omega-3 fatty acids, which reduce the formation of inflammatory compounds.) These simple dietary approaches have shown remarkable effectiveness in these conditions.

Food Allergies

Food allergies are an underlying factor in many cases of poor immune function. It's essential that you identify and deal with any food allergies, especially if you scored high on the hyperimmunity assessment. Strange as it sounds, the biggest source for antigens in the body (substances that trigger an immune response) is the food we eat.

If you are allergic to a food, your body reacts to it as if it were a dangerous invader. The white blood cells migrate in large numbers to the mucous membranes and the lining of the intestinal tract. There they release allergic and inflammatory compounds in an attempt to kill the false invader. All this inflammation causes the intestinal tract to become more permeable. As I discussed on pages 38–39, intestinal permeability—"leaky gut"—can allow large, harmful molecules to be absorbed into the bloodstream. The immune system rightfully recognizes these large molecules as foreign and develops antibodies against them. The result of this immune response can be a range of unpleasant conditions, including asthma, eczema, psoriasis, and even severe inflammatory conditions such as rheumatoid arthritis.

Table 5-2: Symptoms and Diseases Commonly Associated with Food Allergy

System	Symptoms and Diseases
Gastrointestinal	Canker sores, celiac disease, chronic diarrhea, duodenal ulcer, gastritis, irritable bowel syndrome, malabsorption, ulcerative colitis
Genitourinary	Bed-wetting, chronic bladder infections, nephrosis
Immune	Chronic infections, frequent ear infections
Mental/emotional	Anxiety, depression, hyperactivity, inability to concentrate, insomnia, irritability, mental confusion, personality change, seizures
Musculoskeletal	Bursitis, joint pain, low back pain
Respiratory	Asthma, chronic bronchitis, wheezing
Skin	Acne, eczema, hives, itching, skin rash
Miscellaneous	Arrhythmia, edema, fainting, fatigue, headache, hypoglycemia, itchy nose or throat, migraines, sinusitis

Tune-Up Tip: Eliminate Common Allergens

Many nutritionally oriented physicians order blood tests to diagnose food allergies. However, in most cases such tests are not really necessary. For patients who have to pay for such tests out of pocket, the tests can be expensive.

In my practice, I often recommend that patients try a simple elimination diet first to see if their symptoms improve. If there is little improvement but I still think food allergy may be a significant factor, then I will order a blood test to identify such allergies.

Start by eliminating the most common allergens:

- Milk and all dairy products
- Wheat
- Corn
- Citrus
- Peanuts and peanut butter

- Eggs
- Processed foods containing artificial food coloring

If your symptoms disappear, you're on the right track.

By slowly reintroducing the various foods into the diet (for example, adding back one food every three days) and paying attention to which ones cause symptoms to return, you can identify the real culprit.

Will you be able to eat that food again? That depends on whether the allergy is cyclic or fixed. *Cyclic* allergies develop slowly and result from repeatedly eating a certain food. After avoiding the allergenic food for a period of time (typically three to four months), it may be reintroduced. Usually the food won't cause symptoms again unless you eat it too frequently or in high amounts. Cyclic allergies account for roughly 80 to 90 percent of food allergies.

Fixed allergies occur whenever a food is eaten, no matter how much time has passed. If you have a fixed allergy, you will remain allergic to the food for life.

Asthma and Hay Fever

Asthma is an allergic disorder characterized by spasm of the bronchi (branched air passageways that connect the trachea to the lungs), swelling of the mucous lining of the lungs, and excessive production of a thick, viscous mucus. The major concern with asthma is that it can lead to respiratory failure—the inability to breathe.

Hay fever (seasonal allergic rhinitis) is an allergic reaction of the nasal passages characterized by a watery nasal discharge, sneezing, itchy eyes and nose. It shares many common features with asthma. Here are my seven tune-up tips for asthma and hay fever:

1. *Reduce exposure to airborne allergens.* Airborne allergens that can trigger asthma, such as pollen, dander, and dust mites, are often difficult to avoid entirely, but measures can be taken to reduce exposure. A great first step is keeping pets outside and removing carpets, rugs, upholstered furniture, and other surfaces where allergens can collect. If this can't be done entirely, make sure that at least the bedroom is as allergy-proof as possible. Encase the mattress in an allergen-proof plastic; wash sheets, blankets, pillowcases, and mattress pads every week in hot water with additive- and fragrance-free detergent;

consider using bedding material made from Ventflex, a special hypoallergenic synthetic material; and install an air purifier. The best mechanical air purifiers are HEPA (high-efficiency particulate-arresting) filters, which can be attached to central heating and air-conditioning systems. These units are available from suppliers of heating and air-conditioning units.

2. *Identify and eliminate food allergies and synthetic food additives.* Many studies have indicated that food allergies and food additives play an important role in asthma. Adverse reactions to food or food additives may be immediate or delayed. Double-blind food challenges in children have shown that immediate-onset allergies are usually due to (in order of frequency) eggs, fish, shellfish, nuts, and peanuts. Foods most commonly associated with delayed-onset sensitivities include (in order of frequency) milk, chocolate, wheat, citrus, and food colorings. Elimination diets have been successful in identifying allergens and treating asthma and are a particularly valuable diagnostic and therapeutic tool in infants. Elimination of common allergens during infancy (the first two years) has been shown to reduce allergic tendencies in children with a strong familial history of asthma.

3. *Eliminate or reduce the intake of animal products* (with the exception of fish; see #4). A long-term trial of a vegan diet (elimination of all animal products) provided significant improvement in 92 percent of subjects in one study. Improvement was noted in lung capacity, the maximum amount of air expired in one second (FEV1), physical working capacity, and laboratory assessments. The researchers also found a reduction in the tendency to contract infectious disease. Most of the patients responded (their asthma was significantly improved or entirely relieved) within four months.

4. *Eat more fish if it is not an allergen.* Population studies have shown that children who eat fish more than once a week have one-third the risk of getting asthma as children who do not eat fish regularly. Several clinical studies have shown that increasing the intake of omega-3 fatty acids (through supplementation with fish oils that contain eicosapentaenoic acid [EPA] and docosahexaenoic acid [DHA]) offers significant benefits in treating asthma. In particular, improvements in airway responsiveness to allergens have been noted, as well as improvements in respiratory function.

5. *Take a high-potency multiple vitamin and mineral formula.* Higher intakes of vitamin B_6, selenium, magnesium, and possibly other nutrients are associated with improvements in asthma and allergies.

6. *Take extra vitamin C.* The major antioxidant for the lungs is vitamin C. Population studies have shown that when vitamin C intake is low, the rate of asthma is high. Asthmatic patients have been shown to have significantly lower levels of vitamin C in their blood. Since 1973 there have been eleven clinical studies of vitamin C supplementation in asthma patients. Seven of these studies showed significant improvements in respiratory measures and asthma symptoms as a result of supplementing the diet with 1,000 to 2,000 mg of vitamin C per day.

7. *Increase the intake of flavonoids.* Flavonoids appear to be key antioxidants in the treatment of asthma. To increase flavonoid consumption, take quercetin or flavonoid-rich extracts such as grape seed, pine bark, green tea, or *Ginkgo biloba.*

Rheumatoid Arthritis and Other Autoimmune Diseases

Autoimmune diseases are conditions in which the body's immune system literally attacks body tissues. What triggers the autoimmune reaction is not clear, but genetic abnormalities, dietary factors, food allergies, bacterial overgrowth, "leaky gut" syndrome, and immunizations have all been suggested as possible causes. The most well known autoimmune disease is rheumatoid arthritis (RA)—a condition where primarily the joints come under attack. Diseases similar to RA that affect connective tissue (collagen structures that support internal organs as well as cartilage, tendons, muscles, and bone) include systemic lupus erythematosus (lupus or SLE), ankylosing spondylitis, scleroderma, polymyalgia rheumatica, and mixed connective tissue disease. There is tremendous overlap among these diseases in terms of underlying causes, symptoms, and treatment. They share many common features with RA, but the autoimmune and inflammatory process is a bit different in each of these other diseases. There are many treatments available to relieve the symptoms of RA and these other autoimmune diseases, but rather than simply prescribing treatment to mask the symptoms, I recommend addressing some of the underlying causes. The two primary factors that I recommend you focus on if you have RA or any other autoimmune disease are (1) identifying and eliminating food allergies and (2) altering the balance of fatty acids in your body by eliminating animal products (with the exception of fish) from the diet.

The most common food allergies in RA are wheat, corn, dairy products, beef, and plants of the nightshade family (tomatoes, eggplants, peppers, etc.). Talk with your health care provider about starting a therapeutic fast or an elimination diet to identify your food allergies.

CASE HISTORY: Kim's Miracle

Kim was a twenty-two-year-old student who had already been struggling with severe rheumatoid arthritis for more than ten years. The disease—and the twenty-one different medications that she was taking—were crushing body, mind, and spirit. She wanted to be rescued both from the ravages of this cruel disease and from its dangerous treatment.

Since Kim was taking prescription medications for her condition, I could not administer a blood test for food allergies. Instead I began her treatment with a low-allergy diet for two weeks. I restricted her dietary intake to fresh carrot juice, pineapple juice, herbal teas, vegetable broths, and three servings of UltraClear, a hypoallergenic meal replacement formula. Our goal was to decrease the absorption of allergenic food components. After two weeks, I would evaluate her symptoms and joint swelling. Any improvement would suggest that food allergies were likely responsible for her symptoms. I also started Kim on the following supplements:

- High-potency multiple vitamin and mineral formula
- Vitamin C: 1,000 mg three times daily
- Vitamin E: 800 IU daily
- Flaxseed oil: 1 tbsp daily
- Bromelain: 400 mg (1,800 to 2,000 mcu [milk clotting units]) between meals three times daily
- Curcumin: 400 mg between meals three times daily

At her return visit two weeks later, she was noticeably improved, so we moved to phase two, during which Kim reintroduced another food item every second day. If she noticed an increase in pain, stiffness, or joint swelling within two to forty-eight hours, she omitted this item from her diet for at least seven days before reintroducing it a second time. If the food caused worsening of symptoms a second time, it was omitted permanently. We identified some real problem foods for Kim: corn, wheat, milk and other dairy products, oranges, strawberries, and peanuts. Those foods were permanently removed from her diet. I also recommended that she stay away from beef, chicken, turkey, and other meats. The only animal foods that I approved for her were fish and wild game such as venison, elk, or buffalo (these meats have lower overall fat content with a higher percentage of omega-3 fatty acids). I also urged Kim to drink up to 24 ounces of fresh vegetable and fruit juice each day.

After three months I started weaning her off some of her drugs. After one year Kim had been able to reduce the number of drugs she was on from twenty-one to three: prednisone, methotrexate, and Plaquenil. Her dosage of prednisone had been as high as 15 mg per day; anything less and she suffered excruciating pain. Three years after first seeing me, Kim is now on prednisone at a dosage of only 5 mg per day. She no longer takes the twenty other drugs she was taking. Her symptoms have cleared up, her disease is in remission (permanently, we hope). Most important, she has gone from someone who is being ravaged to a ravishing young woman full of life.

Once you've identified any foods that trigger allergies, you should eat a diet that is rich in whole foods, vegetables, complex carbohydrates, and fiber, and low in sugar, meat, refined carbohydrates, and animal fats. It's especially important to take flaxseed oil and eat lots of cold-water fish, such as mackerel, herring, halibut, and salmon. These provide omega-3 fatty acids, which promote healthy cells and suppress production of inflammatory compounds. They also reduce your body's response to allergens.

Also make sure your antioxidant intake is up to par. In addition to taking extra vitamins C and E, I strongly recommend that you increase your intake of fresh fruit and vegetable juice. Autoimmune diseases such as RA and lupus are associated with a tremendous amount of inflammation, much of which is due to free-radical damage. Since antioxidants protect against oxidative damage, low levels of antioxidants in the diet appear to increase the risk for these inflammatory diseases. A recent study that followed patients for fifteen years found that the people most at risk of developing autoimmune diseases were those who had lower levels of vitamin A, beta-carotene, and selenium.

Herbal products can also be used to reduce inflammation. Those that I feel have the most use in rheumatoid arthritis are curcumin (200 mg three times daily), bromelain (200–400 mg three times daily on an empty stomach), and ginger (200 mg of 20 percent gingerol extract three times daily). Another herbal product that is showing promise in rheumatoid arthritis is cat's claw (*Uncaria tomentosa*). In the last few years, there has been considerable medical interest in this South American plant. Most of the clinical research has focused on its possible benefits in AIDS, but there have also been studies in patients with autoimmune disorders such as multiple sclerosis, Sjögren's syndrome, and rheumatoid arthritis. In one double-blind study conducted at the University of Innsbruck (Austria) in forty patients with rheumatoid arthritis, a special cat's claw extract (Saventaro) at a dosage of three capsules daily was shown to produce significant improvements in the number of swollen joints and the amount of swelling.

Tune-Up Tip: Turn on the Juice

One of the best things you can do for health is to drink fresh juice, the liquid extracted from fresh fruits and vegetables. Fresh juice provides high-quality nutrition that is easily absorbed. It also provides a wide assortment of compounds that are extremely beneficial to health, including enzymes; pigments such as carotenes, chlorophyll, and flavonoids; and numerous other antioxidant components. Here is my all-time favorite recipe for relief of rheumatoid arthritis and other autoimmune diseases. Juice the following: 1/2 medium-sized pineapple cut into slices (skin and all if your juicer can handle it); 1/2 cup of blueberries; and a 1/2-inch slice of fresh ginger.

The blueberries offer benefit because of their high flavonoid content. Fresh pineapple contains bromelain, an anti-inflammatory enzyme. Fresh ginger possesses significant anti-inflammatory action.

In order to juice you are going to need two things: fresh organic produce free from pesticides and surface sprays, and a good juicer. I think the best home juicer available is the one that I own, the Juiceman II from Salton.

HEY, COPPER!

For many years, wearing copper bracelets has been a popular folk remedy for rheumatoid arthritis. Does it work? Some evidence exists to suggest that it may. Atoms of copper are slowly absorbed through the skin. Once inside the body, copper binds with another compound that works to reduce inflammation.

Copper and its partner zinc are components of a form of superoxide dismutase (SOD), an important antioxidant. Having adequate copper thus helps reduce tissue damage by free radicals. A form of aspirin that contains copper, copper aspirinate, may be more effective than standard relieving RA.

You can get too much of a good thing, though. Excess copper with peroxides and damage joint tissues.

Tune-Up Tip: DHEA for RA and Lupus

Defective manufacture of testosterone and dehydroepiandrosterone (DHEA) has been proposed as a potential predisposing factor for lupus as well as rheumatoid arthritis. Studies at Stanford Medical Center have shown that supplementation with DHEA offers moderate therapeutic benefits in patients with lupus. In the most recent double-blind study, twenty-one patients with severe lupus received DHEA (200 mg/day) or a placebo for six months. Both patient groups continued conventional treatment with corticosteroids and/or other drugs that suppress the immune system. Significant improvements were noted in seven of the nine patients on DHEA. DHEA supplementation also protected against the bone loss (osteoporosis) so typical of long-term corticosteroid use. Although the dosage of DHEA was very high, mild acne and disruption of normal menstrual cycles were the only side effects noted.

If you have lupus or RA, talk to your physician about these studies and about a trial of high-dosage DHEA. In my own clinical experience, I have found that dosages of 50 mg per day are usually sufficient in cases of RA or lupus in people less than fifty years of age; higher dosages are usually required in older subjects.

Tune-Up Tip: Laugh Hard and Often

Our mood and attitude have a tremendous bearing on the function of our immune system. When we are happy and up, our immune system functions much better. Conversely, when we are depressed, our immune system tends to be depressed. It was easily accepted by conventional medical authorities that negative emotional states adversely affect the immune system, but for some reason the medical community initially scoffed at the notion that positive emotional states can actually enhance immune function.

By the end of the 1970s, several studies had shown that negative emotions suppress immune function. But in 1979 Norman Cousins' popular book *Anatomy of an Illness* caused a significant stir in the medical community. Cousins's book provided an autobiographical anecdotal account that positive emotional states can cure the body of even a quite serious disease (he had scleroderma, an autoimmune disease). Cousins watched *Candid Camera* and Marx Brothers films and read humorous books.

Originally physicians and researchers scoffed at Cousins's account. Now, however, it has been demonstrated in numerous studies that laughter and other positive emotional states can in fact enhance the immune system. In addition, the use of guided imagery, hypnosis, and other meditative states have been shown to enhance immune system function.

Obviously, if you want to have a healthy immune system, you need to laugh often, view life with a positive eye, and put yourself in a relaxed state of mind on a regular basis. By laughing frequently and taking a lighter view of life, you will find that life is much more enjoyable and fun. Here are eight tips to help you get more laughter in your life.

Tip #1: Learn to laugh at yourself. Recognize how funny some of your behavior really is—especially your shortcomings or mistakes. We all have little idiosyncrasies or behaviors that are unique to us that we can recognize and enjoy. Do not take yourself too seriously.

Tip #2: Inject humor anytime it is appropriate. People love to laugh. Get a joke book and learn how to tell a good joke. Humor and laughter really make life enjoyable.

Tip #3: Read the comics to locate a comic that you find funny and follow it. Humor is very individual. What I may find funny, you may not, but the comics have something for everybody. Read them thoroughly to identify a comic strip that you think is particularly funny and look for it every day or week.

Tip #4: Watch comedies on television. With modern cable systems, I am amazed at how easy it is to find something funny on television. When I am in need of a good laugh, I try to find something I can laugh at on TV. Some of my favorites are the old-time classics like *The Andy Griffith Show, Gilligan's Island, The Mary Tyler Moore Show,* and so on.

Tip #5: Go to comedies at the movie theater. My wife and I love to go to the movies, especially comedies. If we see a funny movie together, I find myself laughing harder and longer than if I had seen the same scene by myself. We feed off each other's laughter during and after the movie. Laughing together helps build good relationships.

Tip #6: Listen to comedy audiotapes in your car while commuting. Check your local record store, bookstore, video store, or library for recorded comedy routines of your favorite comic. If you haven't heard or seen many comics, go to your library first. You'll find an abundance of tapes to investigate, and you can check them out for free.

Tip #7: Play with kids. Kids really know how to laugh and play. I am truly blessed with two great kids whom I find hilarious to play with. If you do not have kids of your own, spend time with your nieces and nephews, or with neighborhood children with whose families you are friendly. Become a Big Brother or Big Sister. Investigate local Little Leagues. Help out at your church's Sunday school and children's events.

Tip #8: Ask yourself this question: "What is funny about this situation?" Many times we will find ourselves in a seemingly impossible situation, but if we can laugh about it, somehow it becomes enjoyable or at least tolerable. So many times I have heard people say, "This is something that you will look back on and laugh about." Well, why wait? Find the humor in the situation and enjoy a good laugh immediately.

Key Steps to Tuning Up Your Immune System

- A healthy lifestyle is essential for immunity. Be sure to eat a healthy diet, get exercise, avoid toxins, maintain your appropriate body weight, and get enough sleep.
- Stress lowers immunity. Take steps to manage stress. Practice techniques to activate the relaxation response, such as breathing exercises, visualization, or meditation.
- Diet is vital for supplying your body with the nutrients it needs to build disease-fighting cells and proteins. Eat plant foods, especially green leafy vegetables. Avoid refined sugars and fats, but make sure you get plenty of protein and essential fatty acids.
- Take a high-potency vitamin and mineral supplement. Vitamins C and E, B vitamins, zinc, and selenium are especially important.
- Light to moderate exercise may produce greater overall benefit to the immune system than more strenuous exercise.
- Support thymus function through a good diet and extra antioxidants. Use calf thymus extracts supplying 120 mg of pure polypeptide fractions. Astragalus root (100–150 mg three times daily) is a good alternative to thymus extract for vegetarians.

- Food allergies can activate your body's immune response. Eliminate common sources of food allergies such as wheat, corn, dairy products, peanuts, eggs, and processed foods with artificial coloring, especially if you have allergies or an autoimmune disease.
- A positive attitude and laughter are powerful immune system boosters.

Lifestyle Tune-Up #5: Eat the Right Balance of Fats

To make sure your car runs smoothly, you need to keep it well lubricated and make sure there's plenty of clean, fresh oil. The same is true of your body. Many of my patients are surprised when I tell them that their lives depend on eating fats. I quickly point out, however, that while certain kinds of fats are essential for healthy body functioning, other kinds are deadly. The goal is to learn which fats are good for you and to consume a diet that provides you with adequate amounts in the right proportion.

For your tune-up, the goal is to *decrease* your total fat intake (especially intake of saturated fats) while *increasing* your intake of essential fatty acids.

To explain these terms, I need to tell you a little more about the way fat behaves. Fat molecules are made of carbon, hydrogen, and a little oxygen. Each of the separate atoms attaches to the others only in certain predetermined ways. For example, carbon atoms have four available "parking places," called bonding sites. Several carbon atoms (C) can link together to form a chain:

$$-\overset{\displaystyle |}{\underset{\displaystyle |}{C}} - \overset{\displaystyle |}{\underset{\displaystyle |}{C}} - \overset{\displaystyle |}{\underset{\displaystyle |}{C}} - \overset{\displaystyle |}{\underset{\displaystyle |}{C}} -$$

Hydrogen (H) and oxygen (O) atoms can then attach to the carbons, like chunks of cheese stuck on toothpicks. A *saturated fat* is a fat molecule in which all of the available "toothpicks" are occupied with an atom. In other words, the carbons are saturated with all of the atoms they can hold:

$$\begin{array}{ccccc} & H & H & H & H \\ & | & | & | & | \\ H - & C - & C - & C - & C - O \\ & | & | & | & | \\ & H & H & H & H \end{array}$$

An *unsaturated fat* is one where there are one or more bonding sites left unoccupied:

$$
\begin{array}{ccccccc}
& H & & & & H & \\
& | & | & | & | & & \\
H - & C & - C & - C & - C & - & O \\
& | & | & | & | & & \\
& H & H & H & H & &
\end{array}
$$

However, molecules don't like to leave these places empty for long. If there is no available atom to fill the site, the two neighboring carbon atoms will take up the slack by forming what is called a double bond:

$$
\begin{array}{ccccccc}
& H & & & & H & \\
& | & & & & | & \\
H - & C & - C & = C & - C & - & O \\
& | & | & | & | & & \\
& H & H & H & H & &
\end{array}
$$

A fat molecule with one double bond is called a monounsaturated fat. Molecules with more than one double bond are called polyunsaturated fats. (*Mono-* means "one"; *poly-* means "many.")

The more saturated the fat, the more dangerous it is to your body. Generally, saturated fats are semisolid or solid at room temperature, such as butter or lard. Unsaturated fats, such as cooking oils, are usually liquid at room temperature. Sometimes, during manufacturing, additional hydrogen molecules are added to a vegetable oil to make it more solid. This process, hydrogenation, changes the oil from a naturally unsaturated one to a saturated fat. Many margarines are made with hydrogenated oils.

Some fats contain one or more special units known as *fatty acids*. These are long chains of carbon and hydrogen atoms with a certain group of molecules, called an acid group, attached at one end. The body manufactures some types of fatty acids. But you need to get other fatty acids from the foods you eat. These are known as *essential fatty acids*—more about them in a moment.

The most common types of fats in the diet are triglycerides. These are molecules made of three units of fatty acids plus a sugar molecule. In the body, enzymes break apart the triglyceride, separating the fatty acids from the glycerol. The body can absorb these "free" fatty acids more easily than it can the bulky triglyceride molecule.

Once absorbed into the body, the free fatty acids and other fats, such as cholesterol, attach to and are transported through the bloodstream by special molecules called lipoproteins. There are three main kinds: high-density lipoprotein (HDL), low-density lipoprotein (LDL), and very low-density lipoprotein (VLDL). LDL and VLDL carry fats from the liver to the body cells, while HDL carries fat back to the liver. The higher the levels of LDL and VLDL, the more fat you have in circulation, and the greater your risk of fat-related illnesses such as atherosclerosis ("hardening of the arteries"). In contrast, HDL protects against these illnesses because it removes fats from circulation and puts them back into storage in the liver. When doctors measure cholesterol levels, they also analyze the ratio of HDL to LDL. The more HDL you have and the less LDL, the better off you are. That's why you'll often hear HDL described as "good" cholesterol and LDL as "bad" cholesterol. (For more information, see Chapter 6.)

By now you may be asking why, if fats are so dangerous, our bodies need them in the first place. To answer that, I need to tell you a little more about how your cells function.

As I explained earlier, every human cell has a protective, permeable membrane. That means that certain substances can enter or leave the cell by passing through the membrane. The membrane is also selective, which means it is choosy about what particles can enter. How efficiently substances pass through the membrane depends on the available supply of key nutrients: proteins and fats.

Membranes contain two layers, each made mainly of proteins, cholesterol, and phospholipids. (Phospholipids are almost the same as triglycerides, except that one of the three fatty acid units has been replaced with a molecule that contains phosphorus.) The fat molecules in the membrane bond together in an orderly fashion, forming a kind of sheet. About half of the molecules in a cell membrane are fats. The rest are proteins, of which there are two main types. One type is long enough to penetrate through both layers of the membrane, like a thread drawn through two thin layers of cloth. These are called integral proteins because they are integrated into the membrane's layers. The other type of protein perches on either the external or internal face of the membrane and does not penetrate through the barrier. Because these are not built into the membrane, they are called peripheral proteins. These surface proteins act as the receptors for hormones and various other chemical transmitters.

Cell membranes can change their shape to become more or less porous. The proteins can shift position to create openings, allowing certain molecules to enter. To accommodate that shift, the fat molecules have to be flexible. The more flexible the membrane, the better your cell is able to take in and expel various molecules and thus the better it can carry out its functions.

How fluid your membranes are depends on what types of phospholipids are used in its construction. And that, in turn, depends on what you eat. Because you can't consume phospholipids in the diet, your body has to construct them, using fatty acids as key ingredients. There are more than forty different kinds of fatty acids found in nature. Your body can synthesize many of these types. But to make the best and most fluid kinds of phospholipids, you need certain kinds of fatty acids that your body can't manufacture and that you must consume in your diet. These are linoleic acid and linolenic acid, known as the *essential fatty acids.*

Not all fatty acids are created equal. For example, under the microscope, a normal molecule of fatty acid has a characteristic C shape. The scientific name for this is a *cis* fatty acid. However, during food processing, polyunsaturated oils are subjected to excessive heat, light, and oxygen. As a result, the molecule straightens out, losing its C shape and becoming unnaturally straight. Such transformed molecules are called *trans* fatty acids. Margarine is an example of a product that starts out as something good, polyunsaturated oil, and during processing gets converted into something harmful: hydrogenated (saturated) fats and trans fatty acids.

There are other differences. The essential fatty acids are molecules that contain eighteen carbon atoms. As explained above, these acids are unsaturated, which means they are missing some hydrogen atoms. In linolenic acid, the location of the missing hydrogen atoms, and thus the site of a double carbon bond, is the third carbon atom from one end of the molecule (known as the omega end). For this reason, linolenic acid is called an omega-3 fatty acid. (There are other double bonds elsewhere in the carbon chain, but the name comes from the site of the first double bond, at position number 3.) Its sister molecule with the nearly identical name, linoleic acid, is an omega-6 fatty acid, which means that its first double bond occurs at the sixth carbon molecule.

Let me recap this important information: Your cells need strong, flexible membranes to function. To build membranes, your cells require a supply of fatty acids. The best ingredients for healthy membranes are two essential fatty acids, linolenic acid (an omega-3 fatty acid) and linoleic acid (an omega-6 fatty acid). Because your body cannot manufacture these substances, you must consume them in your diet. Without enough fatty acids, your cells may become damaged, leading to adverse health conditions ranging from heart problems to loss of mental function. It may take some time to see improvement (usually one to three months), but stick with it.

Symptoms Associated with Deficiency of Essential Fatty Acids

Aching joints	Dry skin
Angina, chest pain	Fatigue, malaise, low energy
Arthritis	Forgetfulness
Cardiovascular disease	Frequent colds and sickness
Constipation	High blood pressure
Cracked nails	Immune weakness
Depression	Indigestion, gas, bloating
Dry, lifeless hair	Lack of endurance
Dry mucous membranes (tear ducts, mouth, vagina)	Lack of motivation

These symptoms are not specific; they can also be caused by other diseases or dietary insufficiencies.

There's more to the story. The essential fatty acids also are necessary for the production of hormonelike substances known as prostaglandins. These chemicals carry out many important tasks in the body. They are important for regulating inflammation, pain, and swelling; they play a role in maintaining blood pressure; and they regulate heart, digestive, and kidney function. Prostaglandins are involved in blood clotting. They participate in the response to allergies, help control transmission of signals along the nerves, and are used in the production of steroids and other hormones. Having adequate levels of essential fatty acids—*in the right proportion*—can protect against heart disease, cancer, autoimmune diseases, skin diseases, and other conditions.

ROLE OF PROSTAGLANDINS AND FATTY ACIDS IN BODY FUNCTION
- Stimulate production of steroids and other hormones
- Regulate fluid pressure in the eye, joints, and blood vessels
- Regulate response to pain, inflammation, and swelling
- Mediate immune response
- Regulate body secretions and their viscosity
- Dilate or constrict blood vessels
- Direct endocrine hormones to reach target cells
- Regulate smooth muscle and autonomic (involuntary) reflexes
- Help in construction, fluidity, and permeability of cell membranes
- Regulate the rate of cell reproduction
- Help in the transport of oxygen to tissues
- Maintain proper kidney function and fluid balance
- Keep saturated fats mobile in the bloodstream
- Prevent blood cells from clumping together
- Regulate nerve transmission
- Provide primary energy for heart muscle

Here's what I mean by the "right proportion." There are three main kinds (series) of prostaglandins. The ones we call prostaglandin 1 and prostaglandin 3 are considered good. The series 2 prostaglandins can be troublesome, because they tend to promote allergies and inflammation. Too much prostaglandin 2 can cause blood particles called platelets to become stickier and more likely to form clots, which in turn raises the risk of heart disease and strokes. Your body makes prostaglandins 1 and 2 by converting omega-6 fatty acids in a series of steps, while prostaglandin 3 (the most beneficial kind) is made from omega-3 fatty acids. By altering the type of oils in your diet, you can affect which types of prostaglandins your body produces. The trick here is to consume the proper ratio of essential fatty acids.

As a tune-up goal, I recommend trying to achieve as close to a 1:1 ratio of omega-6 oils to omega-3 oils within body tissues as possible. However, because omega-6 fatty acids are added to many processed foods, most of us eat too many of them. I recommend a combined approach: Reduce the amount of omega-6 fatty acids and increase the intake of omega-3 fatty acids. A typical ratio of omega-6 to omega-3 fatty acids in the American diet is as high as 20:1, and that's way off balance. For one thing, high ratios of omega-6 to omega-3 fatty acids are a significant risk factor for breast cancer. In my opinion, the best way to achieve the right balance is:

- Eliminate foods that contain hidden sources of omega-6, especially salad dressings containing soy, safflower, sunflower, or corn oil.
- Cook with canola or olive oil.
- Increase the intake of fish (not fried), particularly cold-water fish such as salmon, halibut, and mackerel.
- Take 1 tbsp flaxseed oil daily.

These steps will help you achieve the optimal ratio of essential fatty acids for healthy cell membranes and balanced and efficient production of prostaglandins.

Here are my recommendations for making sure you get the right amounts of the right kinds of fats.

1. Reduce the amount of saturated fats and total fat in the diet. Be aware of the fat content of foods. In general, animal products are high in fat, while most plant foods are very low in fat. While most nuts and seeds are relatively high in fat, the calories they supply come mostly from polyunsaturated essential fatty acids. When possible, choose foods that contain monounsaturated or, better still, polyunsaturated fats.
2. Eliminate margarine and other foods containing trans fatty acids and partially hydrogenated oils. These "unnatural" forms of fatty acids interfere with the body's ability to utilize important essential fatty acids.
3. Take 1 tbsp of flaxseed oil daily. Organic, unrefined flaxseed oil is the key to restoring the proper level of essential fatty acids. Flaxseed oil is unique because it contains both essential fatty acids—linolenic (omega-3) and linoleic (omega-6)—in high amounts. Flaxseed oil is the richest source of omega-3 fatty acids—a whopping 58 percent by weight, more than twice the amount of omega-3 fatty acids found in fish oils. Flaxseed oil can be used as a salad dressing, mixed with yogurt or cottage cheese, or used to dip bread in.
4. Limit total dietary fat intake to no more than 30 percent of calories (400–600 calories a day from fat, based on a standard 2,000-calorie-a-day diet). Make a strong effort to incorporate healthful fats in the form of essential-fatty-acid-rich oils such as flaxseed oil in place of dangerous trans, hydrogenated, and saturated fats.

Watch for these "stealth fats" by reading food labels carefully before you buy.

5. Reduce the intake of meat and dairy products while increasing the intake of fish. Particularly beneficial are the cold-water fish such as salmon, mackerel, herring, and halibut, because of their high levels of omega-3 fats.

CHAPTER 6

Tuning Up Your Cardiovascular System

E very second of every minute of your life, your heart beats. The force of this sturdy pump pushes blood, carrying its load of oxygen from the lungs and nutrients from the digestive system, to every one of your tissues and organs. The blood returns to the heart, where the process repeats. When your cardiovascular system works well, every other part of your body—including your brain—functions better.

Unfortunately, millions of people operate at a deficit. Millions more are at risk of dying too soon from damage to the heart and blood vessels. Cardiovascular diseases—heart attacks and strokes—are the leading cause of premature death in this country, accounting for more than 40 percent of all deaths in the United States. It doesn't have to be this way. Heart disease can be prevented. What's more, prevention doesn't require costly drugs or dangerous medical procedures. You can tune up your heart through simple, but effective, natural methods.

A QUICK LANGUAGE LESSON

Cardiac comes from the Greek word for "heart," while *pulmonary* comes from the Latin word for "lungs." The term *cardiopulmonary* thus refers to both the heart and the lungs. We get our word *vessel* from the Latin word *vas*. The vascular system, then, is your network of blood vessels. The word *cardiovascular* refers to the heart and its vessels.

The Heart

Each day the human heart beats 100,000 times and pumps up to 5,000 gallons of fluid. In an average lifetime, the heart will beat 2.5 billion times and pump 100 *trillion* gallons of blood.

Your heart is actually two pumps that work side by side, sending blood through two separate circulatory paths. The right side pumps blood that lacks oxygen. After leaving the heart, the blood from the right side travels to the lungs through two pulmonary arteries. Inside the lungs, blood picks up its oxygen supply. Then it travels back to the left side of the heart through the pulmonary veins. This blood route is called the pulmonary circuit. The left pump sends the blood out through the main artery (the aorta) and into circulation in the body. This route is called the systemic circuit, because it travels through your body's entire system (except for the lungs).

Each side of the heart has two chambers. The top chamber is called the *atrium* and the bottom is the *ventricle*. Passage out of each chamber is controlled by valves; thus your heart has four valves, two on the right and two on the left. The valves ensure that blood travels in only one direction.

Here's how it works: Blood entering the heart first fills the atrium, putting pressure on the valve. The valve opens, and blood pours into the ventricle below. The atrium also contracts to squeeze the remaining blood into the lower chamber. The valve then shuts. Next, the ventricle contracts, which forces its own valve to open and pushes the blood through the valve and out into circulation. The ventricular valve shuts, preventing blood from flowing back into the heart. This sequence happens on the right and left sides at the same time. Both atria fill, then send their blood into the ventricles, and then both ventricles contract simultaneously. You've no doubt listened to the *lub-dub* of your heartbeat through a stethoscope: *Lub* is the sound of your atrial valves closing, and *dub* is the sound of your ventricular valves closing. *Dub* is louder, because the ventricles have to work a lot harder and the valves are much thicker.

These contractions must occur in the right sequence and with the right pressure. Valves have to open and close fully at just the right moments. Also, because the heart is mostly muscle, it must rest between each beat. Otherwise it would wear out pretty quickly. All this heart activity is controlled by electrical signals. The signals have to travel through the muscles at the right pace and at the right strength. Electrical activity is coordinated by a cluster of cells, known as a pacemaker, in the upper right part of the heart.

As you can see, your heart is a complex organ. By tuning up your heart, you provide it with the support it needs, in the form of nutrients and exercise, to keep it going strong for the rest of your life.

HEART RATE

The typical human heart beats somewhere between 60 and 100 times a minute while resting. But the rate changes constantly throughout the day. Simply breathing in tends to increase the rate, and breathing out slows it down. Even when you sleep, your heart rate changes as you pass from one stage of sleep (such as REM sleep, when you dream) to another.

During exercise, your heart beats faster and more strongly so it can send more blood to the muscles. The blood delivers more oxygen and nutrients, which the muscles need to do their work. It also removes the carbon dioxide and waste products that result from all that cell activity.

Stimulants such as caffeine and nicotine raise heart rate. Stress also causes the release of hormones and neurotransmitters, such as epinephrine (adrenaline). Such chemicals crank up the electrical output by the heart's pacemaker.

Heart rate depends on the size and efficiency of the organ. A small heart beats faster to serve the body's needs, while a large heart can beat at a more leisurely pace and still deliver the goods. If you're physically fit, your heart beats slower but more strongly. Well-trained athletes may have a resting heart rate of less than 60 beats per minute. Many people become less fit as they grow older, and so their heart rate tends to increase.

The Blood Vessels

Let's look now at what happens to the blood when it leaves the heart. There are two main types of blood vessels. Arteries carry blood away from the heart, and veins carry blood toward the heart. If all the blood vessels in your body were laid end to end, that vessel would stretch more than sixty thousand miles! Incredible, but true.

Blood vessels have different diameters, depending on their function. The largest vessels are those that transport blood into and away from the heart. Their job is to ship as much blood to its destination as possible. As the vessels spread out through the body, they become smaller and smaller. The smallest vessels are called capillaries, whose walls are quite permeable. This means that important substances, including chemicals, particles (such as nutrients), and gases (oxygen and carbon dioxide), can pass through them. The term *blood pressure* refers to the force with which your blood flows through the vessels. Pressure depends on several factors: how hard your heart is pumping, how much oxygen your body needs at a given moment, how much fluid (water) there is in your blood, and how flexible or resistant your vessels are. The pressure resulting from heart contractions is called *systolic* pressure. The pressure when the heart is at rest is *diastolic* pressure. Systolic pressure is higher than diastolic pressure.

BLOOD PRESSURE: WHAT THE NUMBERS MEAN

When you have your blood pressure measured, you are told it is "140 over 90" or "180 over 100" (written 140/90 or 180/100). The first number represents systolic pressure, the second diastolic. The numbers mean that the amount of pressure in your vessels would be enough to push mercury, the liquid metal, up a tube to a certain height in millimeters. The scientific abbreviation for mercury is *Hg*. Thus, a systolic reading of 140 mm Hg means your pressure could push mercury up the tube to a height of 140 mm.

Nowadays doctors don't have to use a mercury-filled column to get a pressure reading. Instead they use a device with the tongue-twisting name of *sphygmomanometer,* also called a blood pressure cuff. The pressure reading appears on a gauge. But your medical chart will still give the results in mm Hg, or millimeters of mercury.

Your body has its own built-in blood pressure monitoring system. Clusters of cells that are sensitive to changes in pressure are located in several vessels, including the aorta and the carotid artery in the neck. These clusters are known as baroceptors (*baro-* means "pressure"). As blood passes by, the baroceptors detect how much pressure there is. The cells then send signals to the brain center in charge of blood pressure. The brain reacts as needed. For example, if the pressure is too high, your brain might order your kidneys to step up the production of urine, so as to lower the amount of water in the blood.

CASE HISTORY: The Breath of Health

My new patient was near tears as she told me why she had come. Anna was seventy-four years old. Her medical doctor had recently told her that her blood pressure was way too high—190/140—and prescribed a drug to bring it down. She told me she absolutely didn't want to take a drug, but when I measured her pressure again, I found it had soared to 210/160—dangerously high. I told her I agreed with her previous doctor that something had to be done, and explained that sometimes drug therapy is the best approach if the benefits outweigh the risks.

She protested tearfully that I didn't understand. Her mother had been in perfect health, except for high blood pressure, well into her eighties. When her mother finally started taking blood pressure medication, her health started a very fast downward spiral. She died soon afterward. Not surprisingly, Anna was deathly afraid of taking drugs for blood pressure.

It was then I noticed that Anna's breathing was shallow and rapid. I started asking her questions about her life: "What are the things you really enjoy? Do you have grandchildren? Where is the most peaceful place you have ever been?" Her breathing started to slow down, but she was still breathing shallowly, using only her upper chest. I spent the next few minutes teaching her diaphragmatic breathing. Then, as I continued to ask questions that conjured up peaceful and relaxed images in her mind's eye, I took her blood pressure. It had fallen to 160/110. I explained to Anna that we could keep her off blood pressure medication, but only if she agreed to do everything I asked of her.

My first prescription was for her to perform diaphragmatic breathing for five minutes every waking hour. The second task was to walk down to her local fire station for a free blood pressure check every afternoon. And finally, I prescribed a special vitamin, mineral, and herbal supplement for high blood pressure, extra potassium, and a high-quality garlic product. It was Wednesday, and I asked Anna to call me on Saturday morning to give me a report.

Saturday at 7:00 A.M. my phone rang. (I learned a valuable lesson here: Always specify the time for a patient to check in!) Anna told me that her blood pressure had dropped to 140/90. A few days later in my clinic I was pleased to find Anna's blood pressure a normal 120/80.

Was it the pills I had given her? I don't think they had had time to work fully yet. I really think it was simply that she had learned how to breathe deeply again.

CARDIOVASCULAR SYSTEM ASSESSMENT

Part A: Heart and Blood Pressure

Circle the number that best describes the intensity of your symptoms on the following scale:

0 = I do not experience this symptom
1 = Mild
2 = Moderate
3 = Severe

Shortness of breath	0	1	2	3
Chest pain while walking	0	1	2	3
Heaviness in legs	0	1	2	3
Cramps in calf muscles while walking	0	1	2	3
Pounding heart	0	1	2	3
Jittery feeling	0	1	2	3
Missed heartbeats or extra beats	0	1	2	3
Swelling of feet and ankles	0	1	2	3
Rapid beating of heart (>80 beats per minute)	0	1	2	3
Feeling of exhaustion with minor exertion	0	1	2	3
Snoring or sleep apnea	0	1	2	3

Add the numbers circled and enter that subtotal here: _____

Circle the number of the answer that applies to you:

Have male pattern baldness	NO = 0	YES = 10
Have diagonal earlobe crease (wrinkle)	NO = 0	YES = 10
Have high blood pressure (>140/90 mm Hg)	NO = 0	YES = 10
Have total cholesterol level above 215	NO = 0	YES = 10

Add the numbers circled and enter that subtotal here: _____
Add the two subtotals and enter that total here: _____

Scoring *11 or more: High priority*
7–10: Moderate priority
1–6: Low priority

Part B: Circulation

Circle the number that best describes the intensity of your symptoms on the following scale:

  0 = I do not experience this symptom
  1 = Mild
  2 = Moderate
  3 = Severe

Cold hands and feet	0	1	2	3
Slurred speech	0	1	2	3
Cramps in calf muscles while walking	0	1	2	3
Headaches	0	1	2	3
Numbness in extremities	0	1	2	3
Poor concentration	0	1	2	3
Ringing in ears	0	1	2	3
Ear canal hair	0	1	2	3
Pain in back of head and neck when getting up in morning	0	1	2	3
Dizziness	0	1	2	3

Add the numbers circled and enter that subtotal here: _____

Circle the number of the answer that applies to you:
                    History of stroke   NO = 0   YES = 10

Enter the number circled as a subtotal here: _____
Add the two subtotals and enter that total here: _____

Scoring   *9 or more: High priority*
          5–8: Moderate priority
          1–4: Low priority

Interpreting Your Score

The questions in Part A assess the overall condition of your heart. Symptoms such as shortness of breath or swelling of the feet may indicate that your heart isn't pumping efficiently enough to remove fluid. Heaviness in the legs or muscle cramping may mean not enough blood is reaching the muscles, especially during exercise. Abnormal heart rhythms result from problems with electrical signals that regulate the beat; these problems can be caused by damaged or constricted blood vessels, stress, or hormonal imbalance. In most cases, heart disease results from the buildup of cholesterol-containing plaque in the blood vessels.

Section B reflects the state of your circulation. For example, if your blood pressure is not high enough to propel blood to your hands and feet, your fingers and toes may feel cold or numb all the time. In contrast, high pressure can cause vessels to burst, leading to stroke.

YOU MAY BE WONDERING . . .
What does the presence of a diagonal earlobe crease have to do with heart disease? The answer: plenty. More than thirty studies have shown that the presence of a diagonal earlobe crease is more predictive of the risk for having a heart attack than an angiogram (a procedure where dye is injected into the coronary arteries to determine blockage). The earlobe is richly veined, and a decrease in blood flow over a period of time is believed to result in collapse of the vascular bed there. This leads to a diagonal crease. Other interesting findings are that the presence of hair in the ear canal, male pattern baldness, and snoring are also very strong predictors of heart disease and strokes.

A Brief Guide to Cardiovascular Disorders

The term *heart disease* is so broad that it frequently causes confusion. Most often doctors use the term to describe *atherosclerosis,* which is a main cause of heart attacks and strokes. Atherosclerosis results from the buildup of a waxy material called plaque (containing cholesterol, fatty material, and cellular debris) along the walls of the blood vessel. Normally your arteries are very flexible, like a rubber tube. Plaque causes them to become stiff and can even block blood flow.

The plaque can also lead to the formation of blood clots—thickened clumps of blood that form when disk-shaped particles called platelets collect at the site of blood vessel damage. The platelets are held in place by stringy protein strands called fibrin, which is made from smaller particles called fibrinogen. Usually what happens is that the clot forms in a large vessel, where it may slow down—but not stop—blood flow. But if a piece of the clot breaks off, it will eventually circulate into a vessel that is too small to allow it to pass. As a result, blood flow to that part of the body stops, and the nearby organ or tissue can die. The bigger the clot, the bigger (and more important) the vessel it can block. The technical term for this condition is *thrombosis*. A thromboembolism is a clot that has traveled away from its site of origin.

A *heart attack* (also called a myocardial infarction) occurs when something blocks the flow of blood to the heart—it can be a clot, a spasm of a coronary artery, or an accumulation of plaque. Like each of your other organs, the hardworking heart needs a steady supply of blood containing oxygen and other nutrients. The coronary arteries feed the heart. If something interrupts the blood supply, the starved muscle tissue begins to die very rapidly. The longer the blockage lasts, the greater the risk that the heart attack will be fatal.

A *stroke* is brain damage that occurs when the blood flow is interrupted or when a vessel bursts, causing blood to spurt into the surrounding tissue. While heart attacks involve coronary arteries, strokes involve arteries feeding to the brain (carotid arteries). When the supply of blood is shut off, nerves in the brain die almost immediately. Sometimes the pressure of blood gushing through a ruptured vessel slices through the delicate nerves, severing their millions of connections. Depending on which part of the brain is affected, damage can include loss of movement, speech, memory, or virtually any other function of the body. Strokes are fatal in about one case out of three.

High blood pressure can play a critical role in the development of heart disease and strokes. In fact, it is generally regarded as the most serious risk factor for a stroke. The higher the pressure, the greater the stress on the arteries and the more rapid the buildup of plaque, leading to atherosclerosis. Your blood contains lots of different chemicals and particles besides red and white cells. Pressure forces these substances past the cells that line the blood vessels, possibly leading to cell damage due to friction, irritation, or inflammation. If the vessel has a weak spot, high pressure can cause the spot to bulge (an aneurysm) or, in the case of some of the small blood vessels in the brain, possibly burst, resulting in a stroke.

Angina pectoris refers to a squeezing or pressurelike pain in the chest. It is usually caused by an insufficient supply of oxygen to the heart muscle. Angina frequently precedes a heart attack. Since physical exertion and stress increase the heart's need for oxygen, they are often the triggering factors. The pain may radiate to the left shoulder blade, left arm, or jaw. The pain typically lasts for one to twenty minutes. Angina can be a sign of a very serious condition that needs immediate medical attention.

An *arrhythmia* is a disruption of the heart's complex pumping action. This action is governed by electrical signals. If those signals are disrupted, the chambers can start contracting in the wrong sequence. When that happens, the heart may become unable to pump enough blood to meet your body's needs.

Congestive heart failure (CHF) refers to an inability of the heart to effectively pump enough blood. Chronic CHF is most often due to long-term effects of high blood pressure, previous heart attack, disorder of a heart valve or the heart muscle, or chronic lung diseases like asthma and emphysema. Weakness, fatigue, and shortness of breath are the most common symptoms of CHF.

Anemia refers to a group of blood abnormalities. Anemia can result if your bones make too few red cells or if they make defective cells, or if your spleen destroys old red cells faster than your bones can make new ones. The most common cause of anemia is iron deficiency. Without iron your body can't make hemoglobin, and without hemoglobin cells can't transport oxygen. Deficiencies of vitamin B_{12}, folic acid, or copper can lead to red cells that are abnormally large and have less capacity to carry oxygen.

Finally, respiratory disorders can also affect your cardiovascular system. Conditions such as asthma or chronic infections can reduce your ability to breathe in enough oxygen or expel enough carbon dioxide. Similarly, cigarette smoking directly damages lung tissue. If the oxygen supply is reduced, your muscles simply can't do as much work. You may get winded just climbing the front stairs. And because carbon dioxide is poisonous at high levels, buildup can be dangerous. Too much of the stuff, combined with too little oxygen, causes respiratory failure, which can lead to fainting, coma, severe damage to tissues including the heart or brain, or even death.

—————— Understanding Atherosclerosis ——————

To get a clearer picture of how atherosclerosis develops, let's take a closer look at the structure of an artery.

Your blood vessels have three major layers. The innermost layer is known as the intima or the endothelium. The cells of this layer are exposed to constant friction as blood and the various particles it contains flow by, often at high pressure. Molecules called glycosaminoglycans (GAGs) line the cells, protecting them from damage and promoting repair. Beneath the surface of endothelial cells is a protective membrane, which also contains GAGs.

The middle layer, or media, is mainly muscle that allows the vessel to widen (dilate) or shrink in diameter, depending on your circulation needs of the moment. The outer layer, the adventitia, is an elastic membrane consisting of connective tissue. These layers also contain GAGs and other substances that provide support and elasticity.

Atherosclerosis begins when something happens to damage the GAG layer that protects the inner lining of the blood vessel. That "something" might be the presence of a pathogen, such as a virus; a drug or environmental toxin; physical damage due to a spasm or high blood pressure; or an overeager immune response.

Like a leak in a dike, even a small amount of damage to the inner lining can set a deadly chain of events in motion. One critical thing that happens is that fat-carrying proteins (lipoproteins), always circulating in the blood, start attaching themselves to the GAGs like unwanted bystanders at a traffic accident. The low-density lipoproteins (LDL) carry cholesterol. Thus their arrival causes cholesterol to build up. When LDL binds to the site, it begins to break down, or oxidize. This releases free radicals, which further damage nearby cells. This is why dietary cholesterol is such a major risk factor for heart disease. The more you have in your blood, the more it can pile up at the site of damage to the blood vessel.

Vessel damage sets off alarms in the immune system, spurring your body's repair mechanism into action. The damaged cells secrete a chemical called growth factor, which stimulates cells to reproduce and replace damaged cells. The cells also release fibrinogen, the sticky, stringy protein that collects platelets so a clot can form to prevent blood from leaking out of the vessel. White blood cells, ever helpful, arrive at the site and attach themselves to the vessel wall, turning into macrophages. These cells are on duty to destroy any harmful particles, such as oxidized LDLs. But once they become stuffed with LDL, they change into useless blobs called foam cells and lose their scavenging ability.

Macrophages also contribute their own supply of growth factor. All this growth factor causes a weird thing to happen: Cells from the smooth muscle layer of the vessel start migrating toward the inner layer. Once there, they begin replicating. They too turn into foam cells. In the process these cells dump cellular debris, such as fiberlike proteins, into the intima, adding more trash to the heap. Soon a kind of scar tissue, called a fibrous cap, appears on the surface of the artery lining. This combination of lipoprotein, cholesterol, fibrous protein, and biological litter forms a stiff patch called plaque. Over time the plaque continues to grow until eventually it blocks the entire artery.

Your blood flow can be reduced by up to 90 percent before you feel any symptoms of atherosclerosis. By then it may be too late. You are a heart attack waiting to happen.

Risk Factors

The good news about heart disease is that it is highly preventable. Be aware of your risk factors for developing heart disease. The higher your risk, the more aggressive you should be in taking steps to tune up your heart. The major risk factors are:

- Smoking
- Elevated blood cholesterol levels
- High blood pressure
- Diabetes
- Physical inactivity

If two or more of these major factors apply to you, your risk increases significantly (see Table 6-1). For example, if you smoke, have high cholesterol, and have high blood pressure, you are more than seven hundred times likelier to have heart disease—and you will probably die twenty to thirty years sooner—than someone without any of these factors.

Table 6-1: Risk of Heart Disease

Condition	Increased Risk of Heart Disease
Presence of one major risk factor	30%
High cholesterol + high blood pressure	300%
High cholesterol + smoking	350%
High blood pressure + smoking	350%
Smoking + high blood pressure + high cholesterol	720%

Any one or more of these other important factors raises your risk even further:

- Low antioxidant status
- Low levels of essential fatty acids
- Low levels of magnesium
- Low levels of potassium
- Increased platelet aggregation
- Increased fibrinogen formation
- Type A personality

To calculate your risk, complete the risk assessment for men or women below. You'll need to ask your doctor for some of the information required. You should also undergo a thorough clinical examination if you have a personal or family history of heart disease.

MEN: DETERMINING YOUR RISK FOR HEART DISEASE AND STROKES

Answering the questions below will help you calculate your risk of having a heart attack within the next ten years. Circle your score for each section, add your total points, and find your risk. Then compare your risk with the average risk for other people your age.

1. Age

Age	Points
30–34	−1

35–39	0
40–44	1
45–49	2
50–54	3
55–59	4
60–64	5
65–69	6
70–74	7

2. Total Cholesterol

Less than 160	−3
160–199	0
200–239	1
240–279	2
280 or more	3

3. HDL Cholesterol

Less than 35	2
35–44	1
45–49	0
50–59	0
60 or more	−2

4. Blood Pressure

Find the point on the chart where your systolic and diastolic blood pressure readings intersect. For example, if your reading is 130 (systolic) over 80 (diastolic), your point score is 1.

	Diastolic				
Systolic	79 or less	80–84	85–89	90–99	100 or more
Less than 120	0	0	1	2	3
120–129	0	0	1	2	3
130–139	1	1	1	2	3
140–159	2	2	2	2	3
160 or more	3	3	3	3	3

5. Diabetes

NO = 0

YES = 2

6. Smoking

NO = 0

YES = 2

7. 10-Year Heart Disease Risk

Add your total points: _____

Total Points	Risk
Less than 0	2%
0	3%
1	3%
2	4%
3	5%
4	7%
5	8%
6	10%
7	13%
8	16%
9	20%
10	25%
11	31%
12	37%
13	45%
14 or more	53% or more

Compare with average and low risk by age:

Age	Average Risk	Low Risk
30–34	3%	2%
35–39	5%	3%
40–44	7%	4%
45–49	11%	4%
50–54	14%	5%
55–59	16%	7%
60–64	21%	9%
65–69	25%	11%
70–74	30%	14%

WOMEN: DETERMINING YOUR RISK FOR HEART DISEASE AND STROKES

Answering the questions below will help you calculate your risk of having a heart attack within the next ten years. Circle your score for each section, add your total points, and find your risk. Then compare your risk with the average risk for other people your age.

1. Age

Age	Points
30–34	−9
35–39	−4
40–44	0
45–49	3
50–54	6
55–59	7
60–64	8
65–69	8
70–74	8

2. Total Cholesterol

Less than 160	−2
160–199	0

200–239   I
240–279   I
280 or more   3

3. HDL Cholesterol

Less than 35   5
35–44   2
45–49   I
50–59   0
60 or more   −3

4. Blood Pressure

Find the point on the chart where your systolic and diastolic blood pressure readings intersect. For example, if your reading is 130 (systolic) over 90 (diastolic), your point score is 2.

Systolic	**Diastolic**				
	79 or less	80–84	85–89	90–99	100 or more
Less than 120	−3	0	0	2	3
120–129	0	0	0	2	3
130–139	0	0	0	2	3
140–159	2	2	2	2	3
160 or more	3	3	3	3	3

5. Diabetes

NO = 0
YES = 4

6. Smoking

NO = 0
YES = 2

7. 10-Year Heart Disease Risk

Add your total points: _____

Total Points	Risk
−2 or less	1%
−1 to 1	2%
2 to 3	3%
4	4%
5	4%
6	5%
7	6%
8	7%
9	8%
10	10%
11	11%
12	13%
13	15%
14	18%
15	20%
16	24%
17 or more	27% or more

Compare with average and low risk by age:

Age	Average Risk	Low Risk
30–34	Less than 1%	Less than 1%
35–39	Less than 1%	1%
40–44	2%	2%
45–49	5%	3%
50–54	8%	5%
55–59	12%	7%
60–64	12%	8%
65–69	13%	8%
70–74	14%	8%

Tune-Up Strategies for Your Heart

The two main strategies for improving your cardiovascular system involve diet and lifestyle.

Dietary Strategies

1. *Reduce the amount of saturated fat, cholesterol, and total fat in the diet.* Most Americans consume far too much fat in their diet. That's because we love our burgers and fries, and because we crave chips, ice cream, and other high-fat snacks. But we pay a price, in the form of heart disease. By being more careful about the foods you choose, you can significantly reduce the amount of fat you consume.

There is a great deal of research linking a diet high in saturated fat and cholesterol to numerous cancers, heart disease, and strokes. Both the American Cancer Society and the American Heart Association have recommended a diet in which fat supplies no more than 30 percent of total calories. The best and easiest way for most people to achieve this goal is to eat fewer animal products and more plant foods (see Table 6-2). Most plant foods are very low in fat. Nuts and seeds are often high in fat, but many of their calories are derived from polyunsaturated essential fatty acids (see Tune-Up Tip below).

Table 6-2: Food Choices for Reducing Dietary Animal Fats

Reduce intake of:	Substitute with:
Red meat	Fish and white meat of poultry
Hamburgers and hot dogs	Soy-based or vegetarian alternatives
Eggs	EggBeaters and similar reduced-cholesterol products, tofu
High-fat dairy products	Low-fat or nonfat products
Butter, lard, other saturated fats	Vegetable oils
Ice cream, pies, cake, cookies, etc.	Fruits
Fried foods, fatty snack foods	Vegetables, fresh salads
Salt and salty foods	Low-sodium foods, salt substitutes
Coffee, soft drinks	Herbal teas, fresh fruit and vegetable juices

Tune-Up Tip: Go Nuts!

Don't be afraid of the fat in nuts. You might think that because of the high oil content of nuts and seeds, eating these foods would increase the rate of obesity. But a study of 26,473 Americans found that the people who consumed the most nuts were actually less overweight than those who did not eat many nuts. A possible explanation is that the nuts produced a feeling of appetite satisfaction and thus reduced the overall calorie intake. This same study also demonstrated that higher nut consumption was associated with a protective effect against heart attacks (both fatal and nonfatal). Particularly beneficial are walnuts (see Tune-Up Tip on page 206).

One of the most crucial steps in your heart tune-up is to reduce levels of cholesterol in your blood. To do so, it helps to understand that there are different kinds of cholesterol (see box below). What's important is the balance between the "good" and "bad" kinds. By reducing intake of animal fat and eating more fresh fruits, vegetables, and whole grains, you can tip that balance in your favor.

CLEARING UP CHOLESTEROL CONFUSION

A lot of my patients say they're confused about cholesterol. That's not surprising. Cholesterol is a natural substance found in your body. Your cells need a certain amount of cholesterol to make flexible, permeable membranes. Also, all of your sex hormones are produced from cholesterol in your body. But your liver usually makes all the cholesterol you need. The cholesterol you ingest in your diet provides excess amounts.

Cholesterol travels from the liver and into your circulation by hitching a ride on protein molecules called low-density lipoprotein (LDL), often called "bad cholesterol." It is carried away from tissues and back to the liver aboard high-density lipoprotein (HDL), frequently called "good cholesterol" or "protective cholesterol." Some people find it easier to remember the difference by labeling LDL "lousy" and HDL "healthy" or "happy."

The more LDL you have, the more cholesterol is in circulation, and the greater your risk of heart disease. Currently, experts recommend that your total blood cholesterol level should be less than 200 mg/dl. The LDL level should be less than 130 mg/dl and the HDL level should be greater than 35 mg/dl. For every 1 percent drop in LDL levels, there's a 2 percent drop in the risk of heart attack. By the same token, for every 1 percent increase in HDL, the risk of heart attack drops 3 or 4 percent.

The ratio of your total cholesterol to HDL and the ratio of LDL to HDL are clues that indicate whether cholesterol is being deposited into tissues or is being broken down and excreted. The ratio of total cholesterol to HDL should be no higher than 4:2, and the LDL-to-HDL ratio should be no higher than 2:5.

Actually, there's a form of LDL that's even worse: lipoprotein(a), or Lp(a). This stuff looks like LDL, but it has an additional molecule of an adhesive protein called apolipoprotein. That protein makes the molecule much more likely to stick to the artery walls. New research suggests that high Lp(a) levels constitute a separate risk factor for heart attack. For example, it appears that high Lp(a) levels are ten times more likely to cause heart disease than high LDL levels. Lp(a) levels lower than 20 mg/dl are associated with low risk of heart disease; levels between 20 and 40 mg/dl pose a moderate risk, and levels higher than 40 mg/dl are considered extremely risky.

2. *Eliminate the intake of margarine and foods containing trans fatty acids and partially hydrogenated oils.* During the process of manufacturing margarine and shortening, vegetable oils are hydrogenated. This means that a hydrogen molecule is added to the natural unsaturated fatty acid molecules of the vegetable oil to make it solid at room temperature—and more saturated. Hydrogenated vegetable oils raise LDL cholesterol, lower HDL cholesterol levels, and interfere with essential fatty acid metabolism. Although butter may be better than margarine in this regard, the bottom line is that they both need to be restricted in a healthy diet.

Tune-Up Tip: Better Butter

If you simply can't live without butter, try this recipe. Soften some butter, mix in an equal amount of flaxseed oil, place in an airtight container, and then refrigerate. Or use a nonhydrogenated spread such as Spectrum Naturals Spread or similar products, available in most health food stores.

3. *Cook with olive oil or canola oil.* These oils contain oleic acid, a monounsaturated oil that is more resistant to the damaging effects of heat and light compared with highly polyunsaturated oils such as corn, safflower, and soy. When the polyunsaturated oils are exposed to heat or light, the chemical structures of the essential fatty acids are changed to toxic derivatives known as lipid peroxides.

Your body makes LDL cholesterol from the oil you eat. If you cook with olive or canola oils, the LDL molecules that result are less susceptible to peroxidation. Several studies have found a reduced risk for heart disease when the intake of oleic acid is high.

4. *Increase your intake of cold-water fish, eat walnuts, and take 1 tbsp of flaxseed oil daily.* There is considerable evidence that people who consume a diet rich in omega-3 oils from either fish or vegetable sources have a significantly reduced risk of developing heart disease. Cold-water fish such as salmon, mackerel, herring, and halibut are good sources of the longer-chain omega-3 fatty acids eicosapentaenoic acid (EPA) and docosahexanoic acid (DHA). These fatty acids, also available in capsules, lower cholesterol and triglyceride levels. However, commercially available fish oil capsules often contain very high levels of lipid peroxides, which can put a lot of stress on your body's antioxidant defense mechanisms. Instead of using fish oils in capsule form, I recommend that you increase the amount of cold-water fish in your diet, eat walnuts, and take flaxseed oil.

Walnuts and flaxseed oil are good sources of alpha-linolenic acid. The population with the lowest rate of heart disease are the inhabitants of the island of Crete, who have three times the concentration of alpha-linolenic acid in their diet and body tissues compared with those who live in other European countries. This is primarily due to Cretans' frequent consumption of walnuts and purslane.

Tune-Up Tip: Eat Walnuts

Walnuts are one of the most nutritious foods on the planet. They provide an excellent source of essential fatty acids and other beneficial oils, protein (20 percent by weight), vitamin E, calcium, iron, and zinc.

Walnuts are often regarded as a "brain food." This probably stems from the wrinkled, brainlike appearance of the nutmeat and its shell, but it also is true because of the brain-nourishing substances the nuts contain. Based upon recent research, walnuts should also be considered "heart food." In addition to population-based studies showing that walnut consumption offers significant protection against heart disease, there are two clinical studies that have shown that moderate walnut consumption lowers LDL by 12 to 16 percent and reduces the ratio of LDL to HDL cholesterol.

Walnuts are best purchased as whole, uncracked nuts. Whole walnuts can be stored in a cool, dry environment for up to one year. Walnuts can be eaten alone as a snack food, or used in recipes.

Dr. Murray's Greens and Walnuts

One of my all-time favorite dishes—simple to prepare but absolutely delicious, and good for your heart too.

2 large bunches greens (such as spinach, kale, mustard greens, chard, etc.), washed, trimmed, and coarsely chopped
2 tbsp olive oil
1 c diced green onion (optional)
1 or 2 cloves of garlic (thinly sliced)
1 c coarsely chopped walnuts
1 tsp balsamic vinegar
Lemon wedges

Heat olive oil and balsamic vinegar in large skillet or wok over medium-high heat. Add greens, green onion, garlic, and walnuts, and sauté until greens are softened. Serve with lemon wedges. Makes 6 servings.

5. *Eat five or more servings a day of a combination of vegetables and fruits, especially green and yellow vegetables and citrus fruits.* Sadly, less than one person out of ten in this country eats even this minimum recommended amount of fruits and vegetables. That's unfortunate, because mountains of evidence show that a high intake of carotene-rich and flavonoid-rich fruits and vegetables reduces the risk of heart disease and strokes. The flavonoids are plant pigments that supply color to food, and because they are powerful antioxidants, they provide remarkable protection against heart disease and stroke.

The best dietary sources of carotenes are green leafy vegetables and yellow-orange fruits and vegetables, especially carrots, apricots, mangoes, sweet potatoes, and squash. Legumes, grains, and seeds are also significant sources of carotenoids. Red and purple vegetables and fruits, such as tomatoes, red cabbage, berries, and plums, contain high levels of pigments without vitamin A activity, including flavonoids. Other good dietary sources of flavonoids include citrus fruits, onions, parsley, legumes, and green tea. Red wine is another source.

RED WINE, GRAPE JUICE, OR VITAMIN C?

The French consume more saturated fat than Americans, yet have a lower incidence of heart disease. This situation is referred to as the "French paradox." Many experts suspect that the French are less vulnerable to heart disease because they consume more red wine. Presumably the protective effect is the result of the flavonoids in red wine, which protect against oxidative damage from LDL cholesterol.

Grape juice also contains flavonoids and may offer similar protection. However, a recent study indicated that grape juice does not provide any significant protection against damage to LDL. In addition, the study also showed that consumption of white wine actually *increased* LDL oxidation. Red wine contains mainly single molecules of flavonoids (primarily quercetin). In contrast, grape juice flavonoids are usually found in complexes with other flavonoids and are bound to various sugars that may reduce bioavailability. Also, the flavonoid content in white wine is significantly lower than red wine.

One or two glasses of red wine per day appears to be a good prescription for a healthy heart. If you cannot tolerate alcohol or prefer not to drink it, don't worry. You can use vitamins C and E instead. Studies have found that vitamins C and E appear to offer even greater protection than either red or white wine. And protection even better than that offered by red wine can be obtained by taking one of the flavonoid-rich extracts such as green tea, ginkgo, bilberry, and grape seed (see page 231 for dosage information).

6. *Increase your intake of fiber.* Dietary fiber, particularly the soluble fiber found in legumes, fruit, oat bran, and vegetables, is effective in lowering cholesterol levels. Many studies have found that high intake of fiber, especially soluble fiber, is associated with a significant reduction in the level of total serum cholesterol. An intake of 20 g or more typically lowers total cholesterol levels by 10 to 20 percent. My recommendation is to try to consume at least 35 grams of fiber a day from a variety of food sources, especially vegetables. To help my patients achieve this goal, I give them a list of foods with the fiber content noted (see Table 6-3) and urge them to consume at least five servings of vegetables each day. Keep a diet diary to calculate your daily fiber intake. Focus on sources of soluble fiber, since it is the most beneficial. Breads, cereals, and pastas that contain bran (from wheat, rice, oat, or corn) supply fiber, but they also supply high amounts of starch and sugar. Again, try to focus on vegetables.

Some warning is necessary if you are not used to eating a high-fiber diet. Increasing your fiber intake can increase the amount of intestinal gas (flatulence). Don't worry, this side effect will not be a problem after your body has had a chance to adjust. I suggest that you increase the amount of dietary fiber gradually. Start with small amounts and build up to the recommended level over the course of a few weeks. You'll know if you're overdoing it if you experience excessive gas or other abdominal symptoms. Cut back until the symptoms resolve, and then proceed more slowly until you reach a level you can tolerate.

Table 6-3: Dietary Fiber Content of Selected Foods

Food	Serving	Calories	Grams of fiber
Fruits			
Apple (with skin)	1 medium	81	3.5
Banana	1 medium	105	2.4
Cantaloupe	1/4 melon	30	1.0
Cherries, sweet	10	49	1.2
Grapefruit	1/2 medium	38	1.6
Orange	1 medium	62	2.6
Peach (with skin)	1	37	1.9
Pear (with skin)	1/2 large	61	3.1
Prunes	3	60	3.0
Raisins	1/4 cup	106	3.1
Raspberries	1/2 cup	35	3.1
Strawberries	1 cup	45	3.0
Vegetables, Raw			
Bean sprouts	1/2 cup	13	1.5
Celery, diced	1/2 cup	10	1.1
Cucumber	1/2 cup	8	0.4
Lettuce	1 cup	10	0.9
Mushrooms	1/2 cup	10	1.5
Pepper, green	1/2 cup	9	0.5
Spinach	1 cup	8	1.2
Tomato	1 medium	20	1.5
Vegetables, Cooked			
Asparagus, cut	1 cup	30	2.0
Beans, green	1 cup	32	3.2
Broccoli	1 cup	40	4.4
Brussels sprouts	1 cup	56	4.6
Cabbage, red	1 cup	30	2.8
Carrots	1 cup	48	4.6
Cauliflower	1 cup	28	2.2
Corn	1/2 cup	87	2.9
Kale	1 cup	44	2.8

Food	Serving	Calories	Grams of fiber
Parsnip	1 cup	102	5.4
Potato (with skin)	1 medium	106	2.5
Potato (without skin)	1 medium	97	1.4
Spinach	1 cup	42	4.2
Sweet potato	1 medium	160	3.4
Zucchini	1 cup	22	3.6
Legumes			
Baked beans	½ cup	155	8.8
Dried peas, cooked	½ cup	115	4.7
Kidney beans, cooked	½ cup	110	7.3
Lima beans, cooked	½ cup	64	4.5
Lentils, cooked	½ cup	97	3.7
Navy beans, cooked	½ cup	112	6.0
Rice, breads, pastas, and flour			
Bran muffins	1 muffin	104	2.5
Bread, white	1 slice	78	0.4
Bread, whole wheat	1 slice	61	1.4
Crisp bread, rye	2 crackers	50	2.0
Rice, brown, cooked	½ cup	97	1.0
Rice, white, cooked	½ cup	82	0.2
Spaghetti, reg., cooked	½ cup	155	1.1
Spaghetti, whole wheat, cooked	½ cup	155	3.9
Breakfast cereals			
All-Bran	⅓ cup	71	8.5
Bran Chex	⅔ cup	91	4.6
Corn Bran	⅔ cup	98	5.4
Corn flakes	1¼ cups	110	0.3
Grape-Nuts	¼ cup	101	1.4
Oatmeal	¾ cup	108	1.6
Raisin bran type	⅔ cup	115	4.0
Shredded Wheat	⅔ cup	102	2.6
Nuts			
Almonds	10 nuts	79	1.1
Filberts	10 nuts	54	0.8
Peanuts	10 nuts	105	1.4

Tune-Up Tip: Mom Was Right Again—Eat Your Oatmeal

People with high cholesterol levels (above 220 mg/dl) often see a reduction in cholesterol ranging from 8 to 23 percent if they regularly consume 3 g of soluble oat fiber per day. This is the amount of fiber in just one bowl of ready-to-eat oat bran cereal or oatmeal. Oatmeal's fiber content (7 percent) is less than that of oat bran (typically 15 to 26 percent). However, oatmeal contains polyunsaturated fatty acids, which contribute as much to the cholesterol-lowering effects of oats as the fiber content.

7. *Reduce the amount of animal protein in your diet.* Your body needs protein, but most of us eat too much of it. Excess protein intake has been linked to several chronic conditions including heart disease, many cancers, high blood pressure, and osteoporosis. In contrast, a vegetarian diet is associated with a reduced risk of these diseases. The best way to control your protein intake is by reducing consumption of meat and dairy products.

The source of the protein makes a difference. In the United States, approximately 72 percent of protein in the diet comes from animal products. Meat, fish, and poultry account for nearly half of this total; another 18 percent comes from dairy products and 4 percent from eggs. In contrast, plant foods account for only 30 percent of the protein intake. We need to double the amount from plant foods for good heart health.

Limit your intake of animal protein to no more than 4 to 6 ounces per day and choose fish, skinless poultry, and lean cuts rather than fatty cuts.

8. *Limit the intake of refined carbohydrates (sugar).* Sugar and other refined carbohydrates are a significant factor in the development of atherosclerosis. Sugar increases triglyceride and cholesterol levels. But the real problem with sugar appears to be that it elevates levels of insulin, the hormone that controls how your cells use sugar. Elevated insulin levels, in turn, are associated with increased cholesterol, higher triglycerides, elevated blood pressure, and greater risk of death from cardiovascular disease.

Limit sources of refined sugar in your diet. Read food labels carefully for clues on sugar content. The words *sucrose, glucose, maltose, lactose, fructose, corn syrup,* or *white grape juice concentrate* mean extra sugar has been added.

9. *Eat breakfast.* Breakfast is the most important meal of the day. But it's not just the meal, it's the food you eat. Serum cholesterol levels are lowest among adults who eat whole-grain cereal for breakfast and highest among those who skip breakfast altogether. Cereals, either hot or cold, preferably made from whole grains, are the best food choices for breakfast. Other healthy choices include fresh whole fruit, cholesterol-free egg products such as EggBeaters, or a protein shake.

Supplemental Strategies

There are several natural compounds you can take to lower cholesterol and reduce your risk of heart disease. As I'll explain, each offers some level of benefit (see Table 6-4). These compounds should be used only as part of an overall program that includes diet and lifestyle changes.

Table 6-4: Comparative Effects of Supplements on Blood Lipids

	Niacin	Garlic	Guggulipid	Pantetheine
Total cholesterol (% decrease)	18	10	24	19
LDL cholesterol (% decrease)	23	15	30	21
HDL cholesterol (% increase)	32	31	16	23
Triglycerides (% decrease)	26	13	23	32

Niacin (Vitamin B₃)

Since the 1950s, scientists have been aware of the cholesterol-lowering power of niacin. This vitamin, also known as nicotinic acid, does all the right kinds of tweaking: It raises HDL but lowers levels of LDL, Lp(a), triglyceride, and fibrinogen, a blood protein that forms long strands (fibrin) that act like a mesh when a blood clot forms. For people who wish to lower cholesterol through supplements, I consider niacin the first choice.

However, niacin can cause bothersome side effects. The most common is "niacin flush," a reddening of the skin that can develop within about thirty minutes. Other less frequent adverse reactions include gastric irritation, nausea, and liver damage. Timed-release niacin formulations only partly address these concerns; they lower the risk of flushing but increase risk of liver toxicity. I suggest you avoid using timed-release niacin. Niacin also can affect blood sugar control, and so it should be used carefully by people with diabetes or hypoglycemia. Nor should it be used by patients who have liver disease or elevated liver enzymes. If you fit any of these categories, consider using other supplemental strategies described below.

The safest form of niacin currently available is inositol hexaniacinate. This product has long been used in Europe to lower cholesterol levels and improve blood flow. It is about as effective as standard niacin (perhaps even a little more effective) but has a lower risk of flushing and other long-term side effects.

If you're taking pure crystalline niacin, start with a dose of 100 mg three times a day and carefully increase the dosage over four to six weeks to the full therapeutic dose of 1.5 to 3 g daily in divided doses. If you choose inositol hexaniacinate, begin with 500 mg three times daily for two weeks and then increase to 1,000 mg. Take these products with meals.

In my practice, I have found that the combination of diet, lifestyle, and niacin supplementation produces consistent reductions of total cholesterol of 50 to 75 mg/dl in patients whose total cholesterol levels started at 250 mg/dl or higher. Effects are seen within two months. If your initial level is above 300 mg/dl, you may not see these results until after four to six months of treatment.

Once your cholesterol level falls below 200 mg/dl, I suggest reducing the dosage of inositol hexaniacinate to 500 mg three times daily for two months. Should cholesterol rise again above the 200 mark, go back to using 1,000 mg three times a day. However, if cholesterol stays low, then I usually recommend stopping inositol and checking levels again after two months.

CASE HISTORY: My Uncle Jim's Cholesterol

About seven years ago, my uncle Jim (he really is my mom's cousin, but I have always called him my uncle) and aunt Elaine were visiting us from Boise, Idaho. Jim was telling me that he was getting tired of taking the drug Mevacor for his high cholesterol level. This drug works by preventing the manufacture of cholesterol in the liver. It often works quite well, but there is some risk of liver damage. Jim was growing more and more uncomfortable taking the Mevacor, especially when his liver enzymes started creeping out of the normal range. He did not like having to go in every six weeks or so to make sure that his liver was still okay. Jim told me that before he started taking the Mevacor his cholesterol level was very high—around 350 mg/dl. After being on the Mevacor for almost a year, that number had dropped to 278 mg/dl.

I tried my best to conceal my concern that 278 was still way too high. You see, Jim's father had died of a heart attack at the age of fifty. Jim's fiftieth was coming up, so I wanted to do everything I could to make sure that Jim would long outlive his father. I try not to give family members advice unless they ask for it directly, but on this occasion I broke my own rule. I told Jim that he needed to get off the Mevacor immediately and try a more natural approach. We also talked about diet, and Jim promised to cut down on his pipe smoking.

We made the switch from the Mevacor to inositol hexaniacinate (hexa-niacin for short) at a dosage of 500 mg three times per day. (Because I was Jim's doctor, I supervised his switch away from the prescription drug. *Never change your prescription regimen without checking with your physician first.*)

Two months after starting the hexaniacin, Jim had a blood test and was alarmed by the results: His cholesterol level had shot up over 300 mg/dl again. I told him not to worry, that I was confident that the hexaniacin was going to work and that his liver was rebounding from the Mevacor's suppressing effect on cholesterol manufacture. I told him that that in two more months his level should be fine, and I increased his dosage to 1,000 mg three times daily. As I predicted, two months later Jim's total cholesterol level was 248 mg/dl and his HDL level was at an all-time high of 58 mg/dl. Jim's cholesterol values were significantly better now than they had ever been on Mevacor. After six months of therapy, Jim's total cholesterol level was below 200 mg/dl.

Over the years we have tried to wean Jim completely off the hexaniacin, but the best we have been able to do is reduce his dosage to 500 mg three times per day. Anything less and Jim's cholesterol levels rise above 200 mg/dl.

I honestly believe that if Jim had continued with the Mevacor, he might not be here today. His strong family history of heart disease and his high cho-lesterol levels made him extremely vulnerable.

It feels great to help any patient, but the feeling is extra special when that patient is also a family member.

Garlic

For years I have worked hard to educate my patients about the bene-fits of garlic. Here I'll focus on its impact on the cardiovascular system.

Overwhelming evidence shows that garlic can lower "bad" cholesterol, increase "good" cholesterol, and help lower blood pressure.

The main effects of this ancient herb derive from what scientists call volatile compounds—substances that give garlic its characteristic odor. The most potent of these for heart health is allicin, which is formed from the compound alliin in fresh garlic when you chop, crush, or soak the garlic in water. However, allicin is also the stuff that produces the bad breath and body odor associated with eating garlic. The question is, how can you get the good effects of garlic and eliminate the unpleasant social consequences? Cooking garlic inactivates the enzyme that produces allicin, which is why cooked garlic doesn't have as strong an odor as raw garlic. But cooking robs garlic of most of its healthful properties.

To solve this problem, companies have developed techniques to stabilize the alliin in specially coated tablets that pass intact through the stomach into the intestine. Once in the small intestine, the special coating dissolves and the alliin is converted to allicin. Because the allicin is being formed deep in the intestinal tract, it rarely causes garlic breath or garlic body odor. However, if you exceed the dosage recommendation, people will likely be able to smell the garlic compounds that escape through the pores of the skin.

Many people ask me about using aged garlic. However, aging significantly reduces the levels of beneficial compounds present in the garlic. Based on scientific evidence, I strongly recommend using products that are as close to fresh garlic as possible. Choose a product that provides an allicin yield of 4,000 mcg, which is roughly equivalent to one or two cloves of fresh garlic.

Results from many double-blind placebo-controlled studies show that patients whose initial cholesterol level is greater than 200 mg/dl benefit from supplementation with commercial preparations providing a daily dose of at least 10 mg alliin or a total allicin potential of 4,000 mcg. In my practice, I have found that garlic typically lowers total serum cholesterol levels by about 10 to 12 percent and LDL and triglycerides by about 15 percent. HDL cholesterol levels will usually increase by about 10 percent.

Guggulipid

This substance is the standardized extract of the guggul (mukul) myrrh tree (*Commiphora mukul*), native to India. Research shows that it works by increasing the breakdown of LDL cholesterol in the liver, thus lowering LDL levels. It also reduces triglyceride levels and raises HDL levels. The substance may also inhibit platelet aggregation and help clots dissolve. Dosage is based on guggulsterone content. Extracts standardized to contain 25 mg of guggulsterone per 500 mg tablet, taken three times per day, produce good results. No significant side effects have been reported with purified guggulipid preparations. However, crude guggul preparations such as gum guggul can cause skin rashes or diarrhea.

Pantethine

Pantethine is a form of vitamin B_5 (pantothenic acid) that has a greater capacity to lower cholesterol than the vitamin itself. A dose of 300 mg three times a day significantly reduces levels of total cholesterol and LDL levels while raising HDL cholesterol, without toxicity. It is also the most effective natural product against serum triglyceride levels. It works by slowing down production of cholesterol in the liver and by boosting the rate at which your metabolism uses fats. Use of pantethine does not cause side effects. It is the best choice for diabetics.

Other Supplemental Recommendations

In addition to the supplements described above to lower cholesterol, I have a very important recommendation for managing blood lipids and preventing heart disease and strokes: Take extra vitamin E and C.

Vitamin E may offer the greatest antioxidant protection against heart disease because of its special role in preventing oxidation of LDL cholesterol. Much of the damage due to atherosclerosis occurs when fatty substances oxidize and form harmful by-products, such as lipid peroxides and free radicals. Vitamin E is more effective than vitamin C in protecting against heart disease because it is fat soluble and thus becomes incorporated directly into the LDL molecule, like a spy infiltrating the enemy camp. The higher the dose of vitamin E, the greater the protection. I usually recommend 400 to 800 IU per day. People who smoke, who have high levels of oxidative stress, such as diabetics, or who have inflammatory diseases (including rheumatoid arthritis and asthma) may take doses in the higher range.

Vitamin C is associated with good cholesterol control. Generally, the higher the level of vitamin C in the blood, the lower the total cholesterol and triglyceride levels and the higher the HDL levels. This effect is seen even in well-nourished individuals with normal levels of vitamin C in their blood. Research is under way to determine if vitamin C therapy also reduces the risk of heart disease by reducing the levels of Lp(a).

MORE CARDIOLOGISTS TAKE VITAMIN E THAN ASPIRIN
TO PREVENT A HEART ATTACK

A survey among members of the American Academy of Cardiology (AAC) revealed that 54 percent routinely took antioxidant vitamins. In fact, more cardiologists took vitamins than low-dose aspirin (a common recommendation to prevent a heart attack or stroke). The most common daily dosages: 400 IU for vitamin E, 500 mg for vitamin C, and 20,000 IU for beta-carotene.

Why are so many cardiologists taking antioxidant vitamins? Studies are showing promising results. For example, among the more recent studies: A study conducted in Canada with 2,313 men demonstrated vitamin supplement use reduced risk for death due to coronary artery disease by 69 percent. Risk for a nonfatal heart attack was lower by 47 percent. And in the Cambridge Antioxidant Heart Study, 2,002 patients with coronary artery disease were given either 400 IU vitamin E, 800 IU, or a placebo for 510 days. Vitamin E supplementation at either dose reduced the number of patients experiencing a heart attack by 77 percent.

Another intriguing finding from the AAC study was that although a large percentage of cardiologists are taking antioxidants, a much smaller percentage recommend antioxidant supplements to their patients. I can only wonder why doctors are keeping the facts about the importance of antioxidants under wraps.

Tune-Up Tip: **Think About That Thyroid**

People with low thyroid function have higher rates of coronary artery disease. That's because insufficient thyroid hormones can cause an increase in "bad" cholesterol and Lp(a) and a decrease in "good" cholesterol. The problem can exist even in those who do not experience symptoms of hypothyroidism. If you are trying to lower cholesterol, be sure your thyroid is functioning properly. For more information, and tips about improving thyroid function, see Chapter 4.

Lifestyle Recommendations

Quit Smoking

People who smoke are three to five times more likely to develop heart disease. The more cigarettes smoked and the greater the number of years you smoke, the greater your risk of dying from a heart attack or stroke. Smoking also increases your risk of other diseases, especially lung cancer. Overall, the average smoker dies seven to eight years sooner than the nonsmoker.

Tobacco smoke contains more than 4,000 chemicals. Some of the most dangerous of these chemicals are carried throughout the body on molecules of LDL cholesterol. They can directly damage the linings of the arteries, or they can damage the LDL molecule, which in turn damages the arteries. Obviously, the higher your cholesterol, the greater the risk of damage from smoking. What's more, smoking actually raises your cholesterol levels by damaging the feedback mechanisms in the liver that control cholesterol production. Smoking also promotes blood clotting by increasing platelet aggregation and levels of fibrinogen.

Nicotine is a stimulant that can contribute to high blood pressure. Nicotine activates the adrenal glands, resulting in higher secretion of epinephrine (adrenaline) to raise blood pressure. Cigarette smoke also contains heavy metals, such as lead and cadmium, both of which are associated with increased blood pressure. In addition, smoking produces free radicals. Your body deploys its stores of antioxidant vitamins and minerals to neutralize these destructive particles. If you continue smoking, though, you will deplete your supply of antioxidants and leave your tissues vulnerable to damage.

Based on the results of published studies, it appears that the best strategy for quitting smoking is to just stop—to go cold turkey. Nicotine replacement therapy (using gum or the skin patch) is effective for about 13 percent of people who try it. Behavioral modification (rewards and punishments) works for only about two people in every hundred. Acupuncture is slightly better. Some people have been able to quit following hypnosis.

Tune-Up Tip: Protect Yourself from Secondhand Smoke

Secondhand smoke, or passive smoking, appears to be an important risk to heart health. In fact, some studies have shown that people who don't smoke themselves but who inhale smoke from the environment are even more susceptible to damage, because their bodies just aren't used to dealing with the toxic load. Studies have found that passive smoking causes the same kind of damage to artery walls, changes in platelet function, and decreased exercise capacity as that occurring in smokers. Each year in the United States, more than thirty-seven thousand deaths from coronary artery disease are attributed to environmental smoke. I am very happy that most public facilities and restaurants are now smoke-free, and I was ecstatic a few years ago when airlines finally banned smoking.

To protect your lungs if you are regularly exposed to secondhand smoke, make sure that you consume at least five servings of fresh vegetables and two servings of fresh fruit each day. Supplement your diet with 500 to 1,500 mg of vitamin C and 400 IU of vitamin E each day, and take one of the flavonoid-rich extracts (grape seed, pine bark, *Ginkgo biloba*, bilberry, green tea, or hawthorn).

Tune-Up Tip: Detox with Curry

The main ingredient of curry is turmeric. In one study, sixteen chronic smokers were given 1.5 g of turmeric daily. At the end of the thirty-day trial, there was a significant reduction in the level of cancer-causing compounds excreted in the urine. These results signified enhanced detoxification processes. The antioxidant activity of the yellow pigment of turmeric, a compound known as curcumin, is up to three hundred times stronger than that of vitamin E. It may be shown to offer even greater protection against heart disease than vitamin E. In one clinical study, the level of oxidized LDL and HDL dropped dramatically after intake of only 20 mg of curcumin per day.

Vegetable Curry

Here is a recipe that not only will provide exceptional protection against secondhand smoke, but will lower your cholesterol level as well. It also tastes great.

2 tbsp olive oil
1 small onion, chopped
2 cloves garlic, crushed
1 tart apple, peeled and diced
1 tbsp curry powder
2 medium carrots, peeled and diced
1 medium potato, peeled and diced
1$\frac{1}{3}$ c diced yellow squash or zucchini
1 tbsp lemon juice
$\frac{1}{2}$ c frozen peas
$\frac{1}{2}$ c coarsely chopped walnuts

In a large heavy saucepan, sauté onion, garlic, apple, and curry in olive oil for 5 minutes. Add carrot, potato, squash, lemon juice, peas, and walnuts. Cook about 5 minutes longer or until vegetables are tender. Makes 4 servings.

Lower Your Blood Pressure

Virtually every medical authority agrees that the best way to lower blood pressure is through diet and lifestyle. Drugs don't always work, and they can cause serious side effects. Besides, once you begin taking a medication for blood pressure, you need to continue taking it for the rest of your life.

Many of the dietary and lifestyle steps already covered in this chapter result in lowered blood pressure. If you reduce fats and cholesterol, you unclog and unstiffen your arteries, so blood can flow at lower pressure. If you lose weight, your heart doesn't have to work so hard to pump blood through vessels. But there are additional steps you can take specifically to lower blood pressure.

Eating more plant foods is a big factor. In general, vegetarians have lower blood pressure levels and a lower risk of cardiovascular disease than people who eat high amounts of meat and dairy products. That's because a vegetarian diet typically contains more potassium, magnesium, calcium, vitamin C, fiber, complex carbohydrates, and essential fatty acids. At the same time, such a diet has less saturated fat, refined carbohydrates, and protein. All of these nutritional factors help keep blood pressure down.

Tune-Up Tip: Try Celery

A small amount of a compound found in celery, 3-n-butyl phthalide, has been found to lower blood pressure in animals by 12 to 14 percent. Humans can get the equivalent dose by eating four ribs of celery daily. If you are concerned about high blood pressure, the celery prescription is certainly worth a try. I have had some patients notice good enough reductions by eating celery that they were able to avoid having to take blood pressure medications.

—————————— **Supplemental Strategies** ——————————

Potassium

Diets that are low in sodium and high in potassium prevent high blood pressure. In people who already have high blood pressure, potassium can help to lower it, especially in those over the age of sixty-five.

If you don't get enough potassium in your diet, it is possible to boost your intake through other means. Supplements are available, and there are salt substitutes or "lite salts" made with potassium chloride (rather than sodium chloride, the formula for table salt). Interestingly, the FDA restricts the amount of potassium available in over-the-counter potassium supplements to a mere 99 mg per dose. Yet salt substitutes, such as NoSalt and Nu-Salt, provide 530 mg of potassium per one-sixth tsp!

Prescription and over-the-counter potassium supplements are either potassium salts (chloride and bicarbonate), potassium bound to various mineral chelates (such as aspartate or citrate), or food-based potassium sources. Potassium chloride preparations are the most popular kind given by prescription and are available in different formulations (timed-release tablets, liquids, powders, and effervescent tablets). Potassium salts are commonly prescribed in doses of 1.5 to 3 g per day. At high levels, potassium salts in pill form can cause nausea, vomiting, diarrhea, and ulcers. I recommend increasing your intake by eating potassium-rich foods (for example, avocados, bananas, and whole grains), taking food-based potassium supplements such as Vital-K or Bio-K, or using salt substitutes such as NoSalt or Nu-Salt.

Magnesium

Magnesium helps control the "sodium-potassium pump," the mechanism by which your cells regulate the balance of these electrolytes. A deficiency of magnesium causes a decrease in potassium inside the cells. This results in excess fluid outside the cells. The blood picks up this fluid, resulting in an increase in blood pressure.

What's more, magnesium helps block the entry of calcium into muscle cells in the heart and blood vessels. As a result, having adequate magnesium levels reduces vascular resistance, lowers blood pressure, and promotes efficient heart function.

The multiple vitamin and mineral supplement that I recommend to all of my patients provides 250 mg of magnesium. That's adequate for most people, but in patients with high blood pressure, arrhythmia, or any other form of heart disease, I generally recommend more. I calculate the dosage for these patients loosely based on body weight: 12 mg per kilogram (2.2 pounds). Thus a patient weighing 150 pounds should take about 800 mg of magnesium a day. Certain forms of magnesium (aspartate, malate, succinate, fumarate, or citrate) are more easily absorbed and used by the body than other forms (oxide, gluconate, sulfate, or chloride).

Coenzyme Q_{10} (CoQ_{10})

An essential component of the mitochondria, the energy-producing units in your cells, CoQ_{10} acts like the spark plugs in your car, helping the mitochondria burn fuel. Nearly four out of ten people with high blood pressure have a deficiency of CoQ_{10}. In my practice, patients with moderately elevated blood pressure who take CoQ_{10} supplements typically see reductions in blood pressure of about 10 percent. Research suggests that CoQ_{10} works by lowering cholesterol and by stabilizing vascular membranes, thus lowering resistance to blood flow. Standard dose is 50 to 150 mg per day, although up to 300 mg per day may be needed for people with severe heart disease. I recommend soft-gelatin capsules that contain CoQ_{10} in a soybean oil base.

Hawthorn (Crataegus monogyna)

Extracts of hawthorn berries and extracts of the flowering tops of hawthorn are widely used by physicians in Europe for their cardiovascular effects. I recommend hawthorn extract for patients with moderate hypertension, used in combination with CoQ_{10} and other strategies. Hawthorn extract should contain 10 percent procyanidins or 1.8 percent vitexin-4'-rhamnoside. Dosage is 250 mg three times per day. Benefits in mild to moderate high blood pressure are usually seen after two to four weeks of use.

Omega-3 Fatty Acids

Increasing the intake of omega-3 fatty acids is a very effective way of lowering blood pressure. Fish oil is one source of fatty acids, but it can be hard to consume high enough amounts to produce the desired effect. Flaxseed oil is the better choice for lowering blood pressure, especially when cost is considered. Along with reducing the intake of saturated fat, I tbsp per day of flaxseed oil typically drops both the systolic and diastolic readings by up to 9 points.

Vitamins

Other important supplemental strategies for lowering pressure include taking vitamin C, vitamin B_6, and calcium. These supplements are helpful for a variety of reasons. An important one in many cases is that they can help remove lead and other heavy metals from the body. As I discussed in Chapter 3, too much lead or any other heavy metal in the body can lead to high blood pressure. So in most of my patients with hypertension I will recommend a hair mineral analysis to rule out heavy metal toxicity. If the lead level is too high, it really pays to get the lead out.

Exercise

For a complete heart and lung tune-up, you must exercise regularly. You don't have to train for the Olympics; taking brisk thirty-minute walks three or four times a week provides many benefits. Exercise is vital for improving all your body functions, but it's particularly important for your cardiovascular system because it accomplishes all the following:

- Lowers resting heart rate
- Strengthens heart function
- Lowers blood pressure
- Improves oxygen delivery throughout the body
- Increases blood supply to muscles
- Enlarges the arteries to the heart

If you have been inactive, consult your physician before you begin a new exercise program. See pages 107–108 for more information about strategies for more effective exercise.

Reduce Stress

For many people, stress is a significant cause of high blood pressure and increases the risk of heart disease. Stress causes the release of hormones that put your body in a state of constant high alert. Among other things, your heart beats faster and more intensely, leading to a rise in blood pressure. Suggestions for reducing stress and promoting the relaxation response include deep breathing, meditation, and progressive muscle relaxation. (Deep breathing exercises appear following Chapter 2 in Lifestyle Tune-Up #2.)

A risk factor for heart disease is the so-called Type A personality. Type A behavior is characterized by an extreme sense of time urgency, competitiveness, impatience, and aggressiveness. People who exhibit these traits are twice as likely to develop coronary artery disease as those who do not.

Particularly damaging to the cardiovascular system is the regular expression of anger. Somewhat surprisingly, studies have found that people who are more aggressive have higher cholesterol levels. Conversely, people who are better able to control anger have lower LDL/HDL ratios. In other words, learning to control anger or to express it in healthier ways leads to a significant reduction in the risk for heart disease.

KEY RECOMMENDATIONS FOR HIGH BLOOD PRESSURE
For mild hypertension (140–160 over 90–104)

- Reduce excess weight
- Eliminate salt (sodium chloride) intake
- Follow a healthy lifestyle: Avoid alcohol, caffeine, and smoking; exercise and use stress-reduction techniques
- Follow a high-potassium diet rich in fiber and complex carbohydrates
- Increase dietary consumption of celery, garlic, and onions
- Reduce or eliminate the intake of animal fats while increasing the intake of vegetable oils
- Supplement the diet with the following:
  - High-potency multiple vitamin and mineral formula
  - Vitamin C: 500–1,000 mg three times per day
  - Vitamin E: 400–800 IU per day
  - Magnesium: 800–1,200 mg per day
  - Garlic: one or two fresh cloves or garlic supplements that provide 4,000 mcg allicin potential
  - Flaxseed oil: 1 tbsp per day

If blood pressure has not returned to normal after following the above recommendations for a period of three to six months, please consult a physician for further recommendations.

For moderate hypertension (140–180 over 105–114)

- Employ all the measures listed for mild hypertension
- Take coenzyme Q_{10}: 50 mg two or three times per day
- Take hawthorn extract (10 percent procyanidins or 1.8 percent vitexin-4'-rhamnoside): 100–250 mg three times per day

Follow these guidelines for one to three months. If your blood pressure has not dropped below 140/105, work with a physician to select the most appropriate medication.

For severe hypertension (160+ over 115+)

- Consult a physician immediately
- Employ all the measures listed for mild and moderate hypertension. A drug may be necessary to achieve initial control. When you achieve satisfactory control over the high blood pressure, work with your physician to see if you can taper off the medication.

CASE HISTORY: Grizzly Bear to Teddy Bear

Jerry was a fifty-two-year-old retired United States Postal Service employee. In the eleven years since he'd turned forty-one, Jerry had undergone seven different heart surgeries—three coronary artery bypass operations and four angioplasties. Despite all of these procedures and all of the drugs he was taking, Jerry had tremendous angina upon exertion.

A fascinating feature in Jerry's case is that he had no risk factors identifiable by conventional testing. His cholesterol levels were perfect, his blood pressure was actually low, he did not smoke, he was not overweight. For years his doctors had been at a loss to explain why he had such severe heart disease.

It didn't take long for me to figure it out. Jerry seemed like a very affable, mild-mannered guy. But when I asked him how he would evaluate his ability to control his temper I could see that he often "went postal." He told me that he was a real hothead and that his temper was a major problem in his life. I once made the mistake of asking him to give me some examples of what made him mad. His face turned red, the veins in his neck and forehead popped out, and his voice became quite loud as he told me a few things that really ticked him off. A few minutes into this tirade he stopped for a second or two to pop a nitroglycerin pill.

At that point I seized the opportunity to help him make the connection between his inability to control his anger and his heart disease. He was quite resistant at first, because he just wanted me to prescribe some natural medicines. I suggested the following regimen:

High-potency multiple vitamin and mineral formula
Vitamin E: 800 IU daily
Vitamin C: 500 mg three times daily
Flaxseed oil: 1 tbsp daily
Coenzyme Q_{10}: 300 mg per day
Magnesium (as aspartate, citrate, succinate, fumarate, or malate): 250 mg
    three times daily
Hawthorn extract (1.8% vitexin-4'-rhamnoside): 250 mg three times daily

But Jerry was completely uninterested in taking a look at his emotional life. In fact, it was not until the next visit one month later that he really opened up and became receptive to my ideas. At our follow-up visit I told Jerry that I wanted him to read a book by my friend Stephen Sinatra, M.D.: *Heartbreak and Heart Disease* (Keats, 1996). It is an excellent account of the role emotions play in heart disease. I also referred Jerry to a psychotherapist for biofeedback training and to a yoga instructor so that he could start taking yoga classes.

Over the course of the next year and a half, Jerry progressively got better. Even more impressive than his incredible improvements in his physical health were the changes in his emotional health and personality. What impressed me most, however, were the changes in Jerry's relationships with his wife and kids.

It has now been over four years since I first saw Jerry. He has gone from popping nitroglycerin tablets practically every time he got up out of his chair to walking nearly four miles per day. He has not had to use the nitroglycerin tablets for over two years now.

So what led to the improvement? Was it the natural medicines I prescribed for Jerry, or the changes he made in his emotional responses? No doubt the supplements improved his physical well-being. But I am convinced that the most important factor for Jerry's remarkable case was the emotional change.

Other Cardiovascular Problems

Cerebral Vascular Insufficiency

While severe disruption of blood and oxygen supply results in a stroke, minor reductions in blood and oxygen supply to the brain—cerebral vascular insufficiency—are characterized by one or more of the following symptoms: short-term memory loss, dizziness, headache, ringing in the ears, depression, blurred vision. It is extremely common among the elderly in the United States due to the buildup of atherosclerotic plaque in the carotid arteries—the main arteries that supply blood to the brain, located on each side of the neck running parallel to the jugular vein. Prevention of strokes and of cerebral vascular insufficiency involves the same guidelines as preventing a heart attack, since all are caused by atherosclerosis.

Anyone who experiences the symptoms of cerebral vascular insufficiency should consult a physician immediately for proper evaluation. In the past, evaluation of blood flow to the brain involved invasive techniques, but it now involves the use of noninvasive ultrasound techniques. These techniques determine the rate of blood flow and the degree of blockage by using sound waves. Symptoms of cerebral vascular insufficiency may indicate the occurrence of "mini-strokes" known as transient ischemic attacks (TIAs).

For people with cerebral vascular insufficiency, the best natural medicine is *Ginkgo biloba* extract. The quality of research on ginkgo in cerebral vascular insufficiency is exemplary. In numerous well-designed studies, ginkgo has produced significant regression of all the major symptoms of cerebral vascular insufficiency without significant side effects. Ginkgo has also been shown to promote a speedier and more complete recovery from a stroke. A typical dosage for *Ginkgo biloba* extract (24 percent ginkgo flavonglycosides) is 80 mg three times per day.

Varicose Veins

One of the most common cardiovascular disorders, especially in women, is varicose veins—twisted and engorged superficial veins of the legs. Blood in veins is on its way back to the heart; it is blue because it lacks oxygen. Normally, valves in the veins prevent blood from falling back down the leg. In some people, though, the valves become weak or "leaky." The blood collects in the veins, causing them to swell. The problem is more of a cosmetic concern than a medical one, but the legs may feel heavy, tight, and tired.

A more serious form of varicose vein involves obstruction and valve defects of veins that lie deeper in the leg. This can lead to thrombophlebitis (vein inflammation), pulmonary embolism (blood clot in the lungs), heart attack, or stroke. Varicose veins affect nearly one out of two middle-aged adults. Women are four times as likely to have them as men.

It is possible to relieve varicose veins through lifestyle methods, including exercise, and through dietary strategies, such as the use of supplements and botanical medicines. The main goal is to strengthen the wall of the vein, improve circulation, and provide your body with nutrients that prevent formation of blood clots. While small spider veins may resolve entirely, large, well-formed varicose veins should not be expected to magically go away. In these cases, elastic compression stockings are occasionally beneficial, but they are a nuisance to put on and take off.

Fortunately, many of my patients with varicose veins have found that by using botanical medicines, they do not have to put up with the hassles of wearing those compression stockings. The most effective botanical medicine is an extract of horse chestnut (*Aesculus hippocastanum*) concentrated for the compound escin. Good clinical studies have found that horse chestnut seed extract (50 mg of the compound escin daily) is as effective as using support stockings. Escin reduces the permeability of the veins, which helps prevent swelling and inflammation. It also improves the ability of the vein to contract. There are other useful herbs. Gotu kola (*Centella asiatica*) contains compounds that enhance the connective tissue structure of the veins to give them additional support and improve blood flow. Daily dose is 60–120 mg of gotu kola extract standardized to contain 100 percent triterpenes. Butcher's broom (*Ruscus aculeatus*) contains ruscogenins, which prevent inflammation and promote vein constriction. Take 100–200 mg of extract standardized to 10 percent ruscogenins three times daily.

Bioflavonoids such as proanthocyanidins and anthocyanidins help support the structure of blood vessels. Increasing your intake of foods containing these chemicals, such as berries, cherries, and grapes, can relieve varicose veins. The flavonoids are also available in extract form. Grape seed extract and pine bark extract are popular and effective. Many of my patients enjoy buckwheat tea *(Fagopyrum esculentum),* which supplies a flavonoid called rutin and which may relieve leg swelling.

Many people with varicose veins have a decreased ability to break down fibrin, the protein involved in blood clots. Fibrin is deposited in the tissue near varicose veins, causing the skin to become hard and lumpy. Inability to break down fibrin (fibrinolysis) increases the risk of blood clots and other serious heart conditions. Herbs that increase fibrolytic activity include capsicum (cayenne), garlic, onion, and ginger. Bromelain, an enzyme in pineapple, acts like a plasminogen activator (a substance that occurs naturally in the body) to promote the breakdown of fibrin and prevent development of hard and lumpy skin.

CASE HISTORY: My Personal Experience with Varicose Veins

For one person out of two, varicose veins result from faulty genes. I apparently was one of these cases. It seems that I had inherited weak valves on my femoral vein, the large vessel that drains blood from the superficial veins of the leg into the groin region. Because these large valves were not functioning properly, the walls and valves of the superficial veins upstream were under a great deal of pressure. When I was in my late twenties, large, gnarly varicose veins began to develop in both legs.

By following my own recommendations, I was able to slow down the progression and was free from the uncomfortable symptoms. But by my late thirties, I knew I had to do something more. I began consulting experts in the field of phlebology—the study of veins. I also went to the medical library and started reading phlebology textbooks and journals. One option was a procedure called surgical stripping—the surgical removal of the entire vein. A vascular surgeon told me that I would be required to spend a night in the hospital and would be laid up for at least six weeks. I knew that treatment was not for me.

So I began investigating a technique called sclerotherapy with segmental stripping. In this procedure, an agent is injected that causes a clot to form and pinch off the vein. Only the most badly diseased segments of vein are stripped away. I had the procedure done by a phlebologist in Dallas who specializes in varicose veins. After the procedure I walked out of her office, and I flew home the next day. Three days later I was able to resume all of my normal activities.

After the procedure I was instructed to wear elastic compression stockings. I wore them virtually every day for two years, and I absolutely hated them. Oh, they worked—they relieved leg aches and prevented the "pins and needles" feeling that would develop in my feet by the end of the day. But they're uncomfortable, they're hard to put on and take off, and they made me feel like an old man.

One day I came across an article in the medical journal *The Lancet* showing that horse chestnut seed extract could be as effective as support hose in relieving varicose vein symptoms. Shortly thereafter I began using a product (VariCare) that contains 125 mg of horse chestnut seed extract (standardized for 20–22 percent escin), 150 mg of butcher's broom extract (standardized for 9–11 percent ruscogenins), and 15 mg of gotu kola phytosome (standardized for 30–35 percent triterpenes). The dosage is two tablets taken twice a day. The results were almost instantaneous. I was able to discard the stockings immediately. But the real test was how my legs felt during and after a long flight—an important issue given the amount of travel that I do. Even with the compression stockings my legs tended to swell and get uncomfortable on airplanes, but now I do not even notice them.

Key Steps to Tuning Up Your Cardiovascular System

- Reduce the amount of saturated fat, cholesterol, and total fat in the diet.
- Eliminate the intake of margarine and foods containing trans fatty acids and partially hydrogenated oils.
- Cook with olive oil or canola oil.
- Increase your intake of cold-water fish, eat walnuts, and take 1 tbsp of flaxseed oil daily.
- Eat five or more servings of a combination of vegetables and fruits, especially green and yellow vegetables and citrus fruits.
- Increase your consumption of fiber.
- Reduce the intake of animal protein in the diet.
- Limit the intake of refined carbohydrates (sugar).
- Eat breakfast.
- Avoid cigarette smoke. Quit smoking, and avoid secondhand smoke.
- Keep cholesterol levels in the proper range. Use garlic, niacin (as inositol hexaniacinate), or pantethine if levels are elevated.
- Take a high-quality multiple vitamin and mineral formula.
- Take additional antioxidants:
  - Vitamin C: 500–1,500 mg per day
  - Vitamin E: 400–800 IU per day

- Take one of the following:
  - *Gingko biloba* extract (24 percent ginkgo flavonglycosides): 40–80 mg three times per day
  - Bilberry extract (25 percent anthocyanidin content): 40–80 mg three times per day
  - Grape seed extract (95 percent proanthocyanidin content): 150–300 mg per day
  - Green tea extract (70 percent polyphenol content): 150–300 mg per day

Lifestyle Tune-Up #6:
Develop Positive Relationships

Positive human relationships sustain us and nourish us, body and soul. They are absolutely critical to heart health. In fact, data from large, well-controlled population studies have shown that loneliness, isolation, unfulfilling jobs and relationships, and a "broken heart" are risk factors as important for heart disease and premature death as smoking, high blood pressure, high blood cholesterol, obesity, and physical inactivity. In contrast, having positive relationships and a support structure is linked to better health, lower absenteeism, lower incidence of cancer and heart disease, and reduced hospital stays. In one study, researchers divided 1,337 medical students into two groups: students who were not close to their parents and were dissatisfied with their personal relationships, and those who had better relationships with their parents and others. The first group was found to have a risk of cancer later in life three to four times higher than the students with better relationships.

The bottom line here is that good scientific research is telling us something that most of us already know: We all need relationships and the love and acceptance that they should bring to us. In fact, the desire to be loved and appreciated is one of the main drivers of human behavior. Unfortunately, many of us do not always act in a manner that allows us to achieve something that is so vital to our existence.

What is the biggest roadblock to positive human relationships? In my opinion, it is poor listening skills. The quality of any relationship ultimately comes down to the quality of its communication. Poor listening skills lead to poor communication. When you truly listen, you are telling other people that they are important to you and that you respect them. Here are seven tips to being a good listener:

- *Be empathetic.* It is amazing how putting yourself in other people's shoes opens up the lines of communication. If you first seek to understand, you will find yourself being better understood.
- *Be an active listener.* This means that you must be really interested in what other people are communicating. Listen to what they are saying instead of thinking about your response. Ask questions to

gain more information or clarify what they are telling you. Good questions open lines of communication.

- *Be a reflective listener.* Restate or reflect back to other people your interpretation of what they are telling you. This simple technique shows them that you are both listening to them and understanding what they are saying.
- *Do not interrupt.* Wait to speak until the people you want to communicate with are listening. If they are not ready to listen, your message will not be heard, no matter how well you communicate.
- *Don't try to talk over somebody.* If you find yourself being interrupted, relax—don't try to out-talk other people. If you are courteous and allow them to speak, eventually (unless they are extremely rude) they will respond likewise. If they don't, point out to them that they are interrupting the communication process. You can do this only if you have been a good listener. Double standards in relationships seldom work.
- *Help other people become active listeners.* This can be done by asking them if they understood what you were communicating. Ask them to tell you what it was that they heard. If they don't seem to be understanding what it is you are saying, keep after it until they do.
- *Don't be afraid of long silences.* Human communication involves much more than human words. A great deal can be communicated during silences; unfortunately, in many situations silence can make us feel uncomfortable. Relax. Some people need silence to collect their thoughts and feel safe in communicating. The important thing to remember during silences is that you must remain an active listener.

Good communication in our relationships usually translates to greater intimacy. Words are not enough, however, in our most intimate relationships. What I mean is that it is not enough to simply feel love in our friendships and intimate relationships; we must express these feelings. We must demonstrate to our loved ones just how important they are to us. We must continually find ways to communicate our deepest feelings through our actions. Have you ever heard the expression "Words are cheap"? I would not go that far, but what I think this expression symbolizes is that we need to *show* our loved ones just how much we love and appreciate them.

One of the key principles of life is that whatever you sow, so shall you reap, but multiplied a hundred times. When you plant a tomato seed, you get a tomato plant that has dozens of tomatoes on it, each of which has dozens of seeds. Nature always gives back more than it receives. And really, it is the same for human beings. We all need and want to be loved and appreciated, but in order to receive these gifts we must first give them. The more you give, the more you receive.

If you truly are not a "people person," here is the next best thing: Get a pet. A relationship with a pet can be almost as positive as a human relationship. Studies have shown that owning or caring for a pet can relieve loneliness, depression, and anxiety, and even promote a quicker recovery from illness.

CHAPTER 7

Tuning Up Your Brain, Nerves, and Senses

Beyond question, the most astonishing structure in the known universe can be found just a little north of your neck: your brain. Merely to look at it, you wouldn't know the brain held such power. The human brain is about the size of a large grapefruit. It's full of folds and fissures, like a walnut. And it has the consistency of cold oatmeal.

Yet this mass of densely packed, interwoven nerve cells, weighing only about three and a half pounds, has thousands of times more calculating power than the largest computer ever built. It regulates every function within your body. It processes and coordinates signals from thousands of nerves to help you perceive, make sense of, and respond to the world around you. It stores your memories so efficiently that you can instantly recall the lyrics and melody of a song you may not have heard for thirty years. Your brain holds the key to your personality and your temperament—some even say it is the seat of the soul.

The brain sends and receives signals along a network of nerves. The main nerve pathway—the true information superhighway—is the spinal cord, a cylinder of nerves about a foot and a half long and about as thick as one of your fingers. The spinal cord, which runs through and is protected by the bones of the spine, is basically an extension of the brain. Together the brain and spinal cord are called the central nervous system.

Branching out from the spinal cord are several main nerves and many smaller nerve fibers. Using tiny jolts of electricity, the nerves collect information from millions of sensory receptors throughout your body. The nerves transmit that information along one set of pathways to the brain, which sends responses back along another set of pathways. The nerves then tell your body—the organs, muscles, and glands—what to do to carry out the brain's commands. Because these nerves reach the outermost tissues of the body, they are called the peripheral nervous system.

Much of this activity is triggered by input from the outside world. The portals through which this information arrives are your senses: the eyes, the nose, the ears, the tongue, and the skin. Strange as it sounds, your eyes don't actually "see," and your tongue doesn't actually "taste." Your brain does those things. Your sense organs merely collect the data and pass it on to your body's central processor. All of this activity happens within milliseconds.

It does, that is, if your nerves are working at their normal pace. Just as poor diet or lack of exercise can interfere with the activity of other organ systems, your nervous system can slow to a relative crawl due to lack of proper nutrients or an unhealthy lifestyle. By tuning up, you can keep your body's electrical connections tight and humming. You can provide your brain with the molecular tools it needs to think, feel, and remember more effectively. And you can keep your senses sharp. The changes you make now will serve you well, both in the short term and for the rest of your life.

BRAIN AND NERVE ASSESSMENT

Circle the number that best describes the intensity of your symptoms on the following scale:

0 = I do not experience this symptom
1 = Mild
2 = Moderate
3 = Severe

Feeling of heaviness in the head	0	1	2	3
Light-headedness/fainting	0	1	2	3
Loss of balance	0	1	2	3
Dizziness	0	1	2	3
Ringing/buzzing in ears	0	1	2	3
Trembling hands	0	1	2	3
Loss of feeling in hands and/or feet (toes)	0	1	2	3
Exhaustion from slightest effort	0	1	2	3
Feeling that limbs are too heavy to hold up	0	1	2	3
Loss of grip strength	0	1	2	3
Tingling pain sensation	0	1	2	3
Lack of coordination	0	1	2	3
Nervousness	0	1	2	3

Proneness to accidents	O	I	2	3
Loss of muscle tone	O	I	2	3
Need for 10–12 hours of sleep	O	I	2	3

Add the numbers circled and enter that subtotal here: _____

Circle the number of the answer that applies to you:

History of convulsions   NO = O   YES = 10

Enter the number circled as a subtotal here: _____
Add the two subtotals and enter that total here: _____

Scoring   *15 or more: High priority*
5–14: Moderate priority
1–4: Low priority

Interpreting Your Score

These questions are designed to alert you to possible problems with the way your brain and nerves are working. Your brain is an energy hog, demanding a disproportionate amount of the body's blood sugar and oxygen to function. If not enough blood reaches the brain, or if the blood contains inadequate supplies of glucose or oxygen, you may experience such symptoms as light-headedness or dizziness. Sleep is also important, because one of its main functions is to allow the brain to process the information it has collected during the day. Healthy sleep also rests the muscles and allows certain functions to occur that do not take place when we are active.

In some ways, your nerves are like very delicate wires that conduct electrical signals. If something blocks the nerve or causes the wires to snap, the signal cannot travel to its destination. Similarly, if the nerves do not receive adequate nutrients, the signals can slow to a crawl. The results of nerve problems include lack of coordination, and tingling or loss of feeling in the hands and feet. Sometimes the electrical system goes haywire, causing signals to fire repeatedly or too strongly. This causes seizures, which can cause tingling or uncontrolled twitching and muscle spasms (convulsions).

The Brain

Your brain accounts for only about 2 percent of your body weight, but it consumes 20 percent of your body's energy and oxygen. Different areas of brain tissue handle specific tasks. There are basically three main parts of the brain:

- The brain stem, the junction between the spinal cord and the rest of the brain, is responsible for the basic functions of life, including breathing and blood pressure.
- The cerebellum, the lower brain center, deals with muscle coordination, balance, and posture.
- The forebrain consists of the cerebrum, the two large hemispheres with their wrinkles and valleys, and a central group of structures that includes the hypothalamus, the pituitary gland, and the limbic system. The cerebrum constitutes nearly 70 percent of the weight of the brain and is responsible for many higher functions, such as speech, writing, mathematical calculations, decision making, and creativity. The central structures are involved in regulating temperature, thirst, appetite, the production of certain hormones, and emotions.

At maturity, the brain contains perhaps ten billion neurons (or a hundred billion; no one seems quite sure). Given all these neurons, each with many branches, your brain has an estimated 100 trillion connections.

Tune-Up Tip: Eat the Right Type of Fats

The next time someone calls you a fathead, take it as a compliment. Your brain is basically a vat of fat. The type of fat that you regularly consume plays a major role in how well your brain functions. Like other cells in your body, nerve cells are enveloped by membranes composed chiefly of essential fatty acids in the form of compounds known as phospholipids. These phospholipids play a major role in determining the integrity and fluidity of cell membranes. What determines the type of phospholipid in the cell membrane is the type of fat consumed.

A nerve cell that is packed full of phospholipids composed of saturated fats or trans fatty acids differs considerably in structure and function from a nerve cell packed full of essential fatty acids. In addition, there are differences between the structure of a membrane composed of omega-3 molecules and one composed of omega-6 molecules. A diet consisting mostly of saturated fats, animal fats, cholesterol, and trans fatty acids produces cell membranes that are much less fluid in nature than the membranes of people who eat optimal levels of essential fatty acids, especially the omega-3 fatty acids.

In fact, a deficiency of omega-3 fatty acids in cellular membranes makes it virtually impossible for the cell membrane to perform its vital functions. Without a healthy membrane, cells lose their ability to hold water, vital nutrients, and electrolytes. They also lose their ability to communicate with other cells and be controlled by regulating hormones. They simply do not function properly. An alteration in cell membrane function is the central factor in cell injury and death.

How this all relates to impaired mental function (cognition) was illustrated in a study published in the *American Journal of Epidemiology*. The study indicated that the intake of linoleic acid (an omega-6 fatty acid) was positively associated with impaired cognition. The major dietary sources of linoleic acid were margarine, butter, vegetable oils (corn, safflower, sunflower, and soy), and cheese. In contrast, fish consumption (a good source of omega-3 fatty acids) was associated with improved mental function. The more fish consumed, the higher the mental function test scores. I was happy to see that my grandmother was right—fish really is a "brain food"!

Seen under a microscope, neurons look like bizarre sea creatures. The main body of the cell is a blob from which emerge many small stringy projections called dendrites. Each dendrite forms one or more branches. Also projecting from the cell body is a long filament that looks like a tail. This tail, called an axon, ranges in length from a fraction of an inch to several feet. The end of the axon also branches into several terminals. These terminals reach out like tentacles toward the dendrites of neighboring cells. The dendrites and axon terminals don't actually touch; between them is a microscopic gap called a synapse.

The job of the neuron is to transmit signals along the axon to the next neuron. Here's how it generally works. Something happens to stimulate the neuron—perhaps a physical event, such as pain or a change in temperature, or a chemical signal from another neuron. In response, the neuron sends an electrical signal whizzing down the axon.

At the end of the axon's terminals are little pockets called vesicles. The vesicles contain chemicals called neurotransmitters. The electrical signal stimulates the vesicles to release their neurotransmitters. The molecules float quickly across the tiny synapse until they reach the dendrites from neighboring neurons. For a brief moment the neurotransmitter attaches to a specially shaped molecule, called a receptor, on the surface of the dendrite. When the neurotransmitter docks at the receptor, it completes an electrical circuit and causes the nerve to fire. The signal travels then along the dendrite, through the neuron, and down the axon . . . and the process continues, creating all of your thoughts, feelings, sensations, movements, and everything else that really makes us tick.

Most axons are protected by a fatty layer of insulating material called myelin. Like the plastic coating of an electrical cord, myelin protects the "wire" along which the signal travels. If the sheath is defective, the signal won't flow as efficiently. In severe cases, a kind of biological short circuit develops, preventing the signal from reaching the end of the axon. Neurotransmitters aren't released, the signal is not passed on to the next neuron, and the process of nerve communication grinds to a halt.

Every day, on average, about fifty thousand brain cells die. Most of the cells in your body reproduce, but neurons are different. While there is new evidence that some neuronal growth occurs throughout life, most neurons cannot replicate. Your brain grows lighter as you age. At first, this sounds strange—how could the body not replace cells so crucial to its functioning? But when you think about it, this idea makes sense. Over its lifetime, each neuron in the brain forms dozens, perhaps thousands, of intricate connections with its neighbors. You can't simply plug in a new cell and expect it to work like the old one.

This ability to form connections is why the brain is so powerful. Every time you have a new experience, new connections are forged between nerve cells. To lock in a memory, the neurons sprout new branches. These branches, or dendrites, extend toward branches from other nerves, creating a link that hadn't existed before. When you expose yourself to a stimulating environment filled with sights, sounds, and sensations, you literally exercise your brain, helping it become more complex and intricate.

Even though you can't grow new neurons, you can nourish and encourage the ones you have. You start out with enough brain cells to last for hundreds of years—far longer than you actually live—so the rate of loss isn't very alarming. However, if you eat a lousy diet, drink too much alcohol, or put other harmful substances into your body, the rate of death is many times higher.

STRESS AND MEMORY

Memory itself is handled by various regions of the brain. Sensory memories (sight, smell, and so on) are stored and processed in the limbic system, the thalamus, and the hypothalamus. Facts—the date of the first moon landing, the words to "The Star-Spangled Banner"—are scattered in cells throughout the brain, depending on their relative importance and how recently you acquired them. When you recall a memory, your brain pulls together bits and pieces from various locations and processes them into a meaningful image or thought. If you keep your brain in tune, it's easier to access the brain's vast memory archive.

You've probably noticed that when you're under stress you have more trouble remembering things. You're right, and there's a physical reason for that. Stress causes your adrenal glands to release powerful hormones. Almost immediately, these hormones begin to reduce the utilization of glucose by the brain. Thus prolonged stress causes a decline in brain energy, especially in the part that controls memory. Over long periods, stress hormones can sever the delicate connections between nerves. When the connection is broken, the piece of information contained in that cell may be lost. The better you manage stress, the better your brain functions.

Your Nervous System Tune-Up

The key strategy for tuning up the nervous system is to provide your body with the nutrients it needs to make healthy nerve cells, to protect them from damage, and to enhance their ability to carry out their functions. The results can be astounding. You can boost your mental alertness, increase concentration, promote learning, enhance both short-term and long-term memory, and keep your senses sharp.

Your brain requires a constant source of high-quality nutrition. The brain is so metabolically active that a deficiency of any of a number of nutrients can lead to poor mental function, depression, or other serious mental disorders. Since the neurons in your brain communicate through neurotransmitters, you need to supply your body with the raw materials needed to keep a constant supply of neurotransmitters available. There are more than fifty known neurotransmitters. Some are found only in the central nervous system, while others are active there and elsewhere in the body. It's worth familiarizing yourself with a few of these neurotransmitters (see box), because some of the most exciting advances in brain health are coming from our increasing knowledge of these compounds.

SIX KEY NEUROTRANSMITTERS

- *Acetylcholine,* the first brain chemical discovered, is one of the most abundant neurotransmitters in the body. One of its most important jobs is to carry messages between neurons and muscles. It also plays a key role in such brain functions as concentration and memory. You can't take a dose of acetylcholine; the molecule wouldn't survive the journey through the digestive system. However, you can tune up your body's ability to produce the substance. Acetylcholine is made from dietary choline (found in substances such as lecithin), with an assist from vitamins B_1, B_5, B_6, and C, as well as the minerals calcium and zinc.

- *Dopamine* is involved in muscle movement, repair and growth of tissues, sex drive, and immune system function. It also triggers the pituitary gland to release growth hormone, which helps your body build muscle, burn fat, and repair tissue damage. Your body needs amino acids, especially phenylalanine and tyrosine, to produce dopamine. Enzymes convert dopamine into two other important neurotransmitters, norepinephrine and epinephrine.

- *Glutamine and the related compounds glutamate and GABA (gamma-aminobutyric acid)* are interchangeable amino acids that are found in high concentrations in the brain. Generally they work to slow things down in your body. They accomplish this effect by blocking neurotransmitters that stimulate activity. GABA is very much involved in relaxation and sleep. Antianxiety drugs, such as Valium, tap into the GABA system to produce their effects. Drinking alcohol also seems to enhance GABA activity, which is why booze slows your reflexes and impairs your muscle control. Glutamine and glutamate have profound effects on neurons responsible for memory. Preliminary studies have shown L-glutamine supplementation to be helpful in improving memory in patients with Alzheimer's disease, and in reducing the cravings for alcohol in alcoholics.

- *Norepinephrine* controls the release of endocrine hormones, which regulate many metabolic activities, including sexual function, appetite, and use of energy. Norepinephrine also is involved in learning and memory and plays a role in regulating our moods. Your body makes norepinephrine from dopamine, a process that also requires the participation of copper and vitamins B_3, B_6, and C.

- *Serotonin* is found in the brain, where it plays a part in regulating mood, eating behavior, and sleep. It also exists in blood platelets because it helps control blood clotting. There are serotonin-rich cells in the digestive system, perhaps because the neurotransmitter regulates sensations of hunger and fullness. Serotonin also acts as a vasoconstrictor. Your body makes serotonin by converting the amino acid tryptophan into another form, 5-HTP, and then changing 5-HTP into serotonin. Some serotonin is later converted to melatonin, a hormone involved in regulating the body's internal clock.

Nutrients for Brain Power

Following is a quick look at the most important nutritional strategies for boosting brain and nerve function.

Balance your electrolytes. The ability of a nerve to fire depends on the presence of electrolytes—minerals such as potassium, sodium, chloride, and magnesium dissolved in water. They are termed electrolytes to signify their critical role in conducting electricity in the human body. If you have too much sodium and too little potassium in your diet, the imbalance can slow down the ability of neurons to conduct signals. Boosting potassium and magnesium while restricting sodium intake is a very important dietary recommendation for tuning up brain and nervous system function. Eating more whole, unprocessed foods and avoiding high-salt processed foods and table salt is all that is needed for most people to get their potassium and sodium in balance.

Take B vitamins, as they are crucial for brain and nerve function. B_1 and B_2 help control the use of glucose by neurons. They also help your body make fatty acids needed to preserve the integrity of nerve cell membranes. Along with vitamin B_5, they are important for making acetylcholine and thus for helping memory function. Vitamin B_3 (niacin) is vital for proper mental function. People who suffer from niacin deficiency often exhibit signs of dementia. Vitamin B_6 (pyridoxine) acts like a biological shuttle service, ferrying amino acids into the brain for its use in making neurotransmitters. Lack of B_6 can cause abnormal brain wave patterns and a decrease in nervous system activity. Vitamin B_{12} helps your brain make use of carbohydrates and proteins. It is also vital for producing the myelin sheath that protects the axons of your nerve cells. Folic acid works as a partner with vitamin B_{12} in many biochemical processes in the brain, including the manufacture of neurotransmitters like serotonin and dopamine. Impaired mental acuity (or dementia) and depression are common symptoms of folic acid or B_{12} deficiency. Deficiencies of these nutrients are common, especially in elderly subjects, and are an often overlooked cause of dementia and depression in this age group. (See Lifestyle Tune-Up #4 for dosage recommendations.)

Boost your antioxidant intake. Vitamins C and E are found in high levels in the brain and nervous system. Because brain cells are high in unsaturated fat, they are especially vulnerable to damage by free radicals. There is mounting scientific and clinical evidence that the higher the intake of antioxidants over time (some studies have lasted over twenty years), the better the mental function later in life. A high intake of these nutrients is also associated with a significantly lower risk for both Alzheimer's and Parkinson's diseases. Taking 500 to 1,500 mg of vitamin C and 400 to 800 IU of vitamin E is recommended.

Boost choline intake. Choline, a B vitamin–like substance, is a crucial ingredient in the membranes found in every one of your cells. Dietary or supplementary choline can boost the production of acetylcholine and thus is important for memory, learning, and mental alertness. Rich food sources of choline include lecithin, peanuts, wheat germ, and soy foods. Choline is also found in good levels in Brussels sprouts, oatmeal, soybeans, cabbage, cauliflower, kale, spinach, lettuce, and potatoes. The best forms of choline for supplementation are phosphatidylcholine, glycerophosphocholine, and cytosine diphosphocholine, but supplementation is usually not necessary if you boost dietary sources.

ANTIOXIDANTS AND BRAIN CANCER

There always seems to be confusion regarding whether certain dietary factors cause specific cancers. Perhaps the reason why so many studies on dietary links to cancer produce uncertain results is that researchers often look at the problem from only one angle. For example, most studies examining whether nitrites from cured and smoked meats cause brain cancer focus entirely on the level of these compounds in the diet. The studies do not take into consideration the level of protective antioxidants that inhibit the formation of nitrosamines and thus prevent cells from becoming cancerous. When studies take the patient's total oxidative status into consideration, the picture becomes much clearer.

A case in point is a recent study that looked at dietary habits among 434 newly diagnosed patients with gliomas (a type of brain tumor) in the San Francisco area between 1991 and 1994. Data were obtained on use of vitamin supplements and weekly consumption of twenty-four foods. For both men and women, the people with cancer had a higher mean consumption of cured meats and other cured foods, a lower consumption of fruits and vegetables high in vitamins A and C, and a higher average intake of beer and other alcoholic beverages compared with the control group. The results of the study support the hypothesis that nitrites in cured and smoked meats might be a factor in brain cancer. They imply even more strongly that brain cancer risk increases when the antioxidant capacity of the brain cannot keep pace with an overwhelming burden of oxidants.

Tune-Up Tip: Eating Blueberries May Make You Smarter

A secret for maintaining a youthful brain may be as close as your local farm or supermarket. In a study conducted at Tufts University in Boston, researchers demonstrated that elderly rats fed the human equivalent of at least half a cup of blueberries a day noted improvements in balance, coordination, and short-term memory. The researchers tested blueberries along with strawberries and spinach, but only the blueberries produced significant improvements. These results indicate that although spinach and strawberries produce similar antioxidant effects, there is something special in blueberries that boosts brain power. The most likely candidates are the purple flavonoids known as anthocyanidins. These compounds are included in many brain-boosting formulas sold in Europe. Bilberry (European blueberry) extracts are available in the United States and are sold primarily for their benefits for the eyes.

The rats in the Tufts study were nineteen months old, the equivalent of sixty-five to seventy years in humans. Typically rats begin showing signs of impaired coordination and memory at around twelve months. When they are nineteen months old, the time they can stay on a narrow rod before losing their balance drops to five seconds from a high of thirteen seconds when they were younger. After they were fed blueberry extract for eight weeks, the elderly rats could stay on the rod for an average of eleven seconds.

These results support the notion that flavonoid-rich foods or extracts such as bilberry, grape seed, pine bark, or *Ginkgo biloba* are extremely important in fighting off the effects of aging on the human brain.

Problems Associated with Aging

—— DHEA for Age-Related Mental Decline ——
and Depression

Typically, as people age there is a significant drop in the production of DHEA. Preliminary studies in animals and later in humans indicate that taking supplemental DHEA appears to offset some of the effects of aging, including age-related decline in mental function and depression. For example, in a recent preliminary study, it was shown that elderly patients with major depression and low DHEA levels respond quite well to DHEA supplementation. The dosage used in the study ranged from 30 to 90 mg per day. Improvements in mood and mental function were directly related to increases in the blood levels of DHEA and DHEA sulfate.

If you are taking DHEA and you are not under the care of a physician, I strongly urge you to get the test kits that measure the level of DHEA in saliva from either BodyBalance, 1-888-891-3061 or www.bodybalance.com, or Aeron LifeCycles, 1-510-729-0375 or www.aeron.com.

Table 7-1 DHEA Supplementation in the Elderly

Benefits
DHEA has been shown in double-blind clinical trials to:
- Improve mood and cognition; relieve depression
- Promote increased sense of well-being
- Improve erectile dysfunction
- Improve blood sugar control in diabetics
- Boost immune function

Higher DHEA levels are also associated with a lower risk for many chronic diseases, including heart disease.

Risk
- May increase the risk for breast and prostate cancer

Tune-Up Tip: Flex Your Brain

You've heard the expression "Use it or lose it"? The idea applies to the brain, because in a way, the brain is like a muscle: If you exercise it, it will develop. Plan to spend at least ten minutes each day giving your brain a challenge. Solve a crossword puzzle, listen to a complex piece of music, read a few pages of a book on a subject that's unfamiliar to you. Visit a gallery and study a few of the artworks. Attend a lecture. Sign up for an adult education class or workshop. The more you expose yourself to new things and immerse yourself in new experiences, the better your brain can function.

CASE HISTORY: A New Passion for Living

My patients Mildred and George are a very interesting pair. When I first met them, they were bored with life. In their late seventies, they both felt they had nothing to live for. They were in good health, especially for their age (I think the fact that they were on a very extensive nutritional and herbal supplement program was a big reason). They simply were consulting me to make sure that they were on the right track with their supplements. I made a few minor adjustments in their regimen. But my main "prescription" was for them to start off each day by discussing three memories from the past, three things they were grateful for, and three things they wanted to accomplish. I also suggested that they get a computer and check out the Internet. We rescheduled a visit in two months.

The transformation was incredible. Their laughter, joy, and passion for living were evident the moment they entered the clinic—I could hear them and my receptionist laughing while I was still in my office down the hall. What happened? I asked. They told me that the little exercise that I had prescribed reminded them of how thankful they are to still be here. It made them reconnect to all of the good things in life again. They also told me that getting a computer and logging on to the Internet has opened up a whole new world for them. They were having loads of fun. In fact, they ended up buying two computers so they would not have to fight over access!

Tune-Up Tip: Exercise Is a Brain Tonic

Exercise is an essential part of your brain tune-up. Besides protecting the arteries and preventing blockage of blood flow, exercise appears to boost production of a substance called brain-derived growth factor (BDGF), which helps keep neurons strong.

Exercise also has several positive effects on mood. To counteract the stress of exercise, your brain releases substances called endorphins, which act like natural morphine. Exercise stimulates thyroid activity, which in turn keeps your metabolism running efficiently. The very act of concentrating on a physical activity relieves anxiety and serves as a temporary distraction from your troubles. Exercise helps you feel and look better, which naturally enhances self-esteem. Studies suggest that the mood-lifting effects of exercise are most likely to occur if you exercise at least thirty minutes each day. Less intense regimens—twenty minutes three to five times a week—are helpful for cardiovascular fitness but may not produce the same impact on brain function as a more vigorous program.

Our reaction time normally slows by about 15 percent as we age. But whether that slowing down significantly affects our ability to function depends on our lifestyle. Studies show that elderly people who have exercised regularly throughout their lives have about the same reaction time as younger people, but those who are sedentary have a much slower reaction time. The sooner you integrate exercise into your tune-up program, the better your nerves will function in old age.

—— Alzheimer's Prevention and Treatment ——

Of the many problems that may afflict us as we age, losing our memory and mental function is perhaps the most frightening. Alzheimer's disease is a condition in which the neurons in the brain degenerate. The brain literally shrinks. As the cells fall apart, the memories they stored are lost. The ability to control many body functions, including the bladder and bowels, disappears. Seen under a microscope, the neurons of a brain affected by Alzheimer's reveal telltale tangles and scars.

The cause of Alzheimer's disease may involve a chronic deficiency of antioxidants and vitamins such as B_{12} and folic acid. Head injury may be a factor as well. Many experts also suspect aluminum could be a culprit, because the nerve tangles of Alzheimer's victims contain excessive levels of this toxic metal.

There is no cure, but it may be possible to take natural steps to prevent Alzheimer's from occurring or at least to slow down its progression. In a recent study it was found that not a single person over the age of sixty-five who had been taking more than 500 mg of vitamin C or 400 IU of vitamin E daily developed Alzheimer's disease. Studies have also found that many elderly people have deficiencies of vitamins and minerals, especially B$_1$, B$_{12}$, and zinc. Whether these deficiencies cause Alzheimer's is not known, but we do know that these substances are critical for healthy nerve and brain function. In addition, the following substances show considerable promise:

- Ginkgo biloba *extract*. This ancient herb is showing great benefit in the treatment of senility, including Alzheimer's. It increases the functional capacity of the brain by improving blood flow. It also appears to enhance neurotransmitter activity by normalizing acetylcholine receptors in the hippocampus, the brain area most affected by the disease. Ginkgo is not a cure, but it may slow or delay mental deterioration during the early stages, allowing the patient to live a normal life for as long as possible. Improvement may take three to six months to appear. (See the next Tune-Up Tip for dosage range.)

- *Huperzine A.* The symptoms of Alzheimer's appear to result from reduced levels of the neurotransmitter acetylcholine. In the brain, acetylcholine is broken down by an enzyme. A compound from club moss (*Huperzia serrata*) known as huperzine A appears to slow down the action of this enzyme and thus may help preserve the supply of acetylcholine and improve memory in Alzheimer's disease without causing side effects. Preliminary studies in China are extremely impressive. The typical dosage is 200 mcg twice daily. Researchers at Georgetown University are currently evaluating the benefits of synthetic huperzine A.

- *L-acetylcarnitine.* Carnitine is a vitaminlike compound that helps your cells make energy. Carnitine attached to an acetyl molecule becomes L-acetylcarnitine, which looks and acts a lot like acetylcholine. Researchers have found that L-acetylcarnitine delays the progression of Alzheimer's disease and helps elderly patients who have depression or impaired memory. The typical dosage is 500 mg three times daily.

- *Phosphatidylserine.* Phosphatidylserine is the major phospholipid in the brain, where it plays a major role in determining the integrity and fluidity of cell membranes. Normally the brain can manufacture sufficient levels of phosphatidylserine, but if there is a deficiency of methyl donors such as SAM-e, folic acid, and vitamin B$_{12}$ or essential fatty acids, the brain may not be able to make sufficient phosphatidylserine. Phosphatidylserine has shown very good results in the treatment of depression and/or impaired mental function in the elderly. The typical dosage is 100 mg three times daily.

Tune-Up Tip: *Ginkgo Biloba* Extract Can Make Your Brain Young Again

Ginkgo biloba extract standardized to contain 24 percent ginkgoflavongly-cosides has demonstrated remarkably beneficial effects on many symptoms associated with aging, especially those linked to reduced blood flow to the brain: dizziness, ringing in the ears, headache, short-term memory loss, and depression. Ginkgo boosts brain metabolism by promoting the synthesis of ATP, the main energy-producing molecule in the cells. With more energy available, the brain is better able to metabolize glucose. What's more, ginkgo acts as an effective antioxidant and promotes the flow of blood to the brain. Ginkgo exerts so many beneficial effects that I strongly encourage everyone over the age of fifty to take it. For prevention, I recommend 40 mg three times per day. When therapeutic effects are required, I boost the recommendation to 80 mg three times daily.

Table 7-2: Key Uses of Ginkgo biloba

Cerebral vascular insufficiency (insufficient blood flow to the brain)	Neuralgia and neuropathy
	Peripheral vascular insufficiency (intermittent claudication, Raynaud's syndrome, etc.)
Dementia	
Depression	Premenstrual syndrome
Impotence	Retinopathy (macular degeneration, diabetic retinopathy, etc.)
Inner ear dysfunction (vertigo, tinnitus, etc.)	Vascular fragility
Multiple sclerosis	

HEAVY METAL ANALYSIS

Numerous studies have demonstrated a relationship between high blood levels of various heavy metals, such as lead, mercury, and cadmium, and Alzheimer's disease, poor mental function, various psychological diseases (especially depression), and childhood learning disabilities, including attention deficit disorder (ADD). Heavy metal toxicity can mimic serious diseases such as amyotrophic lateral sclerosis (Lou Gehrig's disease) and multiple sclerosis.

If you are suffering from any of these conditions, or if you are employed in a profession with extremely high exposure to heavy metals (battery makers, gasoline station attendants, printers, roofers, solderers, dentists, and so on), please get a hair mineral analysis performed, and see pages 69–71 for more information.

A Word About Parkinson's Disease

Parkinson's disease results from damage to the nerves in the area of the brain that is responsible for controlling muscle tension and movement—the basal ganglia. The damaged cells are the ones needed to produce the neurotransmitter called dopamine. The disease usually begins as a slight tremor of one hand, arm, or leg. In the early stages the tremors are more apparent while the person is at rest, such as while sitting or standing, and are less noticeable when the hand or limb is being used. A typical early symptom of Parkinson's disease is "pill rolling," in which the person appears to be rolling a pill back and forth between the fingers. As the disease progresses, symptoms often get worse. The tremors and weakness affect the limbs on both sides of the body. The hands and the head may shake continuously. The person may walk with stiff, shuffling steps. In many cases, the disease causes a permanent rigid stooped posture and an unblinking, fixed expression.

There is no cure for Parkinson's, but symptoms are often improved by drug therapy. The most popular drug used is Sinemet, which contains two key ingredients: levodopa and carbidopa. Levodopa, or L-dopa, is the "middle step" in the conversion of the amino acid tyrosine into dopamine. L-dopa, but not dopamine, crosses the blood-brain barrier. Carbidopa is a drug that works by ensuring that more L-dopa is converted to dopamine within the brain, where it is needed, and not within the other tissues of the body. Other drugs used include Eldepryl (selegiline), bromocriptine, and amantadine. Certain medications can also help control tremors.

The value of a low-protein diet in enhancing the action of L-dopa has been demonstrated in several clinical studies, and such a diet is now a well-accepted supportive therapy. The usual recommendation is to eliminate major sources of dietary protein from breakfast and lunch in order to keep protein intake below 7 g until the evening meal. This simple method can effectively reduce tremors and other symptoms of Parkinson's disease during working hours.

Population-based studies have indicated that high dietary intakes of antioxidant nutrients, especially vitamin E, may help prevent Parkinson's disease and may also offer some therapeutic effects as well. In one double-blind study, patients with early Parkinson's disease given 3,000 mg of vitamin C and 3,200 IU of vitamin E each day for a period of seven years fared better than the placebo group. Although all patients eventually required drug treatment, the patients receiving the vitamins were able to delay the need for medication for up to three years. These results are quite promising, but a ten-year study with vitamin E at a lower daily intake, 2,000 IU, failed to show any real benefit in slowing the progress of the disease.

I also recommend that people with Parkinson's disease take ENADA. This supplement contains stabilized niacinamide adenine dinucleotide (NADH), the activated form of vitamin B_3 (niacin). NADH is required by the brain to make various neurotransmitters and to produce chemical energy. Typically, the level of NADH declines as one ages. Correcting this state of low NADH leads to significant improvement in mental function. NADH is especially effective in raising the level of dopamine within the brain and so is extremely beneficial in the treatment of Parkinson's disease. The typical dosage for ENADA is 5 to 20 mg daily, depending upon the severity of the symptoms. *Ginkgo biloba* extract may also be helpful.

Mood Regulation

Depression results from an imbalance of the brain chemicals that normally regulate mood. Approximately seventeen million Americans suffer true clinical depression each year, and over twenty-eight million Americans take antidepressant drugs or anxiety medications.

Depression and anxiety often owe their origin to low levels of the neurotransmitter serotonin. Not only is serotonin important in controlling your moods and behavior, but it also acts as a kind of chemical traffic cop, regulating the activity of many other neurotransmitters. The level of serotonin present in your brain can have a tremendous impact on how you think, feel, and behave. Having an adequate supply produces what is sometimes called the "serotonin effect"—a feeling of calmness, mild euphoria, and relaxation. Having too little serotonin can lead to the opposite situation—feelings of depression, anxiety, and other problems associated with serotonin deficiency syndrome.

Table 7-3: The Effects of Different Levels of Serotonin

Optimal Level of Serotonin	Low Level of Serotonin
Hopeful, optimistic	Depressed
Calm	Anxious

Optimal Level of Serotonin	Low Level of Serotonin
Good-natured	Irritable
Patient	Impatient
Reflective and thoughtful	Impulsive
Loving and caring	Abusive
Able to concentrate	Has a short attention span
Creative, focused	Blocked, scattered
Able to think things through	Flies off the handle
Responsive	Reactive
Does not overeat carbohydrates	Craves sweets and high-carbohydrate foods
Sleeps well with good dream recall	Has insomnia and poor dream recall

The lower your level of serotonin, the more severe and widespread the potential impact on your brain and body. For example, low levels of serotonin can cause overwhelming sugar cravings. Research has shown that many people with bulimia, an eating disorder that causes uncontrollable eating binges, have insufficient supplies of serotonin.

Table 7.4: Conditions Associated with Low Serotonin Levels

- Aggression
- Alcoholism
- Anxiety
- Attention deficit disorder
- Bulimia
- Carbohydrate cravings
- Chronic pain disorders (such as fibromyalgia)
- Depression
- Epilepsy
- Headaches (migraines, tension headaches, chronic headaches)
- Hyperactivity
- Insomnia
- Myoclonus (muscle twitching)
- Obesity
- Obsessive-compulsive disorder
- Panic disorders
- Premenstrual syndrome
- Schizophrenia
- Seasonal affective disorder ("winter depression")
- Suicidal thoughts and behavior

The problems arising from serotonin deficiency may vary from person to person. For example, in some people, low levels of serotonin may cause depression, while in others the same level might produce regular disabling headaches or a voracious appetite for sweets and carbohydrates. These variations in the effects of serotonin reflect human biochemical individuality. Although we all have the same basic electrochemical wiring system in our brains, there are major differences in how we respond to the signals sent along that system in terms of mood and behavior.

Unfortunately, you can't boost your serotonin level by taking a serotonin pill. Serotonin can only be manufactured *inside* the body, especially inside the brain. Like a factory, the brain needs an adequate supply of raw materials that it can modify to produce the final result: molecules of serotonin. The best natural ways to boost serotonin levels are to take 5-hydroxytryptophan (5-HTP) and to take St. John's wort extract—two valuable natural medicines best known for their effects in treating depression. In addition, the role of 5-HTP in treating virtually all conditions linked to low serotonin has been extensively documented.

HOW TO TAKE 5-HTP

For depression, weight loss, headaches, and fibromyalgia, the dosage should be started at 50 mg three times per day. If the response is inadequate after two weeks, increase the dosage to 100 mg three times per day. Starting at a low dose will greatly reduce the mild symptoms of nausea often experienced during the first few weeks of 5-HTP therapy. Using enteric-coated capsules or tablets (pills prepared in a manner so that they will not dissolve in the stomach) significantly reduces the likelihood of nausea. 5-HTP can also be taken with food. But if you are taking 5-HTP for weight loss, I recommend taking it twenty minutes before meals.

For more information on 5-HTP, please consult my book *5-HTP: The Natural Way to Overcome Depression, Obesity, and Insomnia* (Bantam, 1998).

In addition to boosting serotonin levels with 5-HTP or St. John's wort, here are some other key considerations in depression:

- It is important to rule out simple organic factors that are known to contribute to low serotonin levels: nutrient deficiency or excess, drugs (prescription, illicit, alcohol, caffeine, nicotine, etc.), hypoglycemia, hormonal imbalance, allergy, environmental factors, and microbial factors.
- Psychological therapy has been shown to be as effective as antidepressant drugs in treating moderate depression.
- Depression is often a first or early manifestation of low thyroid function.
- Elimination of sugar and caffeine has been shown to produce significant benefits in clinical trials.
- Increased participation in exercise, sports, and physical activities is strongly associated with decreased symptoms of anxiety, depression, and malaise.

—— St. John's Wort Extract: Nature's Prozac ——

St. John's wort (*Hypericum perforatum*) is a shrubby perennial plant with numerous bright yellow flowers. The term *wort* is an old English term for "plant." Its being named after St. John was based on the claim that red spots, symbolic of the blood of St. John, appeared on the leaves of the plant on the anniversary of the saint's beheading. St. John's wort is cultivated worldwide, but it grows quite well in northern California and southern Oregon.

The clinical effectiveness of St. John's wort has been demonstrated in over thirty double-blind studies, including studies comparing it with standard antidepressant drugs. The bottom line is that St. John's wort extract is as or more effective as these drugs, but is safer and has fewer side effects. At this time, St. John's wort is most appropriate for the treatment of mild to moderately severe depression. For the severely depressed patient, the best recommendation appears to be standard drugs until there is more research on the role of St. John's wort for this group.

In general, I view St. John's wort as a "crutch" until dietary, lifestyle, and attitude changes have had a chance to really take hold. My experience is that only about 25 percent of people require more than six months of herbal therapy; these patients possibly have a genetic predisposition to depression. Given the excellent safety profile of St. John's wort and the concern over the long-term safety of antidepressant drugs, I would much rather see patients using the herbal extract for an indefinite period than drugs such as Prozac, Paxil, Zoloft, and others. Most patients begin reporting a benefit from the herb within the first two weeks. With St. John's wort, as with most antidepressant agents, maximal benefits are typically seen after six to eight weeks of continued use.

The dosage of St. John's wort preparations are based upon the hypericin content. The overwhelming majority of the studies in depression have used St. John's wort extract standardized to contain 0.3 percent hypericin at a dosage of 900 mg daily.

– Clinical Note: Tapering Off Antidepressant Drugs –

I have used St. John's wort and 5-HTP successfully and without incident in patients taking Prozac, Zoloft, Paxil, Effexor, and various other antidepressant drugs. The real concern when mixing antidepressant drugs with St. John's wort or 5-HTP is producing what is referred to as the "serotonin syndrome," characterized by confusion, fever, shivering, sweating, diarrhea, and muscle spasms. Although this syndrome has never been produced when St. John's wort extract or 5-HTP have been given alone, it is theoretically possible that combining St. John's wort or 5-HTP with standard antidepressant drugs could produce this syndrome. My recommendation is that when you are using St. John's wort or 5-HTP in combination with standard antidepressant drugs, you should be closely monitored by your doctor for any symptoms suggestive of the serotonin syndrome. If these symptoms appear, discontinuation of one of the therapies is indicated.

How best to taper off an antidepressant drug and switch to either 5-HTP or St. John's wort really depends on the patient and the severity of the pretreatment depression. First of all, it is extremely important always to work with your doctor if you want to make the switch. In mild cases of depression, I will have the patient start the St. John's wort extract while halving the daily drug dosage. After two weeks, the drug is totally eliminated. For more severe cases, I recommend keeping the dosage of the antidepressant as it is and adding the St. John's wort extract. We then evaluate at the end of one month and begin tapering off the drug if sufficient mood-elevating effects have been noted. If additional support is necessary, I usually add 5-HTP at a dosage of 50 mg three times daily. I have found the combination of 5-HTP and St. John's wort to work particularly well in patients with depression who also have signs and symptoms of fibromyalgia (see page 303).

WARNING   If you are currently on a tranquilizer or antidepressant and want to start taking 5-HTP or St. John's wort, you will need to work with a physician to get off the drug. Stopping the drug on your own can be dangerous; you absolutely must have proper medical supervision.

Dealing with Anxiety

Anxiety is almost as common as depression, as over fourteen million Americans suffer from anxiety, defined as an unpleasant emotional state ranging from mild unease to intense fear. Anxiety differs from fear in that while fear is a rational response to a real danger, anxiety usually lacks a clear or realistic cause. Though some anxiety is normal and, in fact, healthy, higher levels of anxiety not only are uncomfortable, but can lead to significant problems.

Anxiety can be the result of either physical or psychological factors. For example, extreme stress can definitely trigger anxiety, and so can certain stimulants such as caffeine. According to Melvyn Werbach, M.D., author of *Nutritional Influences on Mental Illness* (Third Line Press, 1999), there are at least six nutritional factors that may be responsible for triggering anxiety:

1. Alcohol
2. Caffeine
3. Sugar
4. Deficiency of the B vitamins niacin, pyridoxine, and thiamin
5. Deficiency of calcium or magnesium
6. Food allergies

By avoiding alcohol, caffeine, sugar, and allergenic foods, a person with anxiety can go a long way toward relieving his or her symptoms. Simply eliminating coffee can result in complete elimination of symptoms. This recommendation may seem too simple to be true, but substantial clinical evidence indicates that in many cases it is all that is necessary. For example, in one study of four men and two women with generalized anxiety or panic disorder who were consuming the amount of caffeine in 1.5 to 3.5 cups of coffee per day, avoiding caffeine for one week brought about significant relief. The degree of improvement was so noticeable, all patients volunteered to continue abstaining from it. Previously, these patients had been only minimally helped by drug therapy. Follow-up exams six to eighteen months afterward indicated that five out of the six patients were completely without symptoms; the sixth patient became symptom free with a very low dose of Valium.

Tune-Up Tip: Kava for Anxiety

The herb kava *(Piper methysticum)* is gaining a good reputation as an alternative to Valium-like drugs often used for anxiety. Based on the results of detailed scientific investigations and favorable clinical studies, several European countries have approved kava preparations as a medical treatment of nervous anxiety, insomnia, and restlessness. Kava appears to be as effective as standard drugs, yet considerably safer. The dosage of standardized kava preparations is based on the level of kavalactones—45 to 70 mg of kavalactones three times daily.

Although no side effects have been reported using standardized kava extract at recommended levels in the clinical studies, several case reports have been presented indicating that kava may interfere with dopamine and worsen Parkinson's disease, exert an additive effect when combined with benzodiazepines, and impair the ability to drive (when consumed in very large dosages). Until these issues are cleared up, kava extract should not be used in Parkinson's patients and should be used with extreme caution and close monitoring in patients taking benzodiazepines (Valium-like drugs).

WARNING   If you are currently on a tranquilizer or antidepressant and want to switch to kava, you will need to work with a physician to get off the drug. Stopping the drug on your own can be dangerous; you absolutely must have proper medical supervision.

The Nerves

You've probably seen what happens to a strand of rope that becomes frayed with use. Well, a similar thing can happen to nerves. Constant pressure or friction can harm the integrity of a nerve cell, slowing or completely destroying its ability to carry electrical signals. This is what happens in conditions known as repetitive stress injuries. The most well known of these is carpal tunnel syndrome. This affliction is common to people who perform repetitive, strenuous work with their hands, such as typists, musicians, or craftspeople. It results from pressure on the nerve that passes between the bones and ligaments of the wrist. Surgery can help—but it can also sometimes make the problem worse.

The best way to address carpal tunnel syndrome is to prevent it from happening. Since your livelihood may depend on your ability to swing a hammer, tickle the ivories, or pound a computer keyboard, that's not always possible. Here are some other solutions to try:

- Researchers have found that taking supplemental doses of vitamin B_6 (no more than 150 mg a day) may help in many cases by raising your pain threshold. It might take three to five months for results to appear. Don't overdo it, because excess B_6 can damage nerves and cause general body pain.
- Bromelain, an enzyme found in pineapple, helps fight inflammation and can reduce pain, swelling, and bruising. Take 200 to 400 mg of bromelain three times daily on an empty stomach.
- Foods with yellow food dyes (e.g., Yellow Dye #5) can make the problem worse; avoid these when possible.
- In some cases, low levels of thyroid hormone can contribute to carpal tunnel syndrome. If you follow the steps for a thyroid tune-up (see Chapter 4), your symptoms may improve.
- Hot and cold water therapy also provides relief. Soak your wrist in hot water for three minutes, then plunge into cold water for thirty seconds. Repeat the cycle three to five times. This technique draws blood to the region, increasing the delivery of nutrients and oxygen, eliminating waste products, and decreasing pain.
- Stretching can also help. Flex the wrists and fists with the arms extended for five minutes. Do this before work starts and frequently throughout the day—at least every hour. Also, use ergonomic desks and chairs that are designed to prevent damage to your body.

Peripheral Neuropathy

Peripheral neuropathy refers to loss of peripheral nerve function in the extremities and is characterized by tingling sensations, numbness, loss of function, pain, and muscle weakness. There are many different causes of peripheral neuropathy, including diabetes and trauma. Whatever the cause of the peripheral neuropathy, natural measures can help.

Jack, a fifty-six-year-old elementary-school principal, consulted me for help with reducing pain after a shingles infection. Shingles refers to irritation, inflammation, and small blisters that erupt in the area of the skin serviced by a nerve that has been invaded by a member of the herpes virus family *(Herpes zoster)*. Jack had undergone chemotherapy and radiation for a lymphoma. As a result, his immune system was weakened and he developed a severe case of shingles. I wish Jack had been my patient before he underwent the chemo and radiation, for I think I could have helped prevent the initial attack by tuning up and boosting his immune function as detailed in Chapter 5. Now, however, he was suffering from the severe pain known as postherpetic neuralgia. The skin lesions were gone, but he still had pain in the area of his rib cage just below his heart.

To deal with pain and other symptoms of peripheral neuropathy, I always recommend topically applied capsaicin. Capsaicin is the active component of cayenne pepper, responsible for its pungent and irritating effects—in other words, it's the stuff that makes red pepper hot. When applied to the skin, capsaicin stimulates and then blocks transmission along small-diameter pain fibers by depleting them of the neurotransmitter substance P. Substance P is thought to be the principal chemical that conducts pain impulses to the nerves. Commercial ointments containing 0.025 percent or 0.075 percent capsaicin are available over the counter. These preparations may offer significant benefit in a number of conditions, including the pain associated with postherpetic neuralgia, diabetic neuropathy, osteoarthritis, and rheumatoid arthritis.

I recommended to Jack that he apply the 0.075 percent cream twice daily to the affected area. It took a couple of weeks, but it eventually worked. The only downside is that in order for it to keep working, Jack has to make sure he is religious in applying it.

Sciatica

Sciatica is a term used to describe irritation of the sciatic nerve, the primary nerve of each leg and the largest nerve of the body. Sciatica is usually associated with radiating pain that extends from the buttocks to the foot. The severity of sciatica can range from mild to excruciating. My recommendations are to consult a good chiropractor and increase your potassium intake.

Ivan, a patient of mine, had sciatica for over twenty-three years. Ivan was very educated about the role of potassium in nerve function (see page 243). Careful dietary assessment (Ivan is an accountant) indicated that he was consuming about 5,000 mg of potassium daily. For most people this may be enough, but people with sciatica appear to require more. I recommended that Ivan boost his potassium intake to over 8,000 mg each day by consuming 24 to 32 ounces of fresh vegetable juice daily along with taking the food-based potassium supplement Bio-K. Within two weeks of following this recommendation, Ivan's sciatica pain completely disappeared and has remained gone. Ivan's case was the most dramatic, but I have seen this simple recommendation work wonders in many other cases.

—— Multiple Sclerosis—A Dietary Approach ——

Multiple sclerosis (MS) is a debilitating syndrome of progressive nervous system disability. The early symptoms of multiple sclerosis may include:

- Muscular symptoms—feeling of heaviness, weakness, leg dragging, stiffness, tendency to drop things, clumsiness
- Sensory symptoms—tingling, "pins and needles" sensation, numbness, dead feeling, bandlike tightness, electrical sensations
- Visual symptoms—blurring, fogginess, haziness, eyeball pain, blindness, double vision
- Vestibular symptoms—light-headedness, feeling of spinning, sensation of drunkenness, nausea, vomiting
- Genitourinary symptoms—incontinence, loss of bladder sensation, loss of sexual function

Dr. Roy Swank, a professor of neurology at the University of Oregon's medical school, has provided convincing evidence that a diet low in saturated fats, maintained over a long period of time (one study lasted more than thirty-four years), tends to halt the progression of MS. Dr. Swank began treating patients successfully with his low-fat diet in 1948. His diet calls for a saturated fat intake of no more than 10 g per day, a daily intake of 40 to 50 g of polyunsaturated oils (margarine, shortening, and hydrogenated oils are not allowed), at least 1 tsp of cod liver oil daily, a normal allowance of protein, and the consumption of fish three or more times a week.

I have treated about a dozen MS patients with a modification of Swank's program (I recommend flaxseed oil over cod liver oil). This approach has benefited every single patient.

The Senses

Your sense organs transform a stimulus into signals that your nerves can then send to the brain for processing. The skin reacts to pressure, heat, and cold (I'll discuss skin in Chapter 9). The nose and tongue respond to molecules that convey aroma and taste. The ears react to sound waves, which arrive as moving air. (The ears also contain vestibular structures, responsible for helping us maintain our balance.) For the eyes, the stimulus is light, which arrives in waves of tiny particles called photons.

Taste and Smell

Both the nose and the tongue respond to molecules of various chemicals. Taste and smell, then, are known as the chemical senses.

Your nose doesn't really do the smelling. Instead the nose serves as the passageway for air, which contains odor molecules. On the roof at the back of the nasal cavity is a layer of cells called the olfactory epithelium. Sticking through this layer are about fifteen million nerve cells called olfactory receptors. The end of each receptor branches into about twenty tiny hairs (cilia). Glands in the epithelium release mucus, which serves to trap odor molecules.

As air passes through the cavity, it deposits odor molecules in the mucus; the mucus causes the molecules to dissolve. The dissolved chemicals stimulate the receptors by binding to proteins on the cilia. The act of binding causes changes in the balance of sodium and potassium. As in other neurons, this activity triggers an electrical signal. The signal travels along nerve fibers connected to a mass of tissue called the olfactory bulb. Neurotransmitters transmit the signals to other nerve fibers, which carry them through the bulb and into the brain.

Compared to most animals, we humans don't have a very keen sense of smell. Only about 2 percent of the air we inhale through the nose passes by the olfactory receptors. If we want to intensify a smell, we sniff. This forces more air to hit the receptors, triggering a more pronounced response.

Some of the signals travel through the limbic system in the brain, which is responsible for our emotional reactions. That's why certain odors can cause such powerful emotional reactions. Smells associated with danger—smoke, natural gas, the scent of a skunk—trigger the flight-or-fight response. Appetizing odors increase salivation and stimulate the digestive tract. Unpleasant odors cause protective reflexes, such as sneezing, choking, or gagging.

Unlike most of the neurons in your body, the olfactory receptors can regenerate. Every two months or so, you produce a new crop of smell cells.

Your senses of taste and smell are intricately related. Your brain combines information on odors with the information on taste to figure out exactly what it is you're eating. In fact, about 80 percent of what you "taste" is actually what you smell. You may remember the old grade-school experiment where the teacher has you shut your eyes and hold your nose and then asks you to bite into a piece of food. Without smell, your tongue can't tell an apple from an onion.

Your tongue contains about two hundred taste buds, which respond to chemical signals from food. A few other taste buds are found in other parts of the mouth. The taste buds aren't as sensitive as the nerve receptors in the nose. We need about twenty-five thousand times more of a substance to taste it than we do to smell it.

Taste happens when a chemical dissolves in saliva, enters the taste pore, and contacts the gustatory hairs. These hairs respond by triggering tiny electrical signals. At the ends of these fibers, the signals trigger the release of neurotransmitters. These neurotransmitters then activate nerve fibers, which collect the information and send it to the brain.

There are four basic kinds of taste: sweet, sour, salty, and bitter. Different regions of the tongue are more responsive to the different tastes. And the tongue also responds to heat, motion, and pain. The reason spicy foods such as chili peppers taste "hot" is that they activate pain receptors.

Tune-Up Tip: The Power of Zinc

Among its other important functions, zinc is essential for the maintenance of vision, taste, and smell. A zinc deficiency results in impaired functioning of these senses. The loss of the sense of taste and smell is a common complaint in the elderly. Zinc supplementation has been shown to improve sensory acuity in these patients.

Several studies have shown that zinc supplementation can also prevent or correct taste abnormalities caused by radiation therapy in patients with cancers of the head and neck region. I tried this approach with Margo, a fifty-nine-year-old woman who had had radiation therapy for a tumor in her neck. Margo had lost about 95 percent of her sense of smell. With zinc supplementation (45 mg of elemental zinc daily), she was once again able to smell the roses in her garden.

Hearing

Your ears can hear an extraordinary range of sound. The outer ear includes the flaps (auricles) that stick out from your head. These capture sound and channel it to the auditory canal. The canal is lined with skin that contains hair and glands that secrete oil and wax. These substances protect the ear from dust and foreign particles, including the occasional curious insect.

The middle ear contains a sensitive membrane called the eardrum. Sound waves cause air to move into the canal and "beat" against the eardrum, which makes it vibrate. Next to the eardrum are three bones, the smallest in your body. The bones are named for their shapes: the hammer, the anvil, and the stirrup. Movement by the eardrum causes the bones to vibrate.

In the inner ear, the stirrup bone is connected to the cochlea, a snail-shaped, fluid-filled tube. Vibrations from the stirrup cause this fluid to push against the membrane of the cochlea, in turn causing it to vibrate. Movement of the cochlear membrane moves hairs in a structure called the organ of Corti; the hairs are connected to thirty thousand nerves. The nerves transmit electrical signals to the auditory centers of the brain, where they are converted into something meaningful.

Here are some tips for keeping your ears in "sound" condition:

- Keep your ears clean; many cases of hearing loss result from a buildup of wax (cerumen) in the ear canal.
- Avoid long exposure to loud noises, since these can wear out the delicate hearing mechanism.
- High blood pressure can cause ringing in the ears (tinnitus), so make sure your blood pressure is under control (see Chapter 6).
- Eat a low-salt diet to reduce excess fluid; doing so helps reduce tissue swelling that can contribute to tinnitus.
- Make sure you get enough zinc and vitamin B_{12}, because the organs in the ear depend on these nutrients to function.

CAUTION: EAR CANDLES   Ear candles are hollow candles that are placed into the external ear canal and lit at the opposite end. The lighted candle is thought to create a vacuum that draws cerumen and other impurities into the hollow candle. A dark brown waxy substance purported to be cerumen is left in the stub of the candle. Ear candling is becoming quite popular, but is it effective and is it safe?

A recent study indicated that ear candling produced no negative pressure in the ear canal. What is more, there was no removal of cerumen from the canal—the brown waxy substance turned out to be candle wax. A survey of 122 otolaryngologists identified twenty-one ear injuries resulting from ear candle use (thirteen cases of burns, seven partial or complete occlusions of the ear canal with candle wax, and one eardrum perforation). These results clearly indicate that ear candling is neither effective nor safe.

CASE HISTORY: Stop the Ringing

Mary, a sixty-seven-year-old retired insurance executive, had been suffering for years with a constant ringing in her ears. The medical term for this symptom is *tinnitus*. If the ringing is due to damage to the eardrum from loud noises, not much can be done. But if the eardrum is not damaged, it usually responds quite well to natural therapies. *Ginkgo biloba* extract is often effective, as is magnesium.

In Mary's case, however, the magic bullet was a special form of vitamin B_{12} known as methylcobalamin. There were two important clues in her case. First of all, she exhibited classic signs and symptoms of decreased stomach acid secretion (weak and brittle nails, numerous digestive disturbances, and so on). As I explained in Chapter 2, many people with low stomach acid do not absorb enough vitamin B_{12}. Second, I had just read an interesting study showing that 47 percent of patients with tinnitus are deficient in B_{12}. Many people with low B_{12} levels experience complete resolution of their tinnitus when given methylcobalamin. Mary was one of those people. In fact, she responded within the first week. I started her off at a dosage of 2,000 mcg twice daily for one month and then reduced it to 1,000 mcg daily as a maintenance dose.

Vision

The way your eyes see is one of the most fascinating of all body functions. Light travels through the clear outer layer (the cornea) through an opening (the pupil) and then through the lens. Both the cornea and the lens focus the beam. The beam travels through the eyeball, a hollow ball filled with fluid, and lands on a patch of cells at the back of the eyeball called the retina.

Your retina—actually a direct extension of your brain—contains two types of specialized cells: rods and cones. Each eye has about 125 million rods, which let us see in dim light and are responsible for our peripheral vision. The cones (6 million per eye) operate in bright light and allow us to see colors and sharp images. The cones are concentrated in the central part of the retina, called the macula, which lies directly behind the lens.

The rods and cones are tubes that contain a stack of tiny disks, like pennies in a coin wrapper. Each disk contains special molecules called visual pigments, which are made from a light-absorbing substance called *retinal* and a protein called *opsin*. Retinal is made from vitamin A, which is why the vitamin is so important for promoting good vision.

Retinal hangs between sections of opsin like a molecular hammock. In the dark, retinal has a bent or kinked shape. But when light of a certain wavelength strikes, retinal straightens out. In the act of straightening, it detaches from the opsin. In response, opsin then triggers a series of events that ultimately results in the production of a tiny electrical signal.

The signals from millions of neighboring eye cells travel along pathways until they reach the main nerve leading out of the eye, the optic nerve. (The "blind spot" in each eye is the place on the retina where the optic nerve forms; there are no light-sensitive cells there, so you can't see light falling on that area.) The optic nerve collects the signals and delivers them to the visual center at the back of the brain. There the brain processes them into a single image, figures out what it means, and responds.

Meanwhile, the retinal molecule that detached is getting a new supply of vitamin A, which converts it back to its original form. In a few minutes it is recycled—stuck back into an opsin molecule—and is ready to let you see again.

Depending on the type of opsin to which it is bound, retinal absorbs different wavelengths of light. The visual pigment in the rods is a deep purple pigment called rhodopsin. It doesn't take very much light to make rhodopsin do its thing. In fact, if you've been standing in total darkness for about twenty minutes, you would be able to see a candle flame five miles away. The cones are different and are more complex. Each one contains a single type of visual pigment that responds to different wavelengths of light: blue, green, or red. There is some overlap in these responses. For example, both red and green cone receptors react to yellow light. When all cones are stimulated equally, we see white. Light has to be more intense to activate the cones. That's why, in dim light such as twilight, all we see are black, white, and shades of gray.

There are several important steps you can take to prevent damage to what many people consider their most precious sense: their sight.

- To preserve acute vision, don't strain your eyes. Always make sure there is adequate light for your task. When working at a computer terminal, look away for a few minutes every fifteen minutes or so. Sit as far back as possible from monitors or TV sets. Never look directly at sources of bright light, including the sun—bright light can literally kill the rods and cones it strikes, leading to blindness.
- Get adequate supplies of vitamin A and carotenes. As I explained earlier, your body makes visual pigments from vitamin A. In fact, another name for vitamin A is retinol, underscoring its importance to vision, especially night vision. The body converts many carotenes into vitamin A. But other carotenes that are not converted are also important to the eyes. Among other things, they help prevent the most common age-related causes of blindness. What your mother told you is true: If you want to see better, eat your carrots (and other carotene-rich plant foods; see Table 7-5).
- Increase levels of antioxidants to avoid free-radical damage to the eyes. Antioxidants play a key role in preventing and treating cataracts, glaucoma, and macular degeneration. Today health food stores offer nutritional supplements specifically designed for the eyes.
- Exposure to free radicals, such as those from cigarette smoke, is a significant source of eye damage. If you smoke, you must stop.
- Because eye health depends on the blood supply to reach the eye, follow the suggestions in Chapter 6 to reduce the risk of cardiovascular disease.

Preventing Cataracts

The lens of the eye is normally crystal clear. But damage to the proteins in the lens can cause it to become cloudy and opaque. The result is a cataract. Cataracts are the leading cause of impaired vision in the United States, affecting more than five million people today. This number is sure to increase dramatically with the aging baby-boomer population, as most people over the age of sixty have some degree of cataract formation.

There are many factors that can contribute to or cause cataracts: eye disease or injury, diseases such as diabetes mellitus, and exposure to toxins and ultraviolet light. Heavy metals, such as cadmium, can cause damage to eye tissues and can prevent antioxidants such as zinc from binding to enzymes. Cigarette smoke is a leading source of cadmium. In many cases, cataracts are simply part of the aging process, the result of years of cumulative free-radical damage.

Many cataracts can be repaired through surgical replacement with an artificial lens. But the best strategy is to prevent cataracts from forming in the first place by tuning up the body's defense mechanisms. The sooner you begin, the better the results. Once a cataract forms, dietary and nutritional strategies can't eliminate the problem, but they can help to slow down the rate at which it progresses.

You can reduce free-radical formation by avoiding fatty foods, especially fried foods. High salt intake also is associated with cataracts. In contrast, a diet rich in vegetables, fruit, calcium, folic acid, and vitamin E provides nutrients that protect against cataracts.

To quench free radicals that do crop up, the tissues in your eye need adequate levels of key antioxidants. The higher your levels of these substances, the lower your risk of cataracts.

Vitamin C supplementation can halt the progression of cataracts and may improve vision. In one study, 450 patients with cataracts were placed on a nutritional program that included 1,000 mg of vitamin C per day, resulting in a significant reduction in cataract development. Though similar patients had previously required surgery within four years, in the patients treated with vitamin C only a small handful required surgery, and in most patients there was no evidence that the cataract progressed over the eleven-year period of the study. The lenses of the eye require much higher concentrations of vitamin C than those found in the blood—at least twenty times more—and by keeping blood vitamin C levels elevated, you make it easier for the body to concentrate vitamin C into the lens. Studies of patients going in for cataract surgery showed that dosages of at least 1,000 mg per day were required to increase the concentration of vitamin C in the lens of the eye.

Tune-Up Tip: Use C to See

In an analysis of 247 nurses between the ages of fifty-six and seventy-one, use of vitamin C supplements at any dosage for longer than ten years was associated with a 77 percent lower rate of cataract formation compared with women who did not take a vitamin C supplement. In other words, 77 out of 100 people who developed cataracts might have prevented them if they had simply taken vitamin C.

Other important factors for preventing cataracts:

- *Glutathione peroxidase* is an enzyme that is normally found in high concentrations in the lens. It neutralizes hydrogen peroxide, a free radical found in the fluid of the eye (the aqueous humor). People with cataracts typically lack sufficient glutathione peroxidase and have hydrogen peroxide levels up to twenty-five times higher than normal. You can boost your glutathione peroxidase supply by making sure you get enough selenium and vitamin E. These nutrients work together as an antioxidant team to neutralize hydrogen peroxide.
- *Superoxide dismutase* is another antioxdant enzyme. Progression of cataracts is also associated with a reduced level of superoxide dismutase (SOD). To function, SOD needs adequate supplies of the cofactor trace minerals zinc, copper, and manganese. In people with cataracts, the lenses have only about 10 percent of the zinc and copper and about half of the manganese they need. Taking SOD as a supplement by itself doesn't seem to work. However, by making sure that you get enough zinc, copper, and manganese, you ensure that SOD has the tools it needs to do its job, in the lens and elsewhere in the body.
- *Flavonoid-rich extracts* can also offer excellent antioxidant protection for the lenses. Among the best are flavonoid-rich extracts from bilberry (*Vaccinium myrtillus*), grape seed (*Vitis vinifera*), and *Ginkgo biloba*. One recent study found that bilberry extract plus vitamin E stopped the progression of cataracts in forty-eight out of fifty patients. (See page 273 for dosages).

Tune-Up Tip: **An Added Shade of Protection Against Cataracts**

Because UV light can cause cataracts, it's a good idea to protect your eyes from sunlight whenever you spend time outdoors. Wear sunglasses with guaranteed UV protection. Put on a hat with a brim that protects your eyes.

Preventing Macular Degeneration

When we look at something, we see sharp detail in the center of our field of vision. Toward the periphery, the image becomes less distinct.

This way of seeing reflects the way the image appears on the retina. The cone-rich part of the retina that handles fine detail in the center of the field of vision is called the *macula*. Sometimes damage occurs to this part of the eye, causing the cells to lose their ability to perceive light. This condition is known as *macular degeneration*. It appears that free-radical damage is one culprit, but a decreased supply of blood and oxygen to the retina also may be involved. Major risk factors include smoking, atherosclerosis, and high blood pressure. More than 150,000 Americans suffer from the condition, and the number of cases will rise as the population ages.

There are two kinds of macular degeneration. The "wet" form involves growth of abnormal blood vessels. Laser surgery is often recommended to stop the growth. The "dry" form is more common, affecting perhaps nine out of ten people with macular degeneration. This form occurs when cellular debris, called lipofuscin, accumulates in retinal tissue and disrupts the cone cells.

There is no known treatment for dry macular degeneration. A tune-up, however, may help you prevent the condition. The strategy is twofold: increase antioxidants and prevent hardening of the arteries. Both of these methods depend on a healthy diet.

The macula is a yellowish tissue. Its color comes from high concentrations of yellow pigments, especially lutein, zeaxanthin, and lycopene. These pigments are carotenes, but the body does not convert them into vitamin A. They function to prevent oxidative damage to the retina, and they play a key role in preventing macular degeneration. See Table 7-5 for foods rich in these carotenes.

Table 7-5: Top Twenty Plant Sources of Lutein, Zeaxanthin, and Lycopene

Corn	Green grapes
Kiwi fruit	Brussels sprouts
Red grapes	Scallions
Squash (zucchini, pumpkin, butternut, etc.)	Green beans
Bell peppers (red, orange, green, yellow)	Orange
Greens (spinach, kale, chard, etc.)	Broccoli
Cucumber	Apple
Peas	Mango
Honeydew melon	Peach
Celery	Tomato paste or juice

Tune-Up Tip: Food or Pills?

Increasing your levels of lycopene, lutein, and zeaxanthin can play a central role in protecting against the development of macular degeneration. Although lycopene and lutein supplements are entering the marketplace, they are relatively expensive, especially when you compare them with food sources. Before you check out at the health food store cash register, check this out:

Lycopene Source	Total Dose of lycopene	Cost
1 ounce tomato paste	16 mg	$0.065
Lycopene supplement (three 5 mg capsules)	15 mg	$1.25

In short, it looks as though the cheapest and healthiest way to boost lycopene (and possibly lutein) levels is through diet. Foods rich in the important carotenes for the eye will also be high in vitamin C and other antioxidants.

Zinc plays an essential role in retinal function. Some (but not all) studies report that elderly persons taking zinc supplements have a lower rate of vision loss than those who do not.

Flavonoid-rich extracts improve eye function and are known to prevent macular degeneration. In my opinion, bilberry, *Ginkgo biloba,* and grape seed extracts are completely interchangeable in this application.

Preventing Glaucoma

Your eyeball is filled with fluid (aqueous humor) under a certain amount of pressure, which helps the eye maintain its shape. The pressure can get too high if the fluid builds up and can't flow out of the eye. This condition is called *glaucoma.* If not corrected, glaucoma can lead to pain, loss of vision, and blindness. Glaucoma affects about two million people in the United States, and another twenty-five million have it but don't know it yet. Plan on seeing your ophthalmologist for an annual eye exam that can detect glaucoma in its earliest stage.

There are two kinds of glaucoma. Acute glaucoma involves sudden increases in pressure, usually on one side only, causing severe throbbing pain and blurred vision. Often the condition causes nausea and vomiting. Acute glaucoma is an emergency requiring immediate medical treatment. Chronic (or open-angle) glaucoma is more gradual; the pressure builds up over years. No symptoms may be apparent in the early stages, but there is a gradual loss of peripheral vision. If it goes untreated, blindness may result. This type of glaucoma usually results from abnormalities in the supportive tissues of the eye. These tissues are made from a protein called collagen.

By tuning up, you can help regulate the pressure in your eye. You can also provide your body the materials it needs to build sturdy collagen. One substance essential for collagen is vitamin C. The vitamin also appears to play a role in lowering fluid pressure in patients with glaucoma. A daily dose as low as 2,000 mg may provide benefits, but some studies report results only with extremely high doses (35,000 mg).

Taking supplements of bioflavonoids supports normal collagen metabolism. The compounds of special interest in this regard are the anthocyanidins, the blue-red pigments found in berries. These substances enhance the effects of vitamin C and improve the integrity of blood vessels. What's more, they improve collagen by preventing free-radical damage, by preventing enzymes from breaking it down, and by linking with collagen fibers to make a sturdier structure. My choice for this purpose is bilberry extract, although *Ginkgo biloba* extract also shows promise in relieving glaucoma. (See page 273 for dosage.)

Other nutrients may be valuable in support of eye health. Magnesium supplementation (600 to 900 mg daily) lowers pressure by blocking calcium, which in turn causes arteries to relax. When the blood vessels relax, fluids flow more normally in and out of the eye. Too, there appears to be a strong association between glaucoma and deficiency of chromium. Maintaining adequate levels of chromium appears to help reduce pressure and improve focusing power. (The recommended daily dosage is 200 mcg.) Animal studies also suggest that omega-3 oils may be important for keeping pressure in the eye at appropriate levels.

Key Steps to Tuning Up Your Brain and Nervous System

- Improve the fatty acid composition of the brain and nerves by boosting consumption of omega-3 fatty acids while reducing the intake of omega-6 fatty acids, animal fats, saturated fats, margarine, and fried foods.
- Increase the intake of high-potassium foods while lowering the intake of salt (sodium).
- Take a high-potency multivitamin and mineral supplement.
- Take additional antioxidants:
  - Vitamin C: 500–1,500 mg per day
  - Vitamin E: 400–800 IU per day
- Exercise your body and your brain.

- Take one of the following:
  - *Gingko biloba* extract (24 percent ginkgo flavonglycosides): 40–80 mg three times per day
  - Bilberry extract (25 percent anthocyanidin content): 40–80 mg three times per day
  - Grape seed extract (95 percent proanthocyanidin content): 150–300 mg per day

Lifestyle Tune-Up #7: Get a Good Night's Sleep

Although we don't completely understand the physiological process of sleep, we know that it is essential for a fully functioning body and mind. Many of the problems that cause people to seek medical care—depression, mental cloudiness, chronic fatigue, overall joint and muscle aches (fibromyalgia)—are in fact the result of, or at least exacerbated by, poor sleep. In my practice, I've found that if I can help patients achieve sound, restful sleep, many of their health-related complaints disappear.

Unfortunately, sleep disturbances are very common. At some point during the course of a year, more than one-half of Americans will experience difficulty falling asleep. For about one-third of the population, insomnia is a regular problem. Each year about ten million prescriptions are written for sleeping aids. Poor or disrupted sleep is dangerous. In one study, healthy male volunteers were deprived of four hours of sleep for a single night. The next day, the activity of certain immune cells (natural killer cells) fell by as much as 30 percent. However, a single good night's sleep restored the cells to their normal level of functioning. Studies on shift workers—those whose job hours change over the course of weeks or months—find that they have more trouble falling and staying asleep. Partly as a result, they suffer more illnesses, have more accidents, and die younger than do people with more stable schedules.

How much sleep you need depends on your individual biological profile. In general, the need for sleep decreases with age. At the age of one year, most babies sleep about fourteen hours a day. Adults average between seven and eight hours. Some of my patients do fine on six hours, while others need nine or more.

Following the general lifestyle recommendations in this book will take you some way toward getting a good night's sleep. For example, learning how to eliminate or cope with stress is important for better sleep. Stress hormones lower your levels of serotonin and melatonin, two important neurotransmitters involved in relaxation and sleep. Avoiding stimulants such as caffeine and nicotine, especially in the evening, takes the buzz out of your system and helps you relax. Exercise also contributes to the quality (duration and depth) of sleep.

Just as your car has a timing mechanism that governs engine activity, inside our brain is a kind of master clock that coordinates the timing of many physiological functions. One important role of sleep is to help orchestrate these various biological rhythms. We achieve optimal health if we keep our rhythms in sync.

Dreams are an important and beneficial component of sleep. Dreaming occurs mostly during the phase of sleep closest to waking. It is marked by rapid eye movements (REM). Experiments have found that people who are deprived of REM sleep, and thus deprived of dreaming, become increasingly irritable, anxious, and depressed. These symptoms disappear when people are once again allowed to enjoy normal sleep.

Here are some suggestions for tuning up the body to improve your quality of sleep.

1. Avoid sleep inhibitors, including caffeine and alcohol.
2. If you eat bedtime snacks, choose whole-grain cereals and breads to keep blood sugar levels steady throughout the night and to increase serotonin levels within the brain.
3. Get regular exercise, but avoid exercising in the two hours before bed.
4. Consider nutritional and supplemental strategies to improve sleep:

   - If you have low levels of melatonin, a hormone that regulates sleep and wakefulness, consider taking melatonin supplements (3 mg at bedtime) or give 5-HTP (50–100 mg at bedtime) a try.
   - Some people benefit by taking plant products known to promote sleep, such as passionflower (300–450 mg of dry powdered extract) or valerian (150–300 mg of powdered extract containing 0.8 percent valerenic acid), forty-five minutes before bedtime.
   - If you have muscle cramps or "restless legs" that disturb sleep, try taking magnesium (250 mg at night) and vitamin E (400–800 IU daily).

CHAPTER 8

Tuning Up Your Bones, Joints, and Muscles

Thanks to our sturdy, flexible musculoskeletal system, we can run along the beach, cuddle a baby, dance the jitterbug. Healthy bones and muscles are crucial for living a full, active life. But too often we neglect these structures. The old adage "Use it or lose it" applies. It's a vicious cycle: If we become inactive as we age, the bones and muscles lose some of their ability to do work. The more capacity they lose, the more inactive we become.

It doesn't have to be that way. There's a lot you can do to tune up your bones, joints, and muscles so that they'll serve you well no matter how long you live. Doing so takes commitment, but the payoffs are worth it: greater strength, more stamina, increased flexibility, and freedom from pain.

The Bones

Bones are not merely inert structures, like the beams or pillars of your house. They are living organs that require nurture and care.

Your bones have several functions. They support the body and protect the soft organs. They permit movement, allowing us to walk, lift, and breathe. Bones also serve as a reservoir for minerals, especially calcium and phosphorus, as well as magnesium and manganese. Like a kind of bank, bones allow us to deposit supplies of minerals and withdraw them later when the body needs them. Finally, and equally important, bone tissue is where most of our blood cells are born.

The human body has 206 bones, ranging from the tiny bones in the ear to the large bones of the upper leg. There are four main kinds of bone: long, short, flat, and irregular. Long bones are found in the arms, legs, and fingers. These bones are covered with a thin membrane containing blood vessels and nerves. Underneath is a hard shell of "ivory" bone. Channels running through the hard bone contain blood vessels, lymph vessels, and nerves. Inside the shell, the bone is soft and spongy. At the center of the bone is a hollow cavity filled with marrow, the fatty tissue in which the red cells, platelets, and most white cells are formed. For this reason, the long bones play a key role in keeping your immune system healthy and functioning.

The other kinds of bone are less complex, containing mostly spongy bone protected by thin layers of hard bone. Short bones are shaped somewhat like dice; you find these in the wrists and ankles. Flat bones are flat, thin, and curved. Ribs and the skull are flat bones. Irregular bones are the vertebrae and hip bones.

Throughout your life, bones constantly add and remove material. This process is called remodeling. Each week you recycle up to 7 percent of your bone mass. Normally, the rate of buildup and breakdown is the same. However, if the amount of bone lost exceeds the amount replaced, the bones become brittle and full of holes. This condition is called osteoporosis, or "porous bones." A similar condition is osteomalacia, or "soft bones." This disorder involves insufficient deposits of calcium, causing the bones to become weak and deformed.

Bone remodeling is controlled in part by hormones, especially parathyroid hormone, secreted by the parathyroid glands, and calcitonin, secreted by the thyroid. Vitamin D stimulates the bones to absorb calcium. Other forces that trigger bone remodeling include stress and gravity. That's why weight-bearing exercise, such as running or weight training, promotes stronger bones.

Osteoporosis

The biggest threat to bone health is osteoporosis, a condition in which the bones lose both their supportive tissue (collagen matrix) and mineral content. Beginning in young adulthood, around age twenty-five, the bones become less efficient at absorbing and holding on to minerals. Normally, after the age of forty, there is a significant decrease in bone mass. The bones become less dense and less flexible, increasing the risk of fracture. Just about any bone in the skeleton can be affected, but bone loss is usually greatest in the hips, spine, and ribs. For women, menopause accelerates this process. By the age of seventy, women may have lost up to 50 percent of their original bone mass and men may have lost 25 percent. (Women have about 30 percent less bone mass to begin with.)

Osteoporosis affects more than twenty million people in the United States. Both men and women are at risk, but the risk for women is higher (see Table 8-1). That's partly due to the fact that during menopause their bodies no longer produce enough estrogen, a hormone involved in maintaining bone mass.

Table 8-1: Major Risk Factors for Osteoporosis in Women

Family history of osteoporosis	Low calcium intake
Gastric or small-bowel resection	Nulliparity (never having been
Heavy alcohol use	pregnant)
Hyperparathyroidism	Postmenopause
Hyperthyroidism	Premature menopause (menopause
Inactivity	before the age of 40)
Leanness	Short stature and small bones
Long-term corticosteroid therapy	Smoking
Long-term use of anticonvulsants	White or Asian race

A diet deficient in calcium can also contribute to the problem. Other causes include hormonal disorders such as Cushing's syndrome, which results in increased production of adrenal hormones, or prolonged treatment with corticosteroid drugs. Smoking and excess consumption of alcohol also increase the risk.

Each year in this country at least 1.5 million fractures result from osteoporosis. The most serious of these are usually hip fractures, of which there are 250,000 annually. These fractures can require long-term care in rehabilitation centers or nursing homes. Hip fracture can be fatal in up to 20 percent of cases. Nearly one-third of women and one-sixth of men will fracture a hip at least once in their lifetime.

ASSESSING YOUR RISK FOR OSTEOPOROSIS

Choose the item in each category that best describes you, and fill in the point value for that item in the space to the right. In categories marked with an asterisk (*), you may choose more than one item; total the point values of the items you choose and write this total in the space to the right.

Frame Size	**Points**
Small frame	10
Medium frame, very lean	5
Medium frame, average or heavy build	0
Large frame, very lean	5
Large frame, heavy build	0
Score	_____

Ethnic Background

Caucasian	10
Asian	10
Other	0
Score	_____

Activity Level

How often do you walk briskly, jog, engage in aerobics/sports, or perform hard physical labor for at least thirty continuous minutes?

Seldom	30
1–2 times per week	20
3–4 times per week	5
5 or more times per week	0
Score	_____

Smoking

Smoke 10 or more cigarettes a day	20
Smoke fewer than 10 cigarettes a day	10
Quit smoking	5
Never smoked	0
Score	_____

Personal Health Factors*

Family history of osteoporosis	20
Long-term corticosteroid use	20
Long-term anticonvulsant use	20
Drink more than 3 glasses of alcohol each week	20

Drink more than 1 cup of coffee per day	10
Seldom get outside in the sunlight	10
Score	_____

For Women Only

Had ovaries removed	10
Premature menopause	10
Had no children	10
Score	_____

Dietary Factors*

Consume more than 4 ounces of meat on a daily basis	20
Drink soft drinks regularly	20
Consume the equivalent of 3–5 servings of vegetables each day	−10
Consume at least 1 cup of green leafy vegetables each day	−10
Take 1,000 mg of supplemental calcium	−10
Consume a vegetarian diet	−10
Score	_____

Total Score

_____

Interpreting Your Score

If your score is greater than 50, you are at significant risk for osteoporosis. However, you can take steps to reduce or eliminate risk factors. Start an exercise program; quit smoking; do not drink alcohol, coffee, or soft drinks (these leach calcium from the bones); take a good calcium supplement; and consume a diet relatively low in protein and high in vegetables. These changes could take as many as 150 points off your total score.

If you are a woman at high risk for osteoporosis, hormone replacement therapy after menopause may be appropriate for you, especially if you experienced an early menopause, had your ovaries surgically removed, or never had children. Both estrogen and progesterone have been shown to protect against bone loss. In women with established bone loss, these hormones may actually increase bone mass.

In my opinion, for women who are at risk of osteoporosis or who have already experienced significant bone loss, the benefits of hormone therapy outweigh the risks. The exception is in women at high risk for breast cancer or women with a disease aggravated by estrogen, such as active liver disease or certain cardiovascular diseases. In these cases, a more natural approach is a better choice. This may involve using black cohosh extract or other approaches detailed in Chapter 10, or using a special flavonoid known as ipriflavone (discussed on page 285). Whatever approach is used, conventional hormone therapy or alternative therapies, it is essential that such women be properly monitored and evaluated for osteoporosis.

Monitoring Bone Loss

I recommend that all women have a baseline bone density study by the age of forty. Of course, there is nothing wrong with getting a bone density test in your twenties, especially if you are at high risk. I use the test in men only if there is some factor that may predispose them to osteoporosis such as long-term use of prednisone or other corticosteroid.

The bone density test assesses how much bone mass you currently have. The test will tell you whether you need to make an even more serious effort to maintain your bone. Information from the test can be used in later years to measure the rate at which bone loss occurs. Of course, a bone density determination may also tell you that you already have osteoporosis.

The technique I recommend is dual-energy X-ray absorptiometry, or DEXA for short. This method is safe, because it involves only low doses of X rays. The information it provides is invaluable.

Once you know your current bone density, the next step is to monitor how fast your bones are breaking down. The easiest way to do this is to measure the products of bone loss in the urine. The tests I recommend are Osteomark-NTX and OsteoCheck. The Osteomark-NTX (also known as urinary cross-linked N-telopeptides of type I collagen) is available through your doctor, while the OsteoCheck is available directly to consumers through BodyBalance. To get this test kit, call 1-888-891-3061, visit www.bodybalance.com, or check to see if your local health food store has it.

I want to stress something here: If you are a woman who cares about her health, it is absolutely essential that you monitor your bone density status and bone turnover.

CASE HISTORY: Saving Karen's Bones

Karen, then forty-nine years old, came to see me because of side effects related to hormone replacement therapy (Premphase) she was taking for menopausal symptoms. She was also concerned that a CT bone density study had demonstrated significant bone loss, even though the Premphase was supposed to protect her bones. She complained of weight gain (12 pounds in the six months since she had been taking Premphase), breast tenderness, and mood instability. I had Karen undergo a baseline Osteomark-NTX, which confirmed that she was losing bone at a rapid rate. I recommended the following program:

- Discontinuation of the Premphase
- A high-potency multiple vitamin and mineral supplement
- Additional calcium and magnesium
- Flaxseed oil, 1 tbsp daily
- Black cohosh extract (Remifemin), two tablets twice daily, with each tablet supplying 1 mg 27-deoxyacteine

Ten weeks after she began my program, Karen came back for a follow-up bone density test. Her results dropped from 44 to 26 units, a highly significant improvement. Karen comes back for bone monitoring every six months. Her results are always below 24, and at one checkup she scored a reassuringly low 21. I attribute this drop primarily to the black cohosh extract, because she was already taking a multiple vitamin and mineral supplement and extra calcium. Remifemin is discussed more fully in Chapter 10.

Preventing Bone Loss

Changes in diet and lifestyle can help you tune up your bones and reduce your risk of osteoporosis. My recommendations are:

- Consume a diet rich in whole, unprocessed foods (whole grains, legumes, vegetables, fruits, nuts, and seeds).
- While consuming enough protein is important, you do not want to overdo it. Protein is a concern in osteoporosis because diets high in protein can accelerate bone loss. Proteins are high in nitrogen and phosphorus. To buffer against these compounds, the body tends to pull calcium from bone. Keep protein intake below 100 g daily.
- Increase consumption of soy foods. Soy contains plant substances, known as phytoestrogens, that act like estrogen in the body. These include genistein and diadzein. These substances enhance the positive effects of calcitonin on calcium metabolism and appear to protect against osteoporosis.
- Eliminate the intake of alcohol, caffeine, and sugar. Intake of these substances speeds up the rate of calcium loss from the body.
- Do not drink sodas or other soft drinks. In addition to their high sugar content, soft drinks are a hazard because they contain phosphates that tend to pull calcium from the bones (see Tune-Up Tip on page 283).

- Get regular exercise. Weight-bearing exercise puts healthy stress on the bones; to cope with the increased load, the bones work to boost their mass. Muscle activity pulls on bones, which increases their strength and vitality. Exercise picks up the pace at which the cardiovascular system delivers nutrients and oxygen to bones and carries away waste. It's never too late to begin exercising. The sooner you start, the better the impact will be on your bones.

Tune-Up Tip: Stay Away from Soft Drinks

One of the best things you can do for your bone health is to stay away from soft drinks. Besides providing unwanted sugar, soft drinks contain phosphates (phosphoric acid). The high phosphate level is required for dissolving the sugar and contributing to the taste. When phosphate levels are high and calcium levels are low, calcium is pulled out of the bones. The phosphate content of soft drinks such as Coca-Cola and Pepsi is very high, and they contain virtually no calcium.

It appears that increased soft-drink consumption is a major factor contributing to osteoporosis. The United States ranks first among countries in soft-drink consumption, with per capita intake in excess of 150 quarts per year, or about 3 quarts per week.

The Great Milk Debate

The main source of calcium in the American diet is dairy products, but it is debatable how effective milk is in strengthening bones. While numerous clinical studies have demonstrated that calcium supplementation can slow down bone loss, it is less certain that high dietary calcium intake from milk prevents osteoporosis and bone fractures. People in countries with the highest dairy intake have the highest rate of hip fractures per capita. Hip fractures most often occur as a result of osteoporosis.

In analyzing data from the Nurses' Health Study, a study involving 77,761 women, researchers found no evidence that higher intakes of milk actually reduced fracture incidence. In fact, women who drank two or more glasses of milk per day had a 45 percent higher risk for hip fracture compared with women consuming one glass or less per week. In other words, the more milk consumed, the more likely a woman would experience a hip fracture. On the whole, despite what the dairy industry tells us, research simply does not support the idea that "every body needs milk." How, then, should you get the calcium you need? Studies support the notion that sources of calcium from plant foods may be much more protective than milk. Plant foods rich in calcium include tofu, kale, spinach, turnip greens, and other green leafy vegetables. These foods also contain vitamin K, which helps a protein in the bone, called osteocalcin, to "join hands" with calcium atoms, thus holding the calcium more securely within the bone. Studies have found that the higher the level of vitamin K, the lower the risk of osteoporosis and hip fracture. The bottom line is that if you want to have healthy bones, do what cows do—eat greens.

Calcium Supplements

Which form of supplemental calcium is best? Calcium bound to citrate or lactate, fumarate, malate, succinate, and aspartate appears to be the best overall in ensuring absorption by the body. However, refined calcium carbonate is also an excellent form for the majority of women. Calcium carbonate is the form of calcium available in Tums, an over-the-counter remedy for excess stomach acid that is also promoted as a good source of calcium for preventing osteoporosis.

The only exception to calcium carbonate being used as a calcium supplement is in people with low output of stomach acid. Studies have found that people with low stomach acid absorb only about 4 percent of an oral dose of calcium carbonate, while a person with normal stomach acid absorbs about 22 percent. In contrast, people with low acid levels absorb up to 45 percent of a dose of calcium citrate. Calcium citrate is also more bioavailable, which means your tissues take up this form more readily.

The better bone-building nutritional formulas combine calcium carbonate and a more easily absorbed form such as calcium citrate. These combinations make sense. Why? Well, first of all, the net absorption of calcium provided by the combination is roughly identical whether you have normal or low stomach acid output. But the real reason manufacturers provide a combination is that doing so literally makes the tablets easier to swallow. Calcium citrate takes up more space in a tablet or capsule than calcium carbonate. You'd have to take four to six times as many tablets to provide 1,000 mg of calcium citrate as you would for carbonate. So, a combination provides the best solution. An effective dosage for supplemental calcium is 600 to 1,200 mg per day for most women. If there is significant bone loss, the dosage needs to be in the 1,000 to 1,500 mg range.

There are some forms of calcium that I strongly urge you to avoid because they tend to have high levels of lead. These forms are natural oyster shell calcium, dolomite, and bone meal products, including microcrystalline hydroxyapatite.

Vitamin D can be helpful in utilizing calcium, especially for elderly

people living in nursing homes, people living farther away from the equa-
tor, and those who do not regularly get outside to get their daily dosage of
vitamin D from sunlight. I recommend a dosage of 400 IU daily. Going
above this level offers no significant benefit and may adversely affect
magnesium levels.

Tune-Up Tip: Ostivone (Ipriflavone)

If you are already showing signs of bone loss or have an elevated
Osteomark-NTX or OsteoCheck, I recommend ipriflavone (Ostivone), an exciting new natural approach to maintaining bone health. Several double-
blind studies have shown that this naturally occurring flavonoid (plant
pigment) can dramatically halt the progression of bone loss when used in
combination with 1000 mg of calcium daily. The typical dosage of ipriflavone
is 200 mg three times a day. While ipriflavone is sold as a dietary supplement
in the United States, it is available as a prescription drug for treatment of osteoporosis in countries such as Japan and Italy. If you have osteoporosis, it is
absolutely essential that you be properly monitored. Your health care provider can discuss with you other options in the treatment of osteoporosis.

The Joints

The places where your bones meet are your joints. Joints help hold the
skeleton together, and they also give it mobility. Because of these dual
functions, the joints are the weakest parts in the skeleton.

Fibrous joints, such as those in the skull, are held together by tough
fibers. These joints have little or no movement. *Synovial* joints are those in
which the bones are separated by a fluid-filled membrane, kind of like a
small water balloon. Most of the body's joints are synovial, including those
in the shoulders, elbows, fingers, hips, knees, and toes. *Cartilaginous* joints
are held together by a smooth, springy, rubbery material called cartilage. The
joint between the ribs and the breastbone and the joints between vertebrae
are of this kind, as are the shoulders, elbows, hips, and knees. Your nose
and outer ears do not contain bones; instead they are made of cartilage.

I'd like to describe cartilage in a little more detail, because it is key to understanding many joint problems. Cartilage contains cells that produce giant molecules. These molecules combine to produce a sturdy, flexible, supportive structure called a matrix. The matrix is made of protein fibers, water, and a fluid material called "ground substance," which helps hold cells and fibers in place. What cartilage does not have, and what it does not need, are nerves and blood vessels.

The most abundant protein in cartilage matrix (indeed, in your whole body) is collagen. The word *collagen* comes from the Greek word for "glue." Collagen is also a vital component of bones, tendons, and connective tissue. The cartilage cells secrete ropelike molecules of collagen into the spaces between cells. The collagen binds to cells and other materials to form a tough, stress-resistant material. I'm not kidding when I say this stuff is tough—collagen is stronger than steel.

Cartilage is resilient—it can spring back after pressure is applied. Pressure forces the fluid in it away. When the pressure is released, the fluid flows back and the cartilage springs back to its original shape. This flow of fluid also nourishes the cartilage in the joints, bringing nutrients to the cells. That's why they don't need blood vessels to survive. It's also why long periods of inactivity weaken cartilage. If you don't apply and release pressure, the tissue doesn't get the fluid and nourishment it needs.

WARNING: For any serious joint injury, consult a physician immediately. See a physician if you have severe pain, injuries to the joints, loss of function, or pain persisting for more than two weeks.

ASSESSING YOUR JOINT HEALTH

Circle the number that best describes the intensity of your symptoms on the following scale:

  0 = I do not experience this symptom
  1 = Mild
  2 = Moderate
  3 = Severe

Back pain	0	1	2	3
Swollen knees/elbows	0	1	2	3

Athletic injury	o	I	2	3
Bursitis	o	I	2	3
Tendonitis	o	I	2	3
Joint pain/arthritis	o	I	2	3
Morning stiffness	o	I	2	3
Decreased range of motion or pain on movement	o	I	2	3
Enlarged joints, especially on hands	o	I	2	3
Cracking and popping of joints when in motion	o	I	2	3

Add the numbers circled and enter that total here: _____

Scoring　*7 or more: High priority*
　　　　　　3–6: Moderate priority
　　　　　　1–2: Low priority

Interpreting Your Score

Chances are if you have problems with your joints, you are well aware of it. The results from your assessment will give you an idea of just how much attention to focus on tuning up your joints. If you are over the age of fifty, more than likely you are showing signs of osteoarthritis.

Osteoarthritis

Arthritis means "inflammation of the joint." To be accurate, arthritis is not a disease by itself. Instead it is a symptom arising in many other health problems.

The most common form is osteoarthritis, also called degenerative joint disease. This condition results from loss of cartilage, the shock-absorbing, gel-like material between joints. Risk of osteoarthritis increases with age. By age fifty, perhaps eight of ten people have it to some extent. The joints most often affected are the hands and the weight-bearing joints, such as the knees, hips, and spine.

Primary osteoarthritis is the degenerative "wear and tear" process that occurs in later life. After years of use, the collagen matrix—the support structure of cartilage—seems simply to wear out. Damage to cartilage causes the cells to release enzymes that destroy surrounding tissues. With age, the body loses its ability to repair the damage and produce normal cartilage.

Secondary osteoarthritis can be traced to some other factor, such as inherited abnormalities, trauma due to injury or surgery, or inflammatory joint disease such as rheumatoid arthritis. It appears that use of aspirin or nonsteroidal anti-inflammatory drugs (NSAIDs) may relieve symptoms of osteoarthritis, but at the same time these drugs may inhibit your body's ability to produce cartilage and can contribute to its destruction. Because the incidence of osteoarthritis is higher among women, hormones, especially estrogen, may be a factor. Low thyroid activity also appears to increase risk.

Osteoarthritis sneaks up on you. You might first notice that your joints are a little stiff when you wake up in the morning. Later, you might feel pain when you move the joint; the pain goes away when you rest. Oddly, X rays might show severe joint damage even though you don't feel much pain. Conversely, you might be in excruciating pain even though X rays show little damage.

The best approach to preventing osteoarthritis, or slowing down its progression, is to enhance repair of the collagen matrix and regeneration by connective tissue cells. Dietary, lifestyle, and supplemental strategies all play a role.

- Your diet should be rich in plant foods. Such a diet will be rich in natural antioxidant compounds that can help fight inflammation.
- Reducing the intake of saturated fat and increasing the intake of omega-3 fatty acids from cold-water fish and flaxseed oil can also be helpful in fighting inflammation.
- Lose excess pounds. Losing weight is usually the most effective strategy for preventing stress on the joints.
- Vitamin C is crucial for maintaining healthy joints. One of the most important roles of vitamin C in the body is the manufacture of collagen. A large and important study, the Framingham Osteoarthritis Cohort Study, found that the group of patients taking high doses of vitamin C were only one-third as likely to develop osteoarthritis as those with average vitamin C intake. In addition, vitamin E stimulates formation of new cartilage components and slows the breakdown of cartilage.
- Your body needs vitamins A and B$_6$, zinc, copper, and boron to make and maintain cartilage. Lack of any one of these may speed up the loss of cartilage, while adequate levels promote cartilage repair and synthesis. Copper, for example, is important in the function of an enzyme called lysyl oxidase, which helps collagen bind with another protein called elastin. There are several reports of people who enjoyed complete or near-complete improvement in osteoarthritis symptoms after taking boron in doses of 6 to 9 mg per day.

- Physical exercise is often very helpful in improving joint mobility and reducing pain in osteoarthritis. The best exercises are isometrics, walking, and swimming. Isometric exercise is a technique in which your effort is directed against a resistant object. (As an example, make "hooks" with all the fingers of both hands. Lock the "hooks" together and try to pull them apart.) These types of exercises increase circulation to the joint and strengthen surrounding muscles without placing excessive strain on joints. Increasing muscle strength around joints affected with osteoarthritis has been shown to improve joint function and reduce pain.

- Physical therapy also helps. Among the various treatments available, short-wave diathermy, a method of administering deep heat, may offer benefit. Combining this with periodic ice massage, rest, and exercise appears to be the most effective approach. I have referred some of my osteoarthritis patients for acupuncture, which often provides a significant degree of relief.

Tune-Up Tip: Shedding Light on Nightshade

Some evidence suggests that compounds found in the nightshade family of plants (tomatoes, potatoes, eggplant, peppers, and tobacco) can inhibit collagen repair or promote inflammatory destruction of the joint. (Cows accidentally fed nightshade plants are known to develop a kind of arthritis.) In my practice, I often recommend that patients with osteoarthritis avoid these foods. After a month or so, they can gradually reintroduce them in the diet and see whether symptoms return.

The Promise of Glucosamine Sulfate

Recently there's been a lot of interest in the use of natural products to support the body's production of collagen. The products that have stirred so much excitement are *glucosamine sulfate* and *chondroitin* (pronounced "kon-DROY-tin") *sulfate*. Let me tell you more about these substances and why glucosamine sulfate is the better choice.

Glucosamine is a simple molecule made of glucose (simple sugar) and an amine. Its role in the joint is to stimulate cartilage cells to produce compounds known as glycosaminoglycans (GAGs). These molecules help hold joint tissue together. Glucosamine sulfate also contributes atoms of sulfur, which makes the collagen substances stickier. The firmer the grip collagen molecules have on their neighboring particles, the stronger your joints. With age, it seems that our bodies are less able to manufacture enough glucosamine. That may be why, over time, cartilage becomes less like flexible, shock-absorbing Jell-O and more like rigid rubber.

I have treated many patients with glucosamine sulfate, and for most of them the results have been extremely good. The standard dose is 500 mg three times per day. It can take time for results to appear. After a month of treatment, most patients report much less pain and much better joint movement. To maintain the benefits, it appears necessary to take the substance continuously. People who are obese or who are taking diuretics may need higher doses; I usually recommend taking a daily dose of 20 mg per kilogram (2.2 pounds). Those who have peptic ulcers should take the dose along with meals.

Research shows that glucosamine sulfate is better in the long run than NSAIDs at relieving pain and inflammation. NSAIDs may relieve the symptoms, but glucosamine actually gets in there and fixes the underlying problem. Unlike NSAIDs, glucosamine does not cause side effects. Some patients don't seem to benefit from the use of glucosamine. On the other hand, I have seen it help people who did not respond to other forms of medical treatment.

CASE HISTORY: The Plumber's Helper

Jack, a fifty-six-year-old plumber, could barely walk into my office because his knee was hurting him so. He told me that he dragged himself in because he had read an article I had written on the advantages of glucosamine sulfate over NSAIDs in the treatment of osteoarthritis.

Jack had learned firsthand how destructive these drugs can be. About ten years before, Jack started experiencing osteoarthritis in his left knee. The only thing his medical doctor had to offer was a prescription for ibuprofen (Motrin). When that didn't work, the doctor prescribed more potent NSAIDs, including Voltaren and Feldene. In the ten years he had taken these drugs, Jack's arthritis only got worse. Adding insult to injury, he developed a severe stomach ulcer.

Two weeks before coming to me, Jack had been hospitalized because his ulcer was bleeding. Because things were so bad with his stomach, he had to stop taking Feldene. When he stopped, his knee hurt worse than ever. The acetaminophen (Tylenol) his doctor now prescribed was simply not working. Jack grew desperate and began looking into other options. That's when he read my article on natural alternatives for dealing with osteoarthritis, but he was such a skeptic that he wanted to hear it directly from the horse's mouth. He simply could not imagine that treating osteoarthritis could be as simple as

I professed. I told him that it did not matter if he believed that glucosamine sulfate would work or not—I knew it would. Jack agreed to try.

When he returned six weeks later, he was ecstatic. He was doing deep knee bends and hopping up and down on his left leg to show me how good he felt. He said it was a miracle. He felt so good that the day before he had gone to his medical doctor's office to show off his progress with glucosamine sulfate. His doctor said it was nothing more than a placebo response. Jack had replied, "Doc, if it was just a placebo, then why didn't you prescribe it to me ten years ago instead of giving me all of those damn drugs?" I think Jack had a good point.

I sent the doctor a packet of information on glucosamine sulfate. A week later I received a very nice letter from him. He thanked me and stated that he was unaware of all the double-blind studies supporting the efficacy of glucosamine sulfate. He was also surprised to learn that glucosamine sulfate is an approved medicine in over seventy countries and has been used successfully by millions of people worldwide.

Make sure that you use glucosamine *sulfate*. This formulation contains sulfur, a key component in providing therapeutic benefit. Using glucosamine without sulfate is like trying to build a house with boards but no nails. Studies have shown that other forms of glucosamine, such as glucosamine hydrochloride or n-acetyl-glucosamine, may be no more effective than a placebo. In contrast to these findings, more than twenty published clinical trials with glucosamine sulfate have demonstrated significant improvement in up to 80 percent in various forms of osteoarthritis. In osteoarthritis of the knee the success rate can be even higher.

Some experts recommend using chondroitin sulfate along with glucosamine sulfate. I strongly disagree. Chondroitin sulfate is one of the GAGs, the same sugar-and-protein molecules that glucosamine helps the body produce. However, as I interpret the data, chondroitin sulfate taken orally is not nearly as effective or as fast-acting as glucosamine sulfate. Virtually all of the dose of glucosamine is absorbed, while no more than 13 percent of a dose of chondroitin sulfate is absorbed. This may be simply a matter of physics: Chondroitin molecules are relatively huge, up to three hundred times larger than glucosamine molecules. There is also absolutely no clinical evidence to suggest that the combination provides any greater benefit than glucosamine sulfate alone. Taking the combination simply drains your pocketbook unnecessarily.

CARTILAGE CONCERNS

You may be wondering, "Can I simply consume cartilage as a supplement?" Certainly many people today are taking cartilage extracts, which come from a number of sources: sharks, cows, sea cucumbers, and the green-lipped mussel.

In my opinion, however, these compounds differ in their degree of purity and in their effectiveness at combating osteoarthritis. Composed largely of chondroitin sulfate, cartilage extracts contain big molecules that are hard for the body to absorb. To sum up: Cartilage extracts are like crude ore—there's good stuff in there, but it's harder for your body to find it and make use of it. For rebuilding cartilage and joints, glucosamine sulfate is as good as gold.

A Word on COX-2 Inhibitors

COX is an abbreviation for *cyclooxygenase*. There are two primary cyclooxygenase enzymes: COX-1 and COX-2. COX-1 helps maintain the health of the stomach lining as well as platelet and kidney function. COX-2 is one of several enzymes that lead to the formation of substances that can cause joint and connective tissue problems. Previously available prescription and over-the-counter NSAIDs such as naproxen, diclofenac, ibuprofen, aspirin, and many others inhibit the COX-2 enzyme, but often cause ulcers, bleeding, and other gastrointestinal side effects because they block the COX-1 enzyme as well. This problem has been resolved by the development of "super aspirins" that inhibit only COX-2.

According to a study published in the *American Journal of Medicine*, experts estimate that 107,000 people are admitted to hospitals annually as a result of complications due to the use of NSAIDs, which in some cases can lead to death. Many researchers feel that these problems could be helped with the use of COX-2-specific inhibitors. However, these drugs are not without side effects, mainly gastrointestinal symptoms (abdominal pain, epigastric pain, heartburn, nausea and vomiting), lower extremity swelling, and elevations in blood pressure. Celebrex and Vioxx are the two COX-2 inhibitors that are on the market.

A natural alternative to these drugs is ginger (*Zingiber officinalis*). Ginger appears to exert specific COX-2 inhibition but is not associated with any side effects when taken at normal levels. Ginger has shown very positive effects in preliminary studies in both rheumatoid arthritis and osteoarthritis. There remain many questions concerning the best form of ginger and the proper dosage. I recommend either fresh gingerroot, 20 g

or ²/₃ ounce (roughly a ¹/₂-inch slice) or a highly concentrated ginger extract (Gingerall). Fresh ginger can easily be incorporated into the diet by
putting it through a juicer when making fresh fruit and vegetable juices.
My recommendation for Gingerall is one or two capsules three times
daily with meals.

Other Botanical Strategies for Arthritis

For thousands of years, people all over the world have sought relief
from osteoarthritis and other causes of joint pain by taking herbal products. Because glucosamine sulfate is so successful for osteoarthritis, I
rarely use these botanical approaches in osteoarthritis—they are better
used in more inflammatory cases such as sports injuries and rheumatoid
arthritis. I also will use them in fibromyalgia.

When I do recommend herbal therapy in osteoarthritis, my first recommendation is usually topical applications of menthol-based preparations (such as Tiger Balm, White Flower Essence, Ben-Gay, or Mineral
Ice) or creams containing capsaicin, the pungent and irritating compound from cayenne pepper (*Capsicum frutescens*). Applied to the skin,
capsaicin first stimulates and then blocks transmission in nerve fibers. It
appears to do so by depleting nerves of the neurotransmitter called substance P. By reducing substance P, capsaicin may relieve the pain and
inflammation of arthritis. Capsaicin creams have to be applied every
day, and benefits may take a week or two to become apparent. In contrast,
the menthol-based preparations can provide immediate benefits on an
as-needed basis.

Oral herbal products that can be helpful in reducing joint inflammation due to osteoarthritis or rheumatoid arthritis include ginger, bromelain, curcumin, Phytodolor, and *Boswellia serrata*. Of these, I think ginger,
Phytodolor, and boswellia are the most effective in osteoarthritis. The
others seem to be more useful in sprains, strains, and more inflammatory
forms of arthritis such as rheumatoid arthritis. Phytodolar is a liquid
preparation of three herbal extracts—common ash (*Fraxinus excelsior*),
aspen (*Populus tremula*), and goldenrod (*Solidago virgaurea*)—that has
been used in Germany since 1963 and is now available in the United
States. Like many herbal products from Germany, Phytodolar has excellent validation of its effectiveness. The dosage that I recommend in most
cases is 50 drops in a glass of water three times daily. Since this product
contains natural forms of aspirinlike substances, it should not be used by
people who are allergic to aspirin.

Boswellia preparations have been used for an even longer period of time than Phytodolor, but now there are newer preparations concentrated for the active components (boswellic acids) that are giving even better results in clinical trials. The standard dosage for boswellic acids in arthritis therapy is 400 mg three times daily. No side effects due to boswellic acids have been reported.

Tune-Up Tip: **Devil's Claw for Lower Back Pain**

Recent studies suggest that devil's claw (Harpagophytum procumbens) — an herb native to Africa that has a long history of use in the treatment of arthritis — may be helpful in patients with low back pain. In a recent double-blind study, two daily doses of H. procumbens extract (600 and 1,200 mg, respectively, containing 50 and 100 mg of harpagosides) were compared with placebo over four weeks in 197 patients with chronic low back pain and current flare-ups that were producing pain worse than 5 on a 0–10 scale. The principal outcome measure was the number of patients who were pain free without medication (Tramadol) for five days out of the last week. The results of the study indicated that devil's claw extract standardized for harpagoside content could reduce the need for stronger medication in low back pain without significant side effects; hence it is both safe and effective.

I would recommend a dosage of 600 mg of devil's claw extract, supplying 50 mg of harpagoside, for individuals with chronic cases that are associated with moderate pain, no radiation of the pain, and no loss of nerve function. In people with more severe cases, I would recommend a dosage of 1,200 mg devil's claw extract, supplying at least 100 mg harpagoside.

Rheumatoid Arthritis

Rheumatoid arthritis (RA) involves severe inflammation that causes the joints to become painful, warm, swollen, and stiff. The joints most often affected are the fingers, wrists, ankles, knees, and toes. In severe cases, the joints can become discolored, severely deformed, and virtually useless. Symptoms may come and go. Usually the same joints are affected on both sides of the body. RA typically begins before middle age and develops gradually. Women are perhaps three times more likely to develop RA than men.

RA is an autoimmune disorder, which means your body's immune system begin to attack cells in the joints as if they were invading enemies. Why this happens is not clear. Probably there are many factors involved, including genetic abnormalities, dietary factors, food allergies, bacterial overgrowth, or other digestive problems such as "leaky gut." Your body normally produces steroid hormones that counteract the effects of inflammation. However, some people with RA may have low levels of DHEA, the molecule from which all steroids are made.

There are many treatments available to relieve the symptoms of RA, but clearly the best strategy is to prevent it from developing by making dietary adjustments to avoid the absorption of toxins and allergens by the digestive system, improving detoxification, and tuning up the immune system. For a fuller discussion of RA, see Chapter 5.

Gout

Gout is a common type of arthritis caused by an increased concentration of uric acid (the final breakdown product of purine metabolism— purine is one of the units of DNA and RNA) in biological fluids. In gout, uric acid crystals are deposited in joints, tendons, kidneys, and other tissues, where they cause considerable inflammation and damage. The first attack of gout is characterized by intense pain, usually involving only one joint. The first joint of the big toe is affected in nearly half of the first attacks, and is at some time involved in over 90 percent of individuals with gout. If the attack progresses, fever and chills will appear.

The first attacks usually occur at night and are usually preceded by a specific event, such as dietary excess, alcohol ingestion, trauma, certain drugs (mainly chemotherapy drugs, certain diuretics, and high dosages of niacin), or surgery.

Subsequent attacks are common, with the majority of gout patients having another attack within one year. However, nearly 7 percent never have a second attack. Chronic gout is extremely rare these days, due to the advent of dietary therapy and drugs that lower uric acid levels. The dietary treatment of gout involves the following guidelines:

- *Elimination of alcohol intake.* Alcohol increases uric acid production by accelerating purine breakdown. It also reduces uric acid excretion by increasing lactate production, which impairs kidney function. The net effect is a significant increase in serum uric acid levels. This explains why alcohol consumption is often a trigger in acute attacks of gout. Elimination of alcohol is all that is needed to reduce uric acid levels and prevent gouty arthritis in many individuals.

- *Low-purine diet.* Foods with high purine levels should be entirely omitted. These include organ meats, other meats, shellfish, yeast (brewer's and baker's), herring, sardines, mackerel, and anchovies. Intake of foods with moderate levels of purine should be limited. These include dried legumes, spinach, asparagus, fish, poultry, and mushrooms.
- *Achievement of ideal body weight.* Weight reduction in obese individuals significantly reduces serum uric acid levels.
- *Reduced consumption of sugar and refined carbohydrates.* Simple sugars (refined sugar, honey, maple syrup, corn syrup, fructose, etc.) increase uric acid production.
- *Low saturated fat intake.* Saturated fats decrease uric acid excretion.
- *Low protein intake.* A high protein intake increases uric acid manufacture.
- *Increased water consumption.* Drinking lots of water—at least 48 ounces each day—keeps the urine diluted and promotes uric acid excretion.

Tune-Up Tip: Cherry Diet Cure for Gout

Consuming half a pound of fresh or canned cherries per day has been shown to be very effective in lowering uric acid levels and preventing attacks of gout. Cherries, hawthorn berries, blueberries, and other dark red-blue berries are rich sources of anthocyanidins and proanthocyanidins. These compounds are flavonoid molecules that give these fruits their deep color and are remarkable in their ability to prevent collagen destruction. In addition, these flavonoids are good antioxidants and inhibit the formation of inflammatory compounds. In addition to consuming flavonoid-rich berries, extracts of bilberry, grape seed, or pine bark can be used, or you can use pills containing the flavonoid quercetin. This flavonoid has demonstrated several effects in experimental studies that indicate its possible benefit to individuals with gout including inhibiting uric acid. For best results, 200 to 400 mg of quercetin should be taken with bromelain between meals three times daily. Bromelain, an enzyme derived from pineapple, may help to enhance the absorption of quercetin as well as exerting anti-inflammatory effects of its own.

—————— **Tendinitis and Bursitis** ——————

The tendons are the connective tissues that link your muscles to your bones. If you stretch a tendon too far, its cells release inflammatory substances. The result is tendinitis, which causes such symptoms as pain, swelling, and redness. The tendons usually affected are those in the ankle, shoulder, thumb, knee, and foot.

The bursa is the membrane sac found in the joints that contains lubricating fluid. Trauma, strain, infection, or arthritis can cause the sac to become inflamed. The result: bursitis. The joints most often affected are the shoulder, elbow, hip, and knee.

Not surprisingly, the people who are most likely to develop these problems are athletes. But trained athletes know they should warm up and stretch before beginning vigorous physical activity. The people most at risk are the weekend sports enthusiasts, whose bodies may not be quite as ready to plunge into a game of pick-up basketball or a sweaty round of tennis. The best way to tune up your tendons prior to exercise is to take at least ten minutes to warm up.

In most cases, tendinitis and bursitis clear up by themselves after a week or two. But if you keep overstretching the tendon or damaging the bursa, the problem can become chronic. Calcium salts may be deposited in the tendon fibers, causing them to become stiff and inflexible.

If you develop these problems, be sure you get adequate levels of vitamins A, C, and E, because these are crucial for proper healing. Along with these vitamins, zinc and selenium are necessary for their antioxidant properties. Vitamin B_{12}, given as an injection in the muscles, may relieve pain and help break up calcium deposits.

The plant pigments called flavonoids reduce inflammation, stabilize collagen, block enzymes that break down collagen, and prevent free-radical damage. Bromelain, an anti-inflammatory enzyme from pineapple, may relieve pain by reducing swelling. I usually use it in combination with curcumin, the yellow pigment in the spice turmeric. Curcumin has potent anti-inflammatory and antioxidant effects. A dosage of 200 to 400 mg of each three times per day is effective. Be sure to take this combination on an empty stomach.

Tune-Up Tip: RICE Is Nice

When you suffer from a sports injury, remember the RICE formula:
- Rest the injured part

- Ice the area of pain
- Compress the area with an elastic bandage
- Elevate the part above the level of the heart

The ice and compress should be applied for thirty minutes. Remove the ice and compress for fifteen minutes to allow blood flow to return. After the acute inflammatory stage (24 to 48 hours), do gentle stretching and flexibility exercises to gradually increase the range of motion. These exercises maintain and improve mobility and prevent adhesions (abnormal scar formation).

The Muscles

The word *muscle* comes from the Latin *mus,* meaning "mouse," because the movement of muscles beneath the skin looked—to some anatomists, anyway—like little mice scurrying around. About half of your body's mass is muscle. Muscle tissue is beautifully designed to carry out its main task: transforming chemical energy into movement.

There are three main kinds of muscles. Skeletal muscles move the bones and thus your body. You have about six hundred different skeletal muscles. Muscles of the internal organs (also called smooth muscles) work to force fluids and other substances through various channels. For example, your blood vessels are wrapped in a muscle layer that permits them to expand and contract. Your intestines depend on rhythmic contractions (peristalsis) to move food along. The air passages also contain smooth muscle. The third type of muscle, cardiac muscle (or myocardium), is found only in the heart.

Each type of muscle has a structure that allows it to do its specific job. Skeletal muscles contain long narrow groups, or bundles, of fibers arranged in an orderly way. Large muscles (such as the one you're sitting on right now) may have hundreds of these bundles, while small ones have only a few. Each bundle contains a smaller set of long muscle fibers. To picture this, imagine that you cut a bunch of rubber bands and lay them out lengthwise. These are the myofibrils. Now wrap some of those in a protective sheet. This is a muscle fiber. Collect a bunch of those wrapped bundles into a group, and *voilà*—a muscle. The wrapping around each fiber and around each bundle is made of collagen.

Smooth muscle is different. It is made of long, tapering cells that are loosely woven together. Many of your hollow organs, such as the intestines, have two layers of smooth muscle. In one layer, the cells run alongside the organ. In the other layer, the cells form a ring around it. Having two layers allows rhythmic contractions that move along the length of the vessel as well as squeezing contractions that occur at specific sites.

Cardiac muscle is similar to skeletal muscle, in that it contains fibers and myofibrils. But the cells are short, branching, and interconnected. This design helps the muscle more effectively distribute the electrical signals that cause the heart to beat.

Movements of the skeletal muscles are under voluntary control. In contrast, you can't control the smooth muscles or the contractions of your heart. That's why these are also called the involuntary muscles.

Muscles respond to signals from nerves. Each single muscle fiber has its own personal nerve ending, giving it a direct connection to the brain. The nerve releases a neurotransmitter called acetylcholine. This stimulates electrical activity in the fluid surrounding the muscle cells. The electrical signals cause muscle fibers to contract. The fibers contain two types of protein filaments, actin and myosin. When they receive an electrical buzz, the myosin filaments slide over the actin filaments, causing the muscle to contract. Other signals tell the filaments to relax. In a way, the filaments resemble a firefighter's ladder, the segments of which can be extended or shortened.

In the body, electrical signals can travel efficiently only if the fluid surrounding the cells has the right balance of sodium, potassium, and calcium. Without enough potassium, signals slow down, leading to muscle weakness. Loss of calcium causes uncontrolled muscle activity, or spasms.

The muscles are attached to the bones by connective tissues called tendons. When the muscle contracts, it pulls the tendon, which in turn pulls the bone.

ASSESSING YOUR MUSCLE HEALTH

Circle the number that best describes the intensity of your symptoms on the following scale:

   0 = I do not experience this symptom
   1 = Mild
   2 = Moderate
   3 = Severe

Muscle spasms	0	1	2	3
Tightness in shoulder muscles	0	1	2	3
Muscle cramps	0	1	2	3
Pain in arms, hands	0	1	2	3
Leg cramps at night	0	1	2	3
Stiffness all over	0	1	2	3
Stiffness in morning	0	1	2	3
Inability to sit straight	0	1	2	3
Pain in neck and/or shoulders	0	1	2	3
Soreness after working out	0	1	2	3
Muscle weakness	0	1	2	3

Add the numbers circled and enter that total here: _____

Scoring   8 or more: High priority
         3–7: Moderate priority
         1–2: Low priority

Interpreting Your Score

If you scored 8 or more, I encourage you to consult a chiropractor or medical doctor who specializes in physical medicine (a physiatrist). A score of 3 to 7 indicates that you need to devote some attention to tuning up your muscles while a score of 1 or 2 indicates that you may only need to follow the most basic recommendations to improve or maintain proper functioning of your muscles.

Exercise: It Is Never Too Late to Start

Exercise benefits just about every one of your body functions. It stimulates the metabolism, promotes good digestion, boosts the immune system, and keeps your cardiovascular system in fine fettle.

But the tissues that benefit most directly are the muscles. When forced to do work, muscle cells respond by becoming larger, longer, and stronger, so that they are better able to handle their tasks. That's why your biceps bulge from weight lifting and your calf muscles expand from running. Your heart, another muscle, grows larger and stronger when you perform regular strenuous exercise. The biggest growth occurs in the left ventricle, the chamber responsible for sending blood to just about every tissue in your body.

The bones also benefit from weight-bearing exercise, because movement ratchets up their ability to absorb calcium, making them stronger and more durable. Astronauts—who are very physically fit—experience bone loss and muscle atrophy during weightless flights, even those lasting just a few days.

Like other cells, muscle cells rely on ATP, the energy molecule. During aerobic exercise, your cells burn a tremendous amount of oxygen—up to twenty times your normal rate—to release the energy from ATP and stored sugar (glycogen). This need for oxygen is one reason why you breathe so hard. The other reason is that your body needs to get rid of the toxic products that result from all this activity, especially lactic acid (the stuff that makes your muscles tingle and itch during a workout). Exercise speeds up the heart rate to circulate more blood to the lungs and skin, so the toxins can be exhaled or sweated away faster.

In contrast, weight lifting and other similar exercises do not require a huge upsurge in oxygen intake. Such exercises are called anaerobic, or isotonic.

It's possible to exercise too much. Stressing muscle cells causes them to break down. Seen under a microscope, overstressed muscle cells show signs of tears and bleeding. No wonder a good workout can leave you feeling sore.

Healing occurs promptly, however, and the repaired cells are stronger than they were. That's why many exercise experts recommend exercising only every other day—your body needs that rest time to repair the muscles. Prolonged vigorous exercise also uses up most of the sugar (glycogen) stored in the muscles, and it takes a while for muscles to build up their energy supply again.

For exercise to be effective, you need to keep at it for the rest of your life. The size and efficiency of muscle cells decrease rapidly once you stop. However, soon after you start exercising again, the muscles quickly return to their former state of fitness.

Tune-Up Tip: Boost DHEA to Increase Muscle Strength

The benefits and risks of DHEA supplementation have been described on page 246. A group of researchers from the University of California at San Diego previously reported that administration of a 50 mg dose of DHEA daily for three months to men and women between the ages of fifty and sixty-five resulted in significant improvement of physical and psychological well-being. One of the findings in men was an increase in muscle strength, thought to be the result of DHEA's elevation of serum levels of insulin-like growth factor I (IGF-I)—an important stimulator of muscle growth and strength. As stated in other chapters, DHEA supplementation should be tailored to the individual. Blood or salivary DHEA determinations can be used in this goal (see page 246 for more information).

Tune-Up Tip: Antioxidants for Muscle Soreness After Exercise

During exercise a great deal of metabolic waste products are produced, including lactic acid, ammonia, and lipid peroxides. These waste products contribute greatly to feelings of muscle soreness. Therefore, in an effort to reduce soreness, the focus is on enhancing the elimination and detoxification of these substances.

In addition to replacing lost water and electrolytes, the foremost strategy in the attempt to reduce muscle soreness is the use of antioxidant nutrients such as vitamins C and E. In a recent double-blind study, 1,000 mg of vitamin C three times daily was shown to reduce muscle soreness after exercise by at least 33 percent in over half of the subjects.

Tune-Up Tip: B Vitamins for Nighttime Leg Cramps

Nighttime leg cramps are extremely common—one survey found that 70 percent of elderly subjects had experienced them at one time or another. According to a recent clinical study, simply taking more B vitamins can bring relief to nearly nine out of ten people. In the study, twenty-eight elderly patients were given a placebo or vitamin B complex (30 mg B_6, 50 mg thiamin, 5 mg riboflavin, and 250 mcg B_{12}) for three months. While 86 percent of the B complex group eliminated the leg cramps, the placebo showed absolutely no benefit.

In addition to the B vitamins, I would also recommend taking magnesium (250 mg) and vitamin E (400 to 800 IU daily). And, if you are over the age of fifty, *Ginkgo biloba* extract (80 mg three times daily) may also be helpful.

— Fibromyalgia and Chronic Fatigue Syndrome —

Many patients come to me complaining of an overall feeling of pain, aches, and fatigue. They have trouble putting their finger on the problem because it sometimes seems as if every muscle and joint in their body is affected. Conventional medicine, frustrated by the vagueness of the symptoms, often assumes that these patients don't really have a medical condition—that the problem is all in their head.

The situation is changing. More and more, doctors are realizing that their patients are struggling with a real condition known as fibromyalgia. The term means "pain in the muscles and connective tissue." Fibromyalgia is common, affecting perhaps 6 percent of the population. In most cases it develops between the ages of twenty and sixty. Three out of four sufferers are women.

Fibromyalgia causes generalized pain usually affecting the neck, shoulders, lower back, hips, shins, elbows, or knees. There are a dozen "pressure points" that are typically affected by the pain of fibromyalgia. The pain is usually worse in the morning. In most cases, the pain is so great that it seriously disrupts sleep. Since sound sleep is crucial for good health, anything that causes sleep disturbances must be addressed. Other possible symptoms include headaches, poor concentration, dizziness, numbness, and tingling.

A related but different condition is chronic fatigue syndrome, or CFS. The main difference is that fibromyalgia involves pain in the skeletal muscles (but not necessarily fatigue), while CFS causes overwhelming fatigue (but not necessarily pain). Some patients with CFS are hardly able to get out of bed in the morning. In certain ways CFS resembles a flulike illness, but we don't yet know whether a virus is the cause. CFS may result from an overeager immune system.

Studies suggest that many patients with fibromyalgia and chronic fatigue have low levels of serotonin. Serotonin is the neurotransmitter involved in regulating mood, sleep, and many other functions. Supplementation with 5-HTP, a form of tryptophan that is converted to serotonin in the body, has shown very good results in improving fibromyalgia. I typically recommend 50 mg of 5-HTP along with 300 mg of standardized St. John's wort and 150 to 250 mg of magnesium three times daily for fibromyalgia.

One of the most important things you can do for your overall health is make sure you get enough sleep. Establish a regular bedtime and stick to it. Avoid stimulants such as caffeine, especially at night.

Again, exercise is important. Of course, tired people with aching muscles seldom feel like exercising, but the health benefits are too great to pass up. Gentle exercise each day is the best—tai chi, "aquacise" (a watery workout that avoids putting too much stress on muscles and joints), yoga, and walking are good choices. I also recommend bodywork (see box) for these patients.

BODYWORK

I have found bodywork to be extremely valuable in helping my patients with fibromyalgia. *Bodywork* is a general term referring to therapies involving touch, including various massage techniques, chiropractic spinal adjustment and manipulation, Rolfing, reflexology, shiatsu, and many more. In most cases, the gentle techniques such as Trager massage, Feldenkrais, and Alexander technique seem to be most helpful.

Trager massage was the innovation of Milton Trager, M.D. According to Trager, we all develop mental and physical patterns that may limit our movements or contribute to fatigue, pain, and tension. During a typical session, the practitioner gently and rhythmically rocks, cradles, and moves the client's body to encourage the client to see that freedom of movement and relaxation are entirely possible. The aim of the treatment is not so much to massage or manipulate, but rather to promote feelings of lightness, freedom, and well-being. Clients are also taught a series of exercises to do at home. Called Mentastics, these simple, dancelike movements help clients maintain and enhance the feelings of flexibility and freedom they experienced during the sessions.

The Feldenkrais method and the Alexander technique involve a practitioner who guides the patient to become aware of posture and habitual limited-movement patterns and to replace them with more optimal movements. The participant learns the difference between muscular tension and relaxation and is shown how different postures feel either restricted or free.

For information on these "gentler" therapies, or to find a practitioner near you, contact:

The Trager Institute
33 Millwood
Mill Valley, CA 94941
1-415-388-2688

North American Society of Teachers of the Alexander Technique
P.O. Box 517
Urbana, IL 61801
1-800-473-0620

Feldenkrais Guild
706 SW Ellsworth Street
Albany, OR 97231
800-775-2118

Key Steps to Tuning Up Your Bones, Joints, and Muscles

Make healthy and strong bones, joints, and muscles a lifelong priority. Begin now by paying careful attention to diet. Talk to your physician about starting an exercise program that's appropriate for you.

- Engage in weight-bearing exercise for at least twenty minutes three times per week.
- Eat a healthy diet, being careful to limit factors that increase calcium excretion, such as salt, sugar, protein, and soft drinks.
- Increase your intake of cold-water fish and take 1 tbsp flaxseed oil per day.
- Lose excess weight.
- Use a high-potency multivitamin and mineral supplement and take additional antioxidants.
- Eat flavonoid-rich foods such as cherries, berries, and citrus, or take flavonoid-rich extracts such as bilberry, grape seed, or pine bark.
- Develop a stretching program (see Lifestyle Tune-Up #8, following this chapter).

306 TUNING UP YOUR BONES, JOINTS, AND MUSCLES

Lifestyle Tune-Up #8: Stretch to Stay Flexible (and Young)

One of the best habits you can develop is stretching: taking your joints through their entire range of motion and stretching the major muscle groups of the body.

My introduction to stretching came in 1980 when a friend of mine gave me the book *Stretching,* by Bob Anderson and Jean Anderson. This husband-and-wife team has been a real driving force in helping people understand the importance of stretching. In 1968, at the age of twenty-three, Bob began a personal physical fitness program, since he felt he was overweight and out of shape. He changed his diet, started eating less, and began running and cycling. His weight went from 190 to 135 pounds over a period of time, and he soon was in much better physical condition. One day, while in a conditioning class, he discovered he could not reach much past his knees in a straight-legged sitting position. After discovering how tight he was, Bob started stretching. In several months he became much more limber; he found that stretching made running, cycling, and other activities easier and more enjoyable and that it eliminated most of the muscular soreness that usually accompanies strenuous physical exertion.

After several years of exercising and stretching with Jean and a small group of friends, Bob gradually developed a method of stretching that could be taught to anyone. Soon he was teaching his technique to others. He began working with professional sports teams, then college teams, other amateur athletes, and a variety of people at sports medicine clinics, racquetball clubs, athletic clubs, and running gear stores throughout the country.

Bob and Jean first published *Stretching* in 1975 and in four years sold over thirty-five thousand copies by mail. The revised version was published in 1980 by Shelter Publications and has now sold over two million copies. Although there are now other excellent books on the market on stretching, I encourage you to get Bob and Jean's book. It is a great guide.

I must admit that even though I knew the value of stretching, I really didn't appreciate it until I turned forty a few years ago. When I started thinking about how I felt at forty compared to twenty or thirty,

I realized that my body did not feel as flexible as it had earlier. I knew that I had to really make stretching more of a priority. I am happy to tell you that it has really paid off.

Another stimulus for paying more attention to stretching was seeing how flexible my two young children are and comparing that to how stiff and inflexible most elderly people are. The older people whom I have had as patients and whom I have known personally who are much younger than their years all had excellent flexibility.

When done properly, stretching can do more than just increase flexibility and make you feel younger. The confirmed benefits of stretching include:

- Contributing to physical fitness
- Enhancing the ability to learn and perform skilled movements
- Increasing mental and physical relaxation
- Enhancing the development of body awareness
- Reducing risk of injury to joints, muscles, and tendons
- Reducing muscular soreness and tension
- Reducing joint pain via stimulation of the production of chemicals that lubricate the joints

To gain the benefits of stretching, it is important to follow these simple guidelines.

- Warm up to stretch. Perform some exercises such as push-ups and jumping jacks, or go for a brisk walk to warm up the muscles before you stretch. It is not a good idea to attempt to stretch before your muscles are warm, as it could lead to pulls and tears in the muscle.
- For maximal results, stretch before and after a period of exercise.
- Isolate the particular muscle you are stretching. For example, you are better off trying to stretch one hamstring at a time, rather than both hamstrings at once. By isolating the muscle you are stretching, you experience resistance from fewer muscle groups, which gives you greater control over the stretch and allows you to more easily change its intensity.
- The stretch must be slow and controlled. Do not bob or jerk when stretching; slow and steady is the approach. Hold the stretch for a minimum of fifteen seconds. As you become more flexible, you will be able to hold the stretch longer. But in the beginning, ten seconds may feel like an eternity.

- Breathe during a stretch. The proper way to breathe during a stretch is to inhale slowly through the nose, expanding the abdomen (not the chest); hold the breath a moment; then exhale slowly through the mouth.

- Do not overstretch. Stretch only to the point of discomfort. You should feel tension in your muscle, but not pain. Do not feel you have to gain or regain flexibility all at once. The tortoise approach definitely wins this race. If you stretch properly, you should not be sore the day after. If you are, then it may be an indication that you are overstretching and that you need to go easier on your muscles by reducing the intensity of some (or all) of the stretches you perform. Overstretching can actually reduce flexibility because it can damage the muscles.

Here is a sample stretching routine to get you started:

Low back stretch. Lie on your back. Hug knees to chest.
Neck stretch. Tilt your ear to your shoulder and hold. Repeat other side.
Lateral side stretch. Extend arm overhead, place opposite hand on hip. Bend sideways at hip. Repeat with the other side.
Calf stretch. Keep your back leg straight and heel on the ground. Move your front foot as far forward as you can while keeping your back heel on the ground. Place both hands on your thigh above your bent knee. Move hips forward. Repeat with the other side.
Hamstring stretch. Stand straight, with one leg supporting your weight. Now place the other leg straight in front of you about six inches. Lift the toe of your forward foot off the floor and reach down with your opposite hand to touch it. Repeat on the other side.
Quadriceps stretch. Standing next to something for balance, such as a wall or heavy chair, bend your knee so that one leg is raised behind you and grab hold of your foot. The upper part of the leg should remain in a vertical position as you pull your foot upward. Repeat with the other side.
Triceps stretch. Place a hand behind your head, with your palm touching the middle of your back. Your elbow points up. Push your elbow down with your other hand so that your hand slides down your back. Repeat with the other side.
Full body stretch. Raise your arms over your head, stand on your toes, and reach for the sky. Flex and extend fingers.

CHAPTER 9

Tuning Up Your Skin and Hair

I magine going into a clothing store and seeing a mannequin wearing a special coat. A sign near the mannequin boasts that the coat is water-proof and washable. It's sturdy, but it's also astoundingly flexible—no matter what size you are, it will always fit you perfectly. This remarkable coat automatically adjusts to the outside temperature—when things heat up, it will cool you down; when things get chilly, it will keep you warm. What's more, it automatically darkens to protect you against sunlight. Amazingly, if it suffers small tears or minor burns, it will mend itself in just a few days. Best of all, the manufacturer guarantees that if you give it a modicum of care, the coat will last you a lifetime.

Sounds good, yes? It probably won't surprise you when I tell you that you already own this coat. You call it your skin. And it will serve you well for years—as long as you keep it in tune.

Collectively, the skin and its associated tissues—oil and sweat glands, hair, and nails—are known as the integumentary system. *Integumentary* means "covering." But the skin is more than just an inert wrapping that holds your body together. It is a complex living organ that serves many functions.

Complete the self-assessment to get a sense of how healthy your in-tegumentary system is. Then we'll look more closely at the main parts of this system and how you can keep them well tuned.

ASSESSING SKIN AND HAIR HEALTH

Circle the number that best describes the intensity of your symptoms on the following scale:

0 = I do not experience this symptom
1 = Mild
2 = Moderate
3 = Severe

Dry, scaly skin	0	1	2	3
Dry hair and scalp	0	1	2	3
Weak, brittle, or cracked nails	0	1	2	3
Cracked or dry lips	0	1	2	3
Acne	0	1	2	3
Thin, translucent skin	0	1	2	3
Buildup of protein in hair follicles on back of arms	0	1	2	3
Easy bruising	0	1	2	3
Dry eyes and/or mouth	0	1	2	3
Lack of radiance of hair and skin	0	1	2	3

Add the numbers circled and enter that total here: _____

Scoring   *8 or more: High priority*
       3–7: Moderate priority
       1–2: Low priority

Interpreting Your Score

Radiant, vibrant, and healthy-looking skin and hair have long been associated with good health. While most people try to improve the appearance of their hair from the outside alone, the real key to healthy skin and beautiful hair is building it from the inside out through good nutrition. Skin and hair follicles are living tissue. And, like all living tissue, they need proper nourishment.

Since hair and nails are derived from skin cells, the nutrients required for healthy skin are the same nutrients required for healthy hair and nails. Adequate levels of B vitamins, minerals, essential fatty acids, and amino acids are all required.

Skin

Skin accounts for about 7 percent of your weight. If you were to peel the skin off an average-sized person and lay it on the ground, it would cover about twenty-one square feet—about the size of the top of a twin mattress. It varies in thickness from one to four mm, or about one-sixteenth of an inch at most.

Thin as it is, the skin is composed of several layers. The outermost portion is the epidermis, which serves as the body's main protective shield. Below that is the dermis, a thicker layer where most of the skin's business goes on. Below the dermis is the subcutaneous tissue, which contains larger blood vessels and fat cells.

The epidermis is itself made of four layers (five in areas with thicker skin). Most of the cells in the topmost layer produce a tough, fibrous protein called keratin. These cells are born in the dermis and migrate upward. By the time they reach the surface they are no longer living. Instead they are like tiny scales that protect the more delicate layers below. Each day you shed millions of these dead cells through washing or abrasion. (Much of the dust in your house is actually dead skin cells.) As you slough them off, new cells rise to take their place. You grow a new epidermis every five to seven weeks. Sweat and oil made in glands in the dermis emerge onto the skin from tiny openings in the epidermis called pores.

The epidermis contains white blood cells (macrophages) as well as cells that connect to nerve endings and that register sensations of touch. Also found in the epidermis are pigment cells (melanocytes). These cells secrete a pigment called melanin. The keratin cells absorb the pigment and turn dark. Melanin acts like a shield to block out the sun's ultraviolet rays, which can penetrate and destroy delicate skin cells. Your skin tans because it is trying its best to control the damage caused from exposure to the sun.

Tune-Up Tip: No Such Thing as a "Healthy Tan"

You need a little bit of sunlight so your body can make its own supply of vitamin D. The cells in your outer skin layer (the epidermis) store the raw materials for making the vitamin. When sunlight penetrates the layer, it starts the conversion process. But you don't need a lot of light for this to happen—fifteen minutes a day should do it.

Too much sunlight is downright dangerous. Ultraviolet light can rip through cells and destroy their membranes, causing them to leak their contents. This leakage is what causes the redness, itching, and irritation of sunburn. If the cells die in massive numbers, the skin peels off in chunks. Such damage—whether it occurs in a few intense episodes or more gradually, over a period of time—puts you at risk of skin cancer, especially the deadly form known as melanoma.

If you plan to spend more than twenty minutes or so outdoors, wear protective clothing, sunglasses, and a hat. And please use sunscreen. The strength of sun-blocking creams and lotions are based on the SPF (sun protection factor). The higher the number, the stronger the protection of your sunscreen. So which rating should you use? SPF 10? SPF 15? SPF 30? These ratings indicate how much longer the sunscreen's use will allow you to be in the sun without getting a sunburn. Example: If you usually start to burn after about twenty minutes, proper use of SPF 2 protects you for about forty minutes and proper use of SPF 15 protects you for about five hours. However, because these figures are derived from a laboratory setting and several important factors—including reflections, altitude, wind, the angle of the sun, the presence on your skin of water or sweat, and so on—reduce the effectiveness of sunscreens as a practical matter, most doctors and the American Academy of Dermatology say the safest approach is for everyone to wear at least SPF 15, even on a cloudy day.

This recommendation makes particularly good sense with children. Here is a sobering statistic: Ninety percent of the sun-related damage that can lead to skin cancer occurs prior to age eighteen. Due to the thinning of the atmosphere's ozone layer, a person born today is twice as likely to develop skin cancer as someone born only a decade ago—and twelve times as likely as someone born 50 years ago!

Tune-Up Tip: Keep an Eye on Your Moles

One of the deadliest skin cancers is melanoma. This cancer arises from moles on the body and is often referred to as black mole cancer. Fortunately, melanoma almost always occurs on the skin surface. You don't see other cancers that may grow undetected inside the body. But you can often spot melanoma—and get treatment before it poses a serious health problem.

To find melanoma, however, you must check yourself routinely, every few months. Report any suspicious moles to your physician or a dermatologist. Look for moles characteristic of these ABCDs:

A: Asymmetrical shape

B: Border is irregular

C: Color varies from one area to another

D: Diameter larger than a pencil eraser

For an illustrated guide on how to recognize suspicious moles during a self-examination, visit the American Academy of Dermatology's Web site: www.aad.org/SkinCancerNews/WhatIsSkinCancer/sclooks.html.

The dermis has fewer layers than the epidermis but is far more complex. It contains miles of nerve fibers, blood vessels, and lymphatic vessels, as well as millions of oil glands and sweat glands.

Most of the dermis consists of flexible connective tissue. The dermis contains a support structure, called a matrix, that is made up of sturdy proteins, especially collagen. (See page 286 for more information about collagen.) Collagen is strong and resilient; it's collagen that prevents most jabs and scrapes from penetrating deeper than they otherwise would. Because collagen binds with water, it helps keep your skin supple and smooth. The dermis also contains elastic fibers called elastin, which allow skin to stretch and return to its original shape. Over time, though, the skin loses some of that elasticity.

A WRINKLE IN TIME

Why does skin wrinkle? The main reason is the cumulative effects of free-radical damage. This damage may be the result of exposure to the elements—sun, wind, and pollution all take their toll—but exposure to internal free radicals is also a major cause. So too is normal aging. Over time, the amount of fat stored in the layer just below the dermis tends to diminish. Thus there is less material to support the skin layer from underneath, causing it to sag. As we age, the collagen in our skin loses its ability to hold its shape, with the fibers becoming fewer and farther between. As the network of collagen shrinks, the skin becomes thinner and less elastic. The glands that secrete natural skin oils wither away, causing skin to become dry and itchy. To prevent wrinkles from forming, eat a diet rich in antioxidants and avoid smoking cigarettes and environmental exposure to free radicals.

You have more than two million sweat glands inside the dermis. One type of gland, called eccrine glands, produces odorless sweat that is 99 percent water; the rest is salt, metabolic wastes, and acids. The other type, apocrine glands, are found mostly in the underarms and in the groin. These glands produce sweat that also contains fatty molecules. When bacteria on the skin break down these materials, an odor results.

The dermis also contains oil glands, which collect fats and debris from dead cells and excrete it through the pores. This oily material is called sebum, and the glands are technically called sebaceous glands. Most of the oil glands actually secrete sebum into the hair follicles. Sebum softens and lubricates hair and skin, preventing hair from becoming brittle, and helps the skin retain moisture. Sebum also helps kill bacteria on the surface of skin. A blocked sebaceous duct swells to form a whitehead. If the trapped material oxidizes and turns dark, it forms a blackhead. Inflamed glands accompanied by swelling produce acne pimples.

The boundary between the dermis and the epidermis is not smooth; instead, it is studded with bumps and ridges. These produce the loops and whorls of your fingerprints. Besides serving as unique identifiers (no two people have identical fingerprints), these ridges actually serve a purpose: They increase fiction and make it easier for your hands to grip objects.

The subcutaneous tissue just below the dermis binds the skin loosely to underlying tissue or bone. This tissue contains fat cells; each of us has fat cells that vary in size and number. There are also sex-related differences in this tissue. In women, the uppermost layer of subcutaneous tissue contains standing fat cell chambers. These chambers look like long balloons arranged side by side. They are separated by walls of connective tissue that are attached to the dermis. In men, this upper layer is thinner, and the fat cells are separated by a network of crisscrossing connective tissue walls. This difference is why many women have fatty deposits, known as cellulite, in some parts of their body. More information about cellulite appears on page 321.

Skin Functions:
More than Skin Deep

The main job of the integumentary system is to protect your body from assault by dangerous forces: bacteria, injury, extremes of temperature, and the effects of harsh chemicals.

As a physical barrier, skin is extremely effective. Because your skin is continuous, there are few breaks where bacteria can enter. Skin is also waterproof. Yes, your fingertips do get a little "pruney" if you spend too long in the bathtub, but water (and any poisons it might contain) can't penetrate beyond the superficial layers of skin. Although waterproof, the skin can release water via the sweat glands when it needs to. However, certain toxic substances can penetrate through the skin, including organic solvents and heavy metals such as lead or mercury.

Your skin also produces chemicals that protect you. Secretions such as sweat and oil make your skin slightly acidic, which keeps bacteria from multiplying too fast. Melanin, the skin pigment, forms an effective shield against UV radiation.

The third line of defense is the immune system, which is active in the skin, as it is elsewhere in the body. Macrophages live in the epidermis, just waiting for the call to action. If bacteria or viruses manage to enter the skin through a cut or tear, the macrophages engulf and destroy them.

Your skin is remarkably good at repairing itself. Because of the high turnover of cells in the epidermis, a minor cut or scrape is as good as new in just a few days. Damaged cells release inflammatory substances. These help destroy invading bacteria and recruit white cells to the scene of the accident. The white cells mop up the invaders, but produce debris (fluid and dead cell particles) as a result, which causes temporary swelling. Meanwhile new epidermal cells migrate up from the dermis to replace the missing cells. Scabs—clots of blood and other material—form a protective cap over the "construction site." Eventually the scab falls away, leaving new skin in its place. If the wound is serious enough, the skin produces large amounts of collagen fibers to link the tissue back together. This material is different from skin. It remains permanently in place and causes a scar.

Another important task of the integumentary system is to regulate your body temperature. It does so by releasing sweat, which dissipates heat collected from the cells as they go about their metabolic duties. Sweat also cools the surface of the skin as the moisture evaporates. Cold temperatures cause the blood vessels in skin to constrict, thus retaining more heat on the inside.

Because it contains nerves, the skin responds to tickles, bumps, pressure, pain, and temperature. This information races to your brain, which immediately figures out how to respond. If the tickle comes from an errant ant wandering along your wrist, you'll casually brush it off. If you touch a hot pan, you immediately jerk your hand away.

Skin also contributes to metabolic activity by synthesizing a precursor to vitamin D, the vitamin your bones need to help them absorb calcium. Sunlight penetrates the epidermis and causes changes in molecules of cholesterol. This modified molecule is then absorbed into the capillaries and transported elsewhere in the body, where ultimately it is converted into vitamin D.

At any given moment, about 5 percent of your blood is circulating through your skin. During exercise, or during the "flight-or-fight response," the blood vessels in the skin constrict, so that blood leaves the skin and travels to the internal organs. Thus your skin serves as a kind of reservoir, keeping a supply of blood ready for use elsewhere.

In addition, skin forms a part of your detoxification system. The skin excretes small amounts of certain kinds of nitrogen-containing waste products, including ammonia and urea. The body detoxifies some metals by attaching them to sulfur atoms and sticking those substances onto hair shafts.

Skin also produces enzymes. Some destroy cancer-causing chemicals before they can harm your cells. Others help get rid of old collagen so that new collagen can take its place. When these enzymes are busy, you are less likely to develop wrinkles.

As you can see, keeping your skin in shape does more than just make you look your best. It keeps you feeling better and helps other body systems work more efficiently.

The best strategy for supporting the skin is to provide it with highest-quality nutrition possible. Eat a generally healthy diet that is high in complex carbohydrates and low in refined or concentrated sugars. Avoid high-fat foods, especially milk and milk products, and those containing other sources of trans fatty acids, such as margarine, shortening, and other hydrogenated oils.

Fiber is important, because fiber binds with toxins in the bowel and eliminates them from the body. If the toxins enter circulation, they can penetrate skin cells and can cause irritation, rashes, and itching.

Make sure you get adequate levels of antioxidant vitamins, especially beta-carotene and vitamins A, C, and E. Antioxidant minerals especially important for healthy skin include selenium and zinc. These key nutrients prevent free-radical damage to skin cells. They also are essential for wound repair.

You also need good levels of omega-3 fatty acids to maintain healthy cell membranes and reduce the production of inflammatory chemicals that can irritate skin tissues.

Because collagen is mostly water, be sure you drink plenty of pure water—at least 48 ounces a day.

The antioxidant enzyme glutathione and the amino acid cysteine are helpful in avoiding wrinkles. Glutathione effectively and quickly repairs damage by free radicals, which prevents skin cells from dying and causing wrinkles. Ways to boost glutathione are discussed on page 78. About a quarter of your collagen is made of cysteine (cysteine contains atoms of sulfur), which forms especially sticky bonds with other neighboring proteins. Without enough cysteine in your diet, you may have brittle nails or thin, dry hair. Good dietary sources of cysteine include nuts, seeds, whole grains, egg whites, and fish.

Tune-Up Tip: Ironing Out Wrinkles

The most popular antiwrinkle and antiaging products contain natural compounds known as fruit acids or alpha-hydroxy acids (AHAs for short). Examples are glycolic, lactic, tartaric, malic, and citric acids. Of these, glycolic acid (from sugar cane) is by far the most common.

First used in 1974, AHAs were quickly adopted as renaissance materials by the cosmetic and dermatology world. Besides ironing out wrinkles, AHA-containing preparations are used as moisturizers in the treatment of dry skin, acne, and age spots. They also help your skin look younger. Dermatologists use AHAs to perform chemical peels of the skin—a procedure where the AHAs literally dissolve or peel away layers of skin. The amount of free acid in the product determines whether it will moisturize, eliminate wrinkles, or act as a chemical peel. The higher the percentage of AHA, the greater the peeling effect. While dermatologists use products with 70 percent free acids, most over-the-counter AHA products contain only 4 percent free acids—the minimum amount needed to produce skin cell renewal.

Use AHA-containing products according to label recommendations. If you use AHAs, be aware that your skin is now even more vulnerable to the negative effects of the sun. Use an effective sun block before exposing your skin to the sun.

It's important to treat your skin gently. Avoid substances that irritate your skin. If your skin gets red or irritated after using a particular soap, cleanser, or cosmetic, try to find a brand that is not irritating. Don't over-wash, since rubbing the skin can irritate it and trigger the release of in-flammatory chemicals. You might want to use a soft natural sponge or a loofah to remove dead cells. Exposure to direct sunlight—but no more than fifteen to thirty minutes a day—can be beneficial.

Tune-Up Tip: A Honey of a Skin Cleanser

You can make a safe, gentle skin cleanser using natural ingredients. Mix equal parts of oat flour, wheat bran, and honey. Then add olive oil and apple cider vinegar in equal measure, enough to make a paste. If you wish, add a drop or two of lavender essential oil. After rinsing your face with warm wa-ter, apply the cleanser. Don't scrub; simply press against the skin and mas-sage gently. Rinse with warm water. Close the pores by splashing gently with cool water.

Stress and emotional tension can worsen many skin problems, includ-ing acne, psoriasis, and dermatitis. One of the best strategies for tuning up skin is to develop smarter ways of coping with, and reducing, stress; for more information, see pages 62–64.

Remember that your skin mirrors your overall health. Poor digestion can rob skin cells of the nutrients they need. Similarly, a malfunctioning detoxification system can allow harmful substances to escape the vigi-lance of the liver and damage skin cells. Low levels of thyroid hormone can cause skin to become dry, rough, and scaly. Hypothyroidism can also lead to dry, brittle, coarse hair or severe hair loss. The nails become thin, brittle, and ridged. A weakened immune system can allow minor wounds or skin infections to worsen and persist. And poor circulation can rob skin and hair of the oxygen and nutrients they need. When you tune up these other systems, you'll tune up your appearance as well.

Targeting Skin Troubles

Your tune-up can help prevent the following conditions from developing. Should they occur, there are many natural steps you can take that provide relief.

Acne

The unsightly blemishes produced by acne are every teenager's nightmare. Although acne typically erupts at puberty, it can develop at any age. Acne is more common among males, because male sex hormones stimulate the production of keratin and sebum. Excess keratin can block pores, leading to blackheads, whiteheads, and cysts. Bacteria trapped in the pores break down the keratin, causing inflammation. Most often, pimples develop on the face, back, chest, and shoulders.

There are four key dietary recommendations to clear up acne. These tips sound simple, but they work.

1. *Eliminate foods containing trans fatty acids* (milk, milk products, margarine, shortening and other hydrogenated vegetable oils).
2. *Eliminate fried foods.*
3. *Stay away from salt and foods with a high salt content,* as the iodine in iodized salts tends to promote pimple formation.
4. *Avoid eating sugar whenever possible;* people who are prone to acne typically do not metabolize sugar properly.

Supplemental strategies are also effective. In your body, the hormone insulin regulates the rate at which cells take in sugar. Chromium is necessary for proper insulin function and normal sugar metabolism. Chromium supplementation (200 to 400 mcg per day of either chromium picolinate or polynicotinate) may improve acne in many cases.

Vitamin A works to reduce sebum production and prevent the buildup of keratin. However, taking high doses of vitamin A poses risks of toxic side effects such as headache, fatigue, emotional instability, and muscle and joint pain. In my opinion, high doses of vitamin A (above 25,000 IU per day) are not necessary if intake of other nutritional factors, especially zinc and vitamin E, is adequate. Because of concern about birth defects, sexually active women of childbearing age should take no more than 5,000 IU per day of vitamin A (as retinol) unless they are using at least two forms of birth control. Many prescription acne medications contain an extremely potent form of vitamin A called tretinoin (Retin-A), which also causes severe birth defects.

Vitamin B_6 is necessary for the proper metabolism of steroid hormones. Lack of B_6 may cause skin cells to be more sensitive to testosterone. This occurs often in women during the last third of their menstrual cycle (the secretory phase). I recommend supplementation of 25 mg of B_6 three times per day. In high doses (2.5 g four times per day) vitamin B_5 (pantothenic acid) can speed up fat metabolism and reduce production of sebum.

Vitamin E and its metabolic partner, selenium, are also important. Vitamin E supports vitamin A in its function and produces antiacne effects of its own. Your body needs selenium to make an enzyme, glutathione peroxidase, that works to control inflammation. (Daily dosage recommendations: vitamin E, 400 to 800 IU; selenium, 200 to 400 mcg.)

Zinc is essential for healthy skin. Low zinc levels increase the rate at which testosterone is converted to DHT (dihydrotestosterone), which in turn increases the risk of acne. Zinc is also necessary for vitamin A function, wound healing, immune system activity, inflammation control, and tissue regeneration. Research suggests that for acne prevention, zinc gluconate or effervescent zinc sulfate may be more useful than other forms. Typical dosage is 45 to 60 mg per day.

Treatment is available should blemishes erupt. Over-the-counter medications typically contain benzoyl peroxide, a skin antiseptic. Prescription medications contain the tretinoin form of vitamin A. While effective, these preparations can cause drying, redness, and peeling. I suggest you use topical products that contain natural substances instead. The most popular formulations are those that contain either tea tree oil, azelaic acid, or sulfur. These natural compounds work by eliminating bacteria and reducing inflammation.

Age Spots

As we get older, large, frecklelike discolorations appear on the skin. These blemishes—commonly called age spots—result from the buildup of lipofuscin, a dark substance produced by your cells. This material is

TARGETING SKIN TROUBLES 321

mostly debris from molecules that have been partially destroyed by free-radical damage. Actually, lipofuscin collects in many tissues throughout your body, including your brain, where it may play a major role in causing age-related memory loss. But the spots are visible only on the skin. The number and severity of age spots is a good indication of the level of oxidative damage that has occurred throughout the body.

It is easier to prevent lipofuscin deposits than to reverse them. The smartest strategy is to avoid excessive sun exposure and to use sunblock. Also make sure your intake of antioxidants, especially beta-carotene, is high. If you are prone to age spots, eat dark green leafy vegetables, carrots, yams, and other foods high in carotenes. You can also take 50,000 IU of beta-carotene per day, preferably from a mixed carotene source such as palm oil or *Dunellia* algae.

If you are really bothered by age spots and want to try a more cosmetic approach, you can use bleaching creams. Creams containing hydroquinone can reduce the darkness of the spots by about 50 percent. Creams containing 10 percent magnesium L-ascorbyl-2-phosphate, a special form of vitamin C, are even more effective; they can completely erase age spots in about 70 percent of cases.

If you have age spots, it's good idea to take *Ginkgo biloba* extract. As a powerful antioxidant, ginkgo may prevent buildup of lipofuscin "age spots" in the brain. Read the label carefully and choose a ginkgo product standardized to contain 24 percent ginkgo flavonglycosides.

Cellulite

With age, the supportive tissue (matrix) in the dermis becomes weaker. When that happens, the fat cells below can start to migrate, pushing up into the layer above. The connective tissue between cells also weakens, allowing the fat cells to become swollen. As a result, the skin over these regions can develop pits and ridges—the so-called mattress phenomenon—and the fatty areas can feel like granules or buckshot. The common name for this condition is *cellulite*.

Cellulite is a cosmetic problem, not a medical one, but because it is unsightly, it can cause great distress in those who have it. Due to sex differences in skin tissue, women are more than nine times as likely to develop cellulite as men. Women who are overweight are far more likely to have cellulite than slender women or athletes. In men, the development of cellulite is likely the result of a deficiency in male hormones, especially testosterone. The regions most often affected are the thighs and buttocks;

less frequently cellulite develops in the lower abdomen, on the nape of the neck, and on the upper arms.

Generally, the number of fat cells in your body is determined by heredity. While you can't control the number of cells you have, to a significant extent you can control how big those cells get. The goal is to maintain a slim subcutaneous fat layer, and the first choice of methods for achieving this should be no surprise: exercise, maintain a healthy weight, and eat a healthy, low-fat diet. Your exercise regimen should provide twenty to thirty minutes of aerobic exercise most days per week.

Follow the general dietary strategies given above. Lose excess weight, but do so gradually, especially if you are a woman over age forty. If weight loss occurs too quickly, the mattress phenomenon can be more apparent, especially in people whose skin and connective tissues are undergoing the normal changes associated with aging.

You can also take steps to improve circulation to the affected area and to increase the integrity of connective tissue. Massage is helpful, because it stimulates better flow of both blood and lymph. You can administer massage yourself, using your hand or a brush. The idea is to gently push against the affected tissue, with strokes moving in the direction toward the heart.

Many cosmetic formulas and herbal preparations claim that they can "cure" cellulite. I am dubious of such claims, because they are usually made without scientific data to back them up. However, research has shown that certain botanical compounds can provide good results for many patients. I recommend using a combination of oral and topical products that strengthen connective tissues.

An extract of centella (*Centella asiatica,* or gotu kola) supports connective tissue metabolism by stimulating the body to produce structural components known as glycosaminoglycans (GAGs). GAGs are the major components of the so-called ground substance, in which collagen fibers are embedded. Use of gotu kola extract helps perhaps six to eight out of ten patients who try it. The dose is 30 mg of a product containing 70 percent triterpenic acids, taken three times per day.

Tune-Up Tip: Biotin for the Diaper Rash That Won't Go Away

Jennifer was desperate to find a cure for her daughter Brittany's diaper rash. Brittany, who was three months old when I saw her, developed the rash two weeks after she was born. It simply would not go away. The poor little kid was miserable, and her mother was at her wits' end.

Jennifer had tried everything Brittany's pediatrician had recommended, to no avail. Frustrated, the doctor encouraged her to consult with me. I suggested that Jennifer add two things to Brittany's formula once a day: ½ tsp freeze-dried *Bifidobacterium bifidum* (the friendly bacteria in infants) and 1 mg of biotin.

Biotin is a B vitamin that functions in the manufacture and utilization of fats and amino acids. Without biotin, body metabolism and skin health are severely impaired. Since a large portion of the human biotin supply is provided by intestinal bacteria, infants are susceptible to biotin deficiency because they have not yet established bacteria in their intestinal tract (breast-feeding results in the establishment of the proper bacterial flora). The medical literature cites several case histories that have demonstrated successful treatment of seborrheic dermatitis (cradle cap) with biotin by giving the mother the biotin if the baby is being breast-fed, or by giving it directly to the infant. Recent reports show that chronic, intractable diaper rash also responds to biotin supplementation.

It sure worked wonders with Brittany—and that's the bottom line on biotin. Of course, be sure to consult your doctor before giving any supplement to your baby.

Eczema

Eczema is a chronic skin inflammation that causes itching, scaling, and blisters. Another name for eczema is dermatitis. Many, but not all, cases may arise due to an allergy to certain foods. If you are bothered by eczema, try to eliminate foods from your diet that are likely to be involved.

ECZEMA AND FOOD ALLERGIES

The first goal in dealing with atopic dermatitis (eczema) is to identify whether a food allergy is involved. Studies show that nearly 90 percent of people with eczema are allergic to one or more of seven foods: milk, eggs, peanuts, wheat, cod, catfish, and cashews. Another study found that milk, eggs, and peanuts accounted for about 81 percent of all cases of childhood eczema. Yet another study found that 60 percent of children with severe eczema had an allergic reaction to one or two foods, including eggs, cow's milk, peanuts, fish, wheat, or soybeans.

To discover if you or your child has a food allergy, use the elimination diet and challenge method. Do not eat any of the most common allergens for a period of at least ten days. Also avoid artificial colors and preservatives.

> Then reintroduce the foods one by one into the diet, two or three days apart. If symptoms return, stay away from that food for at least a year. It often happens that people "outgrow" an allergy after that time.

When the problem results from contact with an allergenic substance, such as poison ivy, the condition is called contact dermatitis. Of course, the solution to contact dermatitis is to avoid whatever it is that causes irritation. Many people are allergic to latex rubber (found in rubber gloves), plant resins, and nickel (found in jewelry).

Essential fatty acids are important for maintaining healthy cell membranes and reducing the "leakage" of substances that can cause inflammation. Many people with eczema may not metabolize essential fatty acids properly. This leads to a greater vulnerability to allergies and inflammation. Although I am a big advocate of flaxseed oil, I believe that for people suffering from eczema, taking fish oil supplements (1.8 g EPA daily) and eating cold-water fish better supplies the kinds of fatty acids needed to control the problem.

Don't forget the zinc, which your body needs to make an enzyme crucial for the metabolism of fatty acids. Be sure you consume at least 30 mg per day; increase the level to 45 or 60 mg per day for active flare-ups.

Many plant products work to control inflammation. Perhaps the most useful in this regard is the flavonoid quercetin, which inhibits the formation and release of histamine. Flavonoid-rich extracts from grape seed, bilberry, *Ginkgo biloba,* and green tea also block allergic activity in the body. Ginkgo also blocks the effects of platelet aggravating factor, a key chemical in the blood that can trigger bouts of eczema.

Licorice (*Glycyrrhiza glabra*) is useful in several ways. Taken internally— for example as a cup of tea—three times daily, it exerts significant anti-inflammatory and antiallergenic effects. Externally, preparations featuring pure glycyrrhetinic acid may work as well as hydrocortisone to relieve rashes, itching, and redness. Other effective topical products are those containing extracts of chamomile or witch hazel. These products are especially good at relieving itch and thus preventing skin damage. Don't use greasy creams or ointments, since these can block pores and make the itching worse.

Reduce skin irritation by avoiding rough-textured clothing, such as wool, or some synthetics. Wear light, absorbent cotton next to the skin. In the laundry, use only mild soaps (no detergents or fabric softeners).

CASE HISTORY: Bob's Incessant Itch

Bob, a seventy-three-year-old retired aircraft engineer, came to see me for some help with something that had been bothering him for years. His skin itched all over. He had tried all sorts of moisturizers, oral antihistamines, and even topical cortisone creams, all to no avail. The medical term for Bob's problem is *idiopathic pruritus*. *Idiopathic* means that the cause is unknown.

In taking Bob's medical history, I uncovered a valuable clue. I asked Bob about his water consumption. "Zero—nada, nothing," he replied. He said he did not want to drink water because he had an enlarged prostate and drinking water made him have to go to the bathroom all the time.

I understood Bob's complaint, but I also knew that the major cause of pruritus in older people is dehydration. When we do not drink enough water, toxic compounds that are normally excreted through the urine or bile build up in the blood. The body wants to remove these toxins, but since the other escape routes are blocked, they are removed through the skin. On their way out of the body, they irritate the cells.

I told Bob that he could take care of his prostate enlargement through natural remedies (see pages 393–394 for more information). I stressed too that he had to start drinking at least six glasses of water per day. He could stop drinking by 7:00 P.M., to prevent excessive nighttime urination.

Bob was the kind of patient who makes my job easier. He followed my instructions carefully. He was a bit uncomfortable at first with the increased water intake, but the level of discomfort was significantly less than the constant itchiness of his skin. After two weeks of diligent water consumption, Bob experienced complete resolution of his pruritus. As a bonus, two months later his prostate symptoms eased up as well.

Psoriasis

Psoriasis is a common skin condition that causes skin cells to multiply too rapidly—up to a thousand times faster than normal skin. The cells accumulate faster than you can shed them. As they accumulate, they form characteristic overlapping silvery scales. Surrounding skin can become red and inflamed.

The rate of cell division is governed by the balance of amino acids inside your cells. This balance can be disturbed by digestive problems that result in incomplete protein digestion or poor absorption of proteins in the intestine. The resulting toxins can lead to uncontrolled cell replication. A diet low in fiber contributes to the problem, since fiber binds with and removes many bowel toxins. A poorly functioning liver may also be involved.

People with psoriasis should follow the general dietary and supplemental strategies described in this chapter. Adequate levels of vitamins A, D, and E, plus zinc, chromium, and selenium, are especially important. Some people benefit from the use of fumaric acid (240–720 mg daily), but I recommend this approach only if other treatments are ineffective, because with fumaric acid side effects such as flushing of the skin, nausea, and diarrhea are common.

Although exposure to UV light is a concern for most people, it can be very helpful as a treatment for psoriasis. A standard medical approach calls for the patient to take a drug called psoralen, which is absorbed into the skin and which becomes active when exposed to UVA radiation. However, studies indicate that exposure to UVB radiation alone can inhibit cell proliferation. The use of heat or ultrasound may also provide relief.

Topical treatments can be very helpful. In addition to licorice and chamomile (see page 324), capsaicin (the active component of cayenne pepper) can relieve pain. It works by depleting nerves of the neurotransmitter known as substance P, which transmits pain signals.

TANNING THERAPY FOR PSORIASIS

The standard medical treatment of psoriasis is called PUVA therapy and involves the use of the drug psoralen (a photosensitizer) plus exposure to ultraviolet A light. Usually the UVA treatment is administered in a dermatologist's office. Dermatologists, taught that commercial tanning beds are ineffective, admonish their patients that nonprescription tanning devices are of no benefit. However, a recent study refutes this contention.

The six-week study involved patients with psoriasis who underwent three to five tanning sessions per week for four weeks. Psoralen was not used. The time of the sessions was calculated to be less than the time required to produce a sunburn in each individual. That's why the dosage varied among the patients. All subjects had significant reduction in the severity of their psoriasis. The only side effect was a mild sunburn in about one-third of the group.

This study showed that commercial tanning beds alone may improve psoriasis and may be considered as an alternative to office-based UVA treatment.

Hair

Compared to other animals, we don't appear to have a lot of hair. One noted anthropologist described humans as "naked apes." Actually, men and women both have millions of hairs scattered around the body. Typically there are about 100,000 hairs on the scalp. A man who shaves must run his razor over about 30,000 hairs every morning. Other patches of hair grow in the pubic region and under the arms. Less obvious hair grows on the arms, legs, trunk, back—everywhere, in fact, except the lips, parts of the genitals, the palms of the hands, and the soles of the feet.

Animals depend on hair for protection from the elements, but human hair is probably more decorative than practical. Hair on our heads protects against minor injury, and it helps retain body heat and protect against sunlight. Eyelashes shield the eyes, and hair in the nose serves as a filter to remove dust particles from the air we breathe. The delicate hairs elsewhere aren't good for much except to enhance sensations of touch.

The root of a hair extends into the dermis, but the cells that line the pit from which hair grows (called the follicle) are actually keratin cells from the epidermis. Keratin in hair is harder than the keratin found in skin cells, making the hair more durable.

The visible part of a hair is called the shaft. Shafts come in three basic styles. Round shafts produce straight hair. Oval shafts produce wavy hair. Shafts that are flattened like ribbons result in kinky hair. The outer layer of a hair shaft is made of keratin cells that overlap like roofing tiles. The tips of the shafts are exposed to friction; if they wear away, they expose inner fibers of the hair and produce the cosmetically annoying split ends.

While a hair on your scalp lives for about four years before it falls out, eyelashes and hair under the arms last only about four months before they are shed and replaced by new hairs.

Your hair has color for the same reason your skin does. At the base of the hair follicle are melanocytes, which secrete a blend of colors (yellow, red, brown, and black). Normally these color-producing cells die off as you age; they contain genes that program them to live only about forty or fifty years. Without color, the hair turns gray or white. Tiny air bubbles also collect in the hair shaft. The more bubbles there are, the less room there is for pigment, and the whiter the hair.

The deep end of the follicle is called the bulb. Wrapped around the bulb is a set of nerve endings. When the hair moves due to light touch, these nerve endings respond. A blood capillary also penetrates the bulb, bringing oxygen and nutrients needed for the hair to grow. Strange as it sounds, hairs are also connected to tiny muscles. When stimulated, for example by fear or cold, the muscles pull on the hairs and cause them to stand up. This action also causes the skin to dimple and produces the little bumps we call goose pimples. Animals use this mechanism to retain additional heat and to make themselves look bigger (and thus perhaps to scare off whatever it is that's making them scared). But for humans goose pimples don't serve much purpose, except to remind you to put your sweater on.

Hair Loss

For many people, a good head of hair is important for self-esteem and a sense of well-being. Unfortunately, hair loss is a predictable, if distressing, trade-off for living a long life. Part of the problem comes from years of using shampoos, conditioners, coloring agents, and other harsh chemicals. Exposure to sun and wind, coupled with constant combing, brushing, and blow drying, doesn't help either.

Tune-Up Tip: Gentle Herbal Rinse

You can make your own herbal rinse for healthier hair. Put one-third cup of dried herb (see list below) into a bowl. Pour in a quart of boiling water and let the mixture steep for fifteen minutes. Strain and pour into a plastic bottle. Apply as a final rinse after shampooing.

Herb	Function
• Chamomile	Adds highlights and gloss
• Ginseng	Replenishes moisture, improves flexibility and sheen
• Lavender	Improves silkiness and shine
• Lemongrass	Conditions
• Nettle	Adds strength and luster
• Rosemary	Detangles; may promote hair growth and control dandruff
• Sage	Hides gray hair
• Yarrow	Improves manageability

In most cases, hair loss is a normal part of aging. By the age of forty or so, the rate of hair growth slows down. The hair follicles just run out of steam, and the new hairs that do appear tend to be finer than the old ones. Both men and women suffer from age-related hair loss, but the problem is more apparent in men.

Hair growth is controlled by hormones, especially male hormones (androgens such as testosterone), but thyroid and adrenal hormones also play a part. The typical "egg-in-the-nest" pattern of baldness seen in men—loss of hair beginning at the temples, followed by further loss along the top of the head—is the result of genetics. For decades the hair grows normally, responding to stimulation from androgens in the hair follicle. But then a gene that has been inactive all this time suddenly switches on, causing changes in the way follicles respond to testosterone. The growth cycle shortens. Hairs don't grow long enough to emerge from the skin before they fall out. The higher a man's testosterone level, the greater the risk of baldness. (This may be the basis for the fact that many women think that bald men are sexier!)

There are other causes for hair loss. Stress alters the hormonal balance in the body. To cope with stress, the body shifts its energy (and its hormones) to other functions that are more important for keeping the body alive. Since protein is needed to make keratin, a diet low in protein can slow production of new hairs. Some women lose hair while breast-feeding their babies because so much of their body's own protein is devoted to the production of milk. Certain skin diseases can destroy hair, and hair loss is a side effect of high fever and of certain medications. Cancer treatments using drugs and radiation often cause hair loss.

Hair Loss in Women

One of the most common complaints from women patients in my clinical practice is hair loss. I don't mean complete baldness, but rather the perception that hair is falling out at an increasing rate. My patients typically complain that other doctors dismiss hair loss as "nothing to worry about"—after all, minor hair loss is hard to measure and it is certainly not a life-threatening disorder. But the patients feel frustrated—it is a big deal to them. Fortunately, there are effective strategies for combating it.

There are five common causes of hair loss in women, which I'll describe in more detail. They are:

- Use of certain drugs and medications
- Nutritional deficiencies

- Hypothyroidism
- Intolerance to gluten
- Excess androgens (male sex hormones).

Drug-Induced Hair Loss

The list of drugs that can cause hair loss is long (see Table 9-1). However, use of one of these drugs is not necessarily enough to cause hair loss by itself. The exceptions are chemotherapy drugs, which are notorious for causing hair to fall out. (The reason is that chemotherapy targets cells that grow the fastest—hair among them.) Usually hair regrows after cancer therapy. When medically appropriate, natural alternatives to suspected culprits of hair loss should be employed.

Table 9-1: Classes of Drugs That Can Cause Hair Loss

Class	Examples
Antibiotics	Gentamicin, chloramphenicol
Anticoagulants	Coumadin, heparin
Antidepressants	Prozac, desipramine, lithium
Antiepileptics	Valproic acid, Dilantin
Cardiovascular drugs	ACE inhibitors, beta-blockers
Chemotherapy drugs	Adriamycin, vincristine, etoposide
Endocrine drugs	Bromocriptine, Clomid, danazol
Gout medications	Colchicine, allopurinol
Lipid-lowering drugs	Gemfibrozil, fenofibrate
Nonsteroidal anti-inflammatory drugs (NSAIDs)	Ibuprofen, indomethacin, naproxen
Ulcer medications	Tagamet, Zantac

Nutritional Deficiency and Hair Loss

A deficiency of any of a number of nutrients can lead to significant hair loss. Low levels of zinc, vitamin A, essential fatty acids, and iron are most likely involved. I typically find that women who suffer from hair loss are deficient in all of these nutrients.

A key sign of low zinc is the presence of white lines on the fingernails, indicating poor wound healing of the nail bed after even the least trauma. I also examine the back of the arms for patches of thick, dry skin (hyperkeratosis), a common sign of vitamin A deficiency. Dry skin also is associated with essential fatty acid deficiency. To evaluate iron status, I recommend a blood test to measure serum ferritin. If values of this protein fall below 30 mcg per liter, the body tries to conserve its iron supply; one way it does so is by slowing down the growth and regeneration of hair.

Biotin, a member of the vitamin B complex, is also important for healthy hair. Apparently biotin works by improving the metabolism of scalp oils.

The treatment of hair loss that results from nutritional deficiency is straightforward: Increase dietary intake of these nutrients and supplement appropriately. Take a high-potency multiple vitamin and mineral formula that contains iron, and take 1 tbsp of flaxseed oil per day. If the serum ferritin level is below 30 mcg/l, then I recommend supplementing with 30 mg of iron (as either iron succinate or iron fumarate) twice daily between meals. If abdominal discomfort develops, take the dose with meals three times daily (the reason the dosage is increased in this case is that iron is not as well absorbed when taken with foods). After two months, have another blood test to measure serum ferritin levels.

One caveat: In many cases, hair loss may result from low secretion of hydrochloric acid (stomach acid). As you learned in Chapter 2, if you can't properly digest foods, your intestines may be unable to absorb the nutrients they need. In these cases, hydrochloric acid supplementation at meals may be all that is needed.

Hypothyroidism and Hair Loss

Up to 4 percent of the adult population has moderate to severe hypothyroidism, and another 10 to 12 percent have mild hypothyroidism. Among women the rate is higher, reaching an estimated 20 percent. Hair loss is one of the cardinal signs of hypothyroidism (see pages 122–123 for others).

Given the importance of adequate thyroid hormone to human health, I tend to be aggressive in recommending supplements and thyroid hormone when lab tests show that thyroid levels are low. See pages 123–127 for more information.

Hair Loss and Gluten Intolerance

The protein gluten and its derivative gliadin are found primarily in wheat, barley, and rye grains. Some people make antibodies to gliadin. Their presence also triggers production of cross-reacting antibodies that attack the hair follicles. This situation can cause alopecia areata, an autoimmune disease characterized by patches of virtually complete hair loss.

Most often the presence of antibodies to gliadin in the blood indicates celiac disease, an intestinal disease characterized by structural abnormalities in the small intestine leading to malabsorption. In many cases, removing gluten from the diet allows the intestine to revert to its normal structure and function. Many people with gluten intolerance do not exhibit overt gastrointestinal symptoms. Instead, they may have indirect signs, such as hair loss. I consider ordering a test to detect antigliadin antibodies in patients with general hair loss, especially if they also have gastrointestinal symptoms.

Androgen-Related Hair Loss

Women, like men, can suffer from androgen-related hair loss. The pattern of loss is more widespread than it typically is in men, so the condition is often referred to as diffuse androgen-dependent alopecia. It is a relatively common condition, affecting perhaps 30 percent of women after age fifty. I offer my patients three recommendations to slow down this process, to which some women are genetically predisposed:

- *Increase antioxidant intake.* Free radicals have been shown to play a central role (along with testosterone) in male pattern baldness. Higher levels of these damaging compounds are found in the hair follicles in men (and presumably women) with male pattern baldness. The reason? Lower levels of the protective antioxidant glutathione. Since vitamin C and E can help preserve glutathione and help slow down the rate of hair loss, I recommend 1,000 to 1,500 mg of vitamin C in divided dosages and 400 IU of vitamin E to both men and women who are concerned about androgen-related hair loss.
- *Use saw palmetto extract.* As discussed on page 395, this herbal medicine is a popular therapy for benign prostatic hyperplasia (BPH) in men. It works by slowing down the enzyme that converts testosterone to a more potent form, dihydrotestosterone (DHT). In women, saw palmetto extract may relieve androgen-related alopecia by reducing the formation of DHT. The dosage for an extract standardized to contain 85 to 95 percent fatty acids and sterols is 320 mg per day.
- *Consider hormone replacement therapy.* The female hormones estrogen and progesterone will counteract the effects of testosterone on hair loss in women, especially in those experiencing hair loss during or after menopause. Of course, this therapy also has its risks, as discussed on pages 359–360.

Nails

Your fingernails and toenails are part of your epidermis. Like hair, they contain hard keratin. Nails look pink, but they are actually white; the pink color comes from the blood vessels underneath. Nails grow from a root beneath the skin. As they push outward, they grow away from the skin to which they are attached, producing the white part (or free edge) that we trim away. The cuticle is a fold of skin that overlaps and protects the corner of the nail. On average, a nail grows about two-hundredths of an inch in a week. The nail on the middle finger grows fastest, the pinkie slower, and the toenails slowest of all. With age, toenail growth tends to slow down considerably, and the nails become thick and ridged.

Tune-Up Tip: Biotin for Strong Nails

As early as 1940, researchers knew about an association between deficiency of B vitamins and nail brittleness. More recent research, especially from the world of veterinary medicine, has focused on the role of biotin, a member of the B vitamin complex, in this common disorder.

Biotin has been shown to increase the strength and hardness of hooves in pigs and horses. Recent human studies have shown that biotin supplementation (2,500 mcg per day) can produce a 25 percent increase in the thickness of the nail plate in patients diagnosed with brittle nails of unknown cause. More than nine out of ten patients taking this dosage will experience definite improvement.

Key Steps to Tuning Up Your Skin and Hair

- What you put inside your body determines what happens on the outside. The best strategy for healthy skin, nails, and hair is to eat a nutritious diet high in fiber and complex carbohydrates and low in refined sugars and fats. Also drink plenty of water.
- Nutrients especially important for maintaining skin and for repairing wounds include:
  - Vitamin A: up to 25,000 IU per day (no more than 5,000 IU for women who are or who may possibly become pregnant)

- Vitamin B_6: 25 mg three times per day
- Vitamin C: 500–1,500 mg per day
- Vitamin E: 400–800 IU per day
- Zinc: 45–60 mg per day

- Avoid overexposure to the sun. Excessive tanning increases your risk of dangerous skin cancer. Wear protective clothing, including a hat and sunglasses, and use sunblock.
- Alpha-hydroxy acids are valuable for reducing wrinkles and rejuvenating skin.
- Make sure your thyroid is functioning normally.
- To slow hair loss due to excess male hormones (androgens), try vitamin C (1,000–1,500 mg per day in divided doses), vitamin E (400 IU per day), and saw palmetto berry extract (320 mg per day of an extract standardized to 85 to 95 percent fatty acids and sterols).

Lifestyle Tune-Up #9: Connect with Nature

Most Americans spend 90 percent of their lives indoors, separated from fresh air, sunlight, and nature. I do not think that this is healthy. There is something extremely refreshing (and calming) about getting in touch with nature, whether it is simply a walk through a park, tending to our lawns, gardening, going on a picnic, or getting out in the wilderness for a weekend of camping. For your lifestyle tune-up, try to engage in at least one outdoor activity a week. Make it a high priority. I try to get outdoors every day. But since I can't always enjoy nature as much as I would like, I try to find other ways to commune with nature. Here are some simple tips:

- Adopt a plant. Plants are not only a way to get in touch with nature, but also phenomenal air filters, especially if you work in an office building. Much of the pollution that is generated in a large office building stems from the outgassing of the materials and machines used in building or in maintaining the structure. There are many sources, including foam insulation, plywood, particulate fibers, plastics, inks, oils, fax machines, and copiers. But when plants are present, the contaminants are sucked into the leaves and migrate into the soil, where microorganisms associated with the roots break them down and turn them into plant food. The more plants you have in an office building or house, the purer the air becomes.
- Listen to sounds of nature. In my office, car, and home, I usually have a recording of sounds of nature playing in the background. The recordings are of beautifully relaxing music intertwined with sounds of nature such as the sounds of an isolated beach, waterfall, or forest. I find that I'm more productive and relaxed when these gentle sounds are playing, and I highly recommend it.
- If you use a computer, use nature scenes as your desktop wallpaper and screen saver. I know that this may seem like a real stretch, but I cannot tell you how much pleasure I get from watching the nature scenes on my computer screen during the course of my day while I am on the phone or not using my computer.

CHAPTER 10

Tune-Up for Women

The female human body is truly a wonder. Like its male counterpart, the female body carries on all the normal, complex functions of living. Beyond that, it is capable of bringing new life into the world and nurturing that life during its critical early months.

But this amazing capacity comes at a price. The hormonal tides that govern sexuality and reproduction can cause real problems: mood swings, weight fluctuations, potentially dangerous changes in the cells. Because of this complexity, a tune-up is essential for balancing a woman's physical and psychological functions.

Here's a quick look at the organs and systems unique to the female body.

The Female System

The ovaries are the main reproductive organs. Besides storing eggs and releasing them for fertilization, the ovaries produce several crucial hormones: estrogens, progesterone, and testosterone. The ovaries are shaped like almonds and are about twice as large.

Inside the ovaries are tiny saclike structures called follicles, each of which contains an immature egg. At birth, the female already has her lifetime supply of eggs—approximately 700,000 of them. Each month during the reproductive years, hormones stimulate one follicle (rarely, more than one) to ripen and release its egg. This process is called ovulation.

The egg then travels along one of two passageways called the fallopian tubes. The tubes open into the uterus, a hollow muscular organ designed to support and nourish a developing baby. If sexual intercourse has occurred and if sperm from the male are present in the fallopian tube, the egg may become fertilized. Shortly after fertilization, the egg begins to divide and produce new cells. After it reaches a certain size it is called an embryo. An embryo can attach itself to the lining of the uterus, where it develops into a fetus.

The lining of the uterus, the endometrium, prepares for the egg by becoming thicker and more endowed with blood vessels and glands. But if a fertilized egg does not arrive, the lining begins to break down. The tissue detaches from the uterine wall and passes out through the vagina along with blood and other fluids. This process is called menstruation.

At its base, the uterus forms a narrow neck known as the cervix. The cervix has an opening that leads into the vagina. Sperm from the male must pass through this opening for fertilization to take place.

The vagina is a thin-walled, flexible tube about four inches long. It is rich in blood vessels and nerves. To accommodate the penis during intercourse, the vagina has many glands that secrete lubricating mucus. During birth, the vagina (sometimes called the birth canal) expands to allow passage of the baby.

Outside the vagina are the external genitalia, or vulva. The labia (from the Latin word for "lips") are two pairs of skin folds that protect the opening to the vagina and the urinary opening (urethra). The outer pair, the labia majora, are thick, fleshy, and covered with hair. The inner pair, the labia minora, are thin and hairless. The labia minora meet to form the hood (prepuce) that covers the clitoris.

The clitoris is a small knob of tissue packed with nerves and blood vessels. When stimulated, the clitoris becomes swollen, erect, and sensitive. In this way, the clitoris serves a function similar to that of the male penis. However, the penis is the conduit through which urine and sperm pass. In the female, the sexual and the excretory functions are completely separate. The only function of the clitoris is to provide sexual pleasure.

Both men and women have breasts, but only in women do the breasts serve a function. Glands inside the breast (known as mammary glands) produce milk to nourish a newborn baby. The milk collects in passageways called ducts and travels through tiny openings in the nipple. This activity is under the control of hormones released during pregnancy and after childbirth. The hormones cause the ducts to develop and thus increase the size of the breast. In women who are not pregnant or lactating, breast size depends on the amount of fatty tissue present.

Tune-Up Tip: Kegel Exercises

One of the best exercises a woman can do is a Kegel—a type of exercise designed to strengthen the muscles attached to the pelvic bone, which act like a hammock to hold your pelvic organs in place. These exercises are often prescribed during pregnancy to make childbirth easier and as a way to treat urinary incontinence (the inability to control the bladder), but all women can benefit from Kegels, as they increase sexual enjoyment, improve vaginal secretions, and help prevent drooping of the pelvic organs. If you have never done one, the first thing that you need to do is feel exactly what a Kegel is. The easiest way to do this is to try to stop the flow of urine during urination, or insert two fingers in the vagina and try to clamp down. Once you know what the sensation of tightening the pelvic muscles feels like, simply tighten the muscle for five seconds and then relax. This is a basic Kegel. To strengthen these muscles, do at least twenty Kegels daily (you can do them while you're on the phone, while sitting in traffic, and so on).

The Dance of Hormones

All of the female body's amazing, life-giving activity is under the control of hormones, powerful chemicals that ebb and flow in rhythmic cycles. Let me give a brief description of the most important of these.

Women experience two main hormonal cycles. The *ovarian cycle* involves hormones that act on, or are produced by, the ovaries. The *menstrual cycle* regulates the changes in the uterus. These cycles are closely linked and involve activity by many of the same hormones.

We'll begin with the ovarian cycle. The process begins in the hypothalamus, a region in the brain. The hypothalamus produces gonadotropin-releasing hormone (GnRH), a sort of master chemical in the process. (*Gonado-* comes from the Greek word for "genitals"; *-tropin* means "turning" or "changing.") GnRH enters the pituitary, a neighboring gland in the brain, where it triggers the release of two other hormones, follicle-stimulating hormone (FSH) and luteinizing hormone (LH). These substances then travel to, and act on, the ovaries.

FSH and LH stimulate the follicle to grow and mature. As the follicle grows, it begins to release estrogen. (Technically, there are several kinds of estrogens, the most important of which is estradiol; I'll use *estrogen* to refer to all of these.) LH also prods the cells to release hormones known as androgens. Androgens, including testosterone, are usually thought of as male hormones, but men and women both produce androgens and estrogen. In women, most of the androgens get changed into estrogen. Small amounts of androgens enter the blood and produce various effects throughout the body.

High estrogen levels cause all sorts of things to happen. The hormone signals the follicles to release even more estrogen. Estrogen also tells the pituitary to quit releasing FSH and LH for the moment and to stockpile a supply of those hormones instead. About halfway through the monthly cycle, the pituitary releases a sudden spurt of the FSH and LH it has accumulated. This flood of hormones causes the follicle to burst and release its egg. LH also causes the ruptured follicle to change into a yellowish tissue, known as the corpus luteum (*luteum,* which is also the root of *luteinizing,* means "yellow"). The corpus luteum is a gland, which goes to work secreting another hormone, progesterone, as well as estrogen.

The combination of progesterone and estrogen signals the pituitary to shut off the supply of LH and FSH. This, in turn, prevents further growth of other follicles. The drop in LH causes the corpus luteum to stop functioning and begin to degenerate. That, in turn, causes a fall in progesterone and estrogen production. Once those hormones are out of the picture, the pituitary gears up to begin producing LH and FSH . . . and the cycle spins again.

Now for the menstrual, or uterine, cycle. The uterus is able to accept an embryo for only a brief period of time, approximately seven days after ovulation. The changes in the endometrium that permit the embryo to implant depend on the levels of ovarian hormones.

The menstrual cycle begins at day 1, when the uterus starts shedding all but the deepest part of its lining, the endometrium. At the start of this, the menstrual phase, GnRH and the ovarian hormones are at their lowest levels. The loss of the endometrium causes bleeding for three to five days. Typically, by around day 5, the follicles in the ovary develop and begin producing estrogen.

The next stage is called the proliferative phase, because it is during this time that the endometrium proliferates, or regrows, due to stimulation by estrogen. The new layer thickens and new blood vessels and glands form. At the same time, estrogen causes cells in the endometrium to produce receptors that are sensitive to progesterone. As the name suggests, progesterone promotes gestation, or development of the fetus. Ovulation occurs at the end of the proliferative phase, around day 14.

During most times of the month, the cervix—the neck between the uterus and the vagina—produces a thick, sticky mucus. During the proliferative phase, however, estrogen causes the mucus to become thinner. This gives any sperm present an easier passage into the uterus for a rendezvous with the egg.

The final stage of the uterine cycle is the secretory phase. Now the endometrium goes into high gear preparing for the arrival of the embryo. Progesterone flooding out of the corpus luteum travels to the endometrium, where it boosts the formation of blood vessels and cells that secrete mucus. Glands begin to develop that will produce nutrients known as glycoproteins, which the embryo needs prior to implanting. Progesterone also causes cervical mucus to thicken again, which helps plug the opening and protect against invasion by bacteria.

You can see the wondrous ingenuity of this system: Ideally, everything works together to produce a mature egg, facilitate its encounter with sperm, and provide a suitable environment for the egg to implant and grow.

Of course, fertilization does not always occur. If the "guest of honor"— the embryo—does not arrive, the cycle begins to wind down. As the corpus luteum degenerates, progesterone levels fall. Without adequate supplies of hormone, the structures of the endometrium break down: The cells die, the blood vessels disintegrate. Bleeding causes the tissue to fragment and slough off. We are back at day 1, with the onset of menstruation.

Obviously, the picture changes if the embryo *does* implant. That process takes about a week, and it usually occurs by two weeks after ovulation—at just the time when the endometrium is most ready for its tiny visitor. Should menstruation occur, the fetus would be swept away. For that reason, the body needs to keep up its supply of progesterone, which maintains the endometrium and prevents menstruation. The hormone that signals the corpus luteum to keep producing progesterone is called human chorionic gonadotropin, or hCG. The source of hCG? The embryo. In an amazing display of self-preservation, the tiny ball of cells that will ultimately become a new human being takes over hormonal control of the uterus during the early stage of development. By releasing hCG, the fetus causes the ovaries to keep up their release of progesterone. (Pregnancy tests—including home test kits—work by detecting hCG, which is present as early as one week after fertilization.)

Let's flash forward nine months, to the time the baby is delivered. This process too is hormonal. During the last few weeks of gestation, estrogens are produced by the placenta, the protective sac that surrounds the fetus. Estrogen causes cells in the uterus to produce receptors that will respond to another hormone, oxytocin. At the same time, estrogen interferes with progesterone, causing the uterus to become "irritable." Just before birth, the mother's pituitary releases oxytocin, which triggers the release of other hormones called prostaglandins. Both hormones work together to trigger contractions of the uterine muscle. Those contractions propel the baby through the cervix, down the birth canal, and into the world.

During the final stages of pregnancy, estrogen, progesterone, and another hormone called lactogen all pay a visit to the hypothalamus. Their arrival causes the hypothalamus to secrete prolactin-releasing hormone (PRH). PRH makes a quick trip to the nearby pituitary, which responds by releasing the hormone prolactin. As its name implies, prolactin stimulates milk production (lactation) by the breast. When the baby sucks on the nipple, nerve signals travel to the brain; the brain signals the pituitary to release oxytocin. This hormone triggers the let-down reflex, which causes milk to eject from the glands and into the baby's mouth.

The hormonal processes I've just described focus on the release of eggs and the creation of a nurturing environment for the development of life. But the hormones involved also produce many powerful effects on other tissues throughout the body.

For example, estrogen is responsible for causing the female reproductive organs to develop and mature. It also manages the development of secondary sex characteristics, such as breast development and the growth of pubic hair. By affecting the distribution of fat, estrogen produces the characteristic "feminine" shape of the body: broader hips, rounded buttocks, a slender waist. Estrogen promotes bone growth, prevents loss of bone minerals, and preserves muscle mass. It raises "good" cholesterol and lowers "bad" cholesterol, thus lowering the risk of heart disease.

As I explained earlier, the main role of progesterone is to promote development of the endometrium. However, it also works with estrogen to stimulate breast growth and milk production. Progesterone helps the body produce urine, and it plays a role in temperature regulation.

A word about testosterone: It may have surprised you to learn that, as I mentioned earlier, testosterone is an important hormone for women as well as men. In fact, testosterone is crucial for normal female function. In women, testosterone is produced by the ovaries and the adrenal glands. In both sexes, one of testosterone's main jobs is to produce sex drive (libido). Women produce lower amounts than men, but it doesn't take a lot to maintain a healthy interest in sex. Testosterone also promotes hair growth; in women, high levels can cause unwanted hair on the face or elsewhere. In the female body, most of the testosterone is converted into estrogen.

Now that we've had a "grand tour" of the female system, let's look at how tuning up can keep things running efficiently. Parts A and B of the self-assessment address common issues for women who are still menstruating, while later in the chapter, Part C focuses on the needs of women in the perimenopausal, menopausal, and postmenopausal years.

FEMALE HEALTH ASSESSMENT • PART A
Premenstrual Syndrome

Circle the number that best describes the intensity of your symptoms on the following scale:

> *0 = I do not experience this symptom*
> *1 = Mild*
> *2 = Moderate*
> *3 = Severe*

Do you experience any of these symptoms within approximately two weeks prior to menstruation?

Monthly weight gain	0	1	2	3
Fatigue, lethargy	0	1	2	3
Depression	0	1	2	3
Moodiness, nervousness, or irritability	0	1	2	3
Bloating and swelling of fingers	0	1	2	3
Uterine cramping	0	1	2	3
Nausea and/or vomiting	0	1	2	3
Headaches	0	1	2	3
Easily distracted	0	1	2	3
Changes in appetite (sugar cravings)	0	1	2	3
Tender and enlarged breasts	0	1	2	3
Low backache	0	1	2	3

Add the numbers circled and enter the total here: _____

Scoring   *9 or more: High priority*
        5–8: Moderate priority
        1–4: Low priority

FEMALE HEALTH ASSESSMENT • PART B
Fibrocystic Problems

*Circle the number that best describes the intensity of your symptoms
on the following scale:*
   0 = I do not experience this symptom
   1 = Mild
   2 = Moderate
   3 = Severe

Breasts painful or sore to the touch	0	1	2	3
Premenstrual breast pain or discomfort	0	1	2	3

Add the numbers circled and enter that subtotal here: _____

Circle the number of the answer that applies to you:

Breast lumps/cysts	NO = 0	YES = 10
Uterine cysts (fibroids)	NO = 0	YES = 10
Mother used DES (a hormone) while pregnant	NO = 0	YES = 10
Family history of breast cancer	NO = 0	YES = 10

Add the numbers circled and enter that subtotal here: _____
Add the two subtotals and enter that total here: _____

Scoring   *9 or more: High priority*
         3–8: Moderate priority
         1–2: Low priority

Interpreting Your Score

Part A addresses the symptoms that can develop in the premenstrual
phase of the monthly cycle. During this time, the body undergoes a series of
hormonal changes that can affect nearly every organ system. Some of the
symptoms are physical, some are emotional, and some are behavioral. Each
woman responds differently to these hormonal tides. Many are able to go
about their daily routines with only minimal disruption. For others, the con-

dition can be so painful and debilitating that they are out of commission for a few days. In the worst cases, some women become so depressed that they think about suicide. As you'll learn below, there are many ways to moderate the symptoms of PMS through careful attention to diet and the use of special natural herbs and supplements.

Sometimes menstrual and premenstrual symptoms result from the presence of abnormal tissue in the female reproductive organs. For example, cysts—sacs or pouches filled with fluid—often develop in breast tissue and may be the result of a blocked duct or infection. In many cases, the breast lumps that can be felt on examination are the result of cysts. Part B reflects the pattern of symptoms associated with these growths, which together are known as fibrocystic breast disease.

Premenstrual Syndrome

PMS is defined as a recurrent condition characterized by troublesome symptoms occurring seven to fourteen days before the onset of menstruation. PMS affects between 30 and 40 percent of women in their reproductive years. Fortunately, most cases are relatively mild. However, for about one woman in ten with PMS, the condition can be severe, causing physical and emotional distress, missed days of work, and other problems. The range of symptoms is wide, showing the influence of hormones on both body and mind.

For years, debate has raged in the medical world about whether PMS is a "real" condition. Because of this foot dragging, many women who suffer from monthly symptoms have not been treated properly. Some physicians prefer to prescribe drugs to address the psychological aspects of PMS, including antidepressants such as Prozac or antianxiety drugs such as Valium. While these powerful medications might relieve some symptoms, they do not address the underlying hormonal changes. Worse, they cause a risk of serious side effects. And they can cost a fortune, especially for women who are told to take them on a monthly basis for perhaps thirty years of their lives.

In my opinion, a more rational approach for long-term health is to identify the specific factors that produce symptoms and to design a targeted treatment involving changes in diet, nutritional supplementation, and exercise. The most common causes of PMS are:

- Excess estrogen
- Progesterone deficiency
- Elevated prolactin levels
- Hypothyroidism
- Stress, low endorphin levels, and adrenal dysfunction
- A diet too high in sugar or saturated fat
- Deficiency of micronutrients (vitamins, minerals, or both)

Usually, the symptoms of PMS arise from a combination of two or more of these factors.

—— Restore the Estrogen-Progesterone Balance ——

An imbalance in the ratio between estrogen and progesterone can cause many related symptoms. Excess estrogen impairs liver function, which in turn can reduce your body's ability to detoxify itself. A deficiency of the B vitamins can make things worse, because your liver needs these nutrients to break down excess estrogen and excrete it in the bile.

The imbalance of hormones can also impair your brain's ability to produce serotonin, which can lead to depression. Similarly, estrogen excess during the luteal phase can reduce levels of your body's own natural pain-killing substances, the endorphins. Studies have shown that low endorphin levels during the luteal phase are common among women affected by PMS. Similarly, excess estrogen can cause mild increases in the level of aldosterone, an adrenal hormone that helps the body retain salt and water. Bloating and water retention are typical complaints of PMS sufferers. Breast tenderness may result from high levels of prolactin, which causes swelling of breast tissue as if the body were preparing to breastfeed. Estrogens, both those that are internally produced and those that are ingested as birth control pills or in drugs such as Premarin, are known to increase prolactin secretion by the pituitary gland.

For PMS relief, take these steps for reducing your estrogen-to-progesterone ratio.

1. *Eat a healthy diet.* See the top six dietary recommendations on pages 348–350.
2. *Establish proper gastrointestinal flora.* The liver eliminates excess

estrogen by attaching it to a molecule called glucuronic acid, which renders the hormone powerless and allows it to be excreted through the intestine. Unfortunately, certain bacteria in the gut secrete an enzyme called beta-glucuronidase, which breaks the bond between the acid and the estrogen. Once free, the estrogen is available to go back into circulation. By promoting the growth of friendly bacteria and thus reducing the population of this unwanted bacteria, you reduce the supply of glucuronidase and eliminate estrogen more efficiently. Try supplementing with probiotics such as *Lactobacillus acidophilus* and *Bifidobacterium bifidum* to encourage the beneficial bacteria. Take a supplement that will provide five to ten billion live bacteria daily.

3. *Check your intake of B vitamins and magnesium.* To detoxify estrogen, you need plenty of B vitamins and magnesium. Take at least ten times the RDA for each B vitamin and 250 to 400 mg of magnesium daily.

4. *Enhance liver detoxification with lipotropics.* In addition to the above steps, consider the use of formulas that contain lipotropic factors. These are substances that hasten the removal or decrease the deposition of fat and bile in the liver. In a sense, lipotropic factors are "decongestants" for the liver. Compounds typically used for this purpose include choline, methionine, folic acid, and vitamin B_{12}. Take a daily dose of 1,000 mg of choline along with 500 mg of methionine or cysteine or both; 400 to 800 mcg of folic acid; and 400 to 1,000 mg of vitamin B_{12}.

5. *Use herbs to regulate estrogen activity.* Chasteberry extract is the best choice for most women with PMS, especially if they are experiencing breast pain, infrequent periods, or ovarian cysts. It appears to affect hormone secretion by the brain's master glands, the hypothalamus and the pituitary. As a result, the extract may lower the output of prolactin-releasing hormone and GnRH, thus lowering the release of prolactin by the pituitary and the release of FSH. The net result: reduced estrogen and a lower risk of breast tenderness.

6. *As a last step, consider progesterone therapy.* You may have been asking, "If one of the primary features of PMS for most women is an elevated estrogen-to-progesterone ratio, why not simply take progesterone to improve the ratio?" Although progesterone administration has been the most common prescription for PMS in conventional as well as alternative medical communities, clinical trials have failed to consistently show the superiority of progesterone therapy over a

placebo. The few studies that show a positive effect have used dosages of progesterone (200 to 400 mg twice daily as a vaginal or rectal suppository, from fourteen days before the expected onset of menstruation until the onset of vaginal bleeding) that raise progesterone levels well above normal; as a result, side effects, although generally mild, are common. The most frequently reported side effects are irregularity of menstruation, vaginal itching, and headache.

I think it is better to help the body naturally improve the estrogen-to-progesterone ratio by addressing the underlying causative factors such as reduced detoxification or clearance of estrogen along with reduced corpus luteum function rather than artificially and drastically tipping the ratio in favor of progesterone. Nonetheless, here are some guidelines if you elect to give a progesterone-containing cream a try:

- First of all, make sure that the level (in mg) of progesterone per dosage unit is provided so that you can calculate how much of the cream is required to achieve the high dosage required (200 mg to 400 mg applied twice daily intravaginally). A distinction must be made between prescription progesterone preparations and some of the over-the-counter progesterone-containing creams, including those misrepresented as "yam concentrates." Mexican yam is a source of a compound known as diosgenin, which can be converted in a laboratory environment to progesterone as well as DHEA. There is no evidence that such a conversion occurs in the human body. Some companies will label a progesterone-containing cream as a yam concentrate as a marketing ploy, while other companies will market a true yam concentrate without any significant progesterone content yet promote it as providing the same benefit as a progesterone-containing cream. In both cases the misrepresentations are wrong.
- Intravaginal administration is more effective than simply applying the cream to anywhere on the skin. In fact, progesterone applied to the skin (instead of to mucous membranes) is poorly absorbed.
- Monitor your progesterone levels with saliva or blood progesterone levels. Saliva tests are available directly to consumers through BodyBalance, 1-888-891-3061 or www.bodybalance.com, or Aeron LifeCycles, 1-510-729-0375 or www.aeron.com.

CAUTION: I Yam Not What I Appear to Be   Many health food stores sell topical creams that contain "yam concentrates" and that are touted as being natural sources of progesterone. These are derived from the Mexican yam, which contains a substance called diosgenin. In the lab, scientists can wave their magic wands and change diosgenin into progesterone. However, the body is not able to do this trick, so such products are worthless as a strategy for raising progesterone levels.

Stress, Exercise, and PMS

As you know, stress is a major cause of many ailments. PMS is no exception. Prolonged or severe stress causes a domino effect, altering the function of the adrenal glands and leading to a big drop in the secretion or activity of endorphins. If depression is among your symptoms, I'm sure you already know that stress can trigger it. Any treatment for PMS must include effective stress-management techniques.

Many studies show that women who exercise regularly experience less frequent and less severe PMS symptoms, especially less deterioration of mood before and during menstruation. Exercise lifts mood, relieves anxiety, improves concentration, lowers the risk of behavioral or personality changes, and reduces pain.

The Anti-PMS Diet

A healthy diet is crucial for reducing the impact of PMS. In my practice, I have found that the worse a woman's diet, the more severe her symptoms. A noted researcher, Guy Abraham, M.D., discovered that, compared with symptom-free women, PMS patients consume:

- 62 percent more refined carbohydrates
- 275 percent more refined sugar
- 79 percent more dairy products
- 78 percent more sodium
- 53 percent less iron
- 77 percent less manganese
- 52 percent less zinc

Here are my top six dietary recommendations for relieving PMS:

1. *Eat a vegetarian or predominantly vegetarian diet and reduce intake of fat.* Because they consume more fiber and less fat, women who eat a vegetarian diet excrete more estrogen in their feces and have lower levels in their blood than meat eaters. Since your body makes estrogen from cholesterol, eating less saturated fat can dramatically reduce circulating estrogen levels. One study looked at what happened when women switched from the standard American diet (40 percent of calories from fat, only 12 g of fiber daily) to a healthier diet (25 percent of calories from fat, 40 g of fiber). Results showed a 36 percent reduction in blood estrogen levels within eight to ten weeks.

2. *Eliminate sugar.* Eating refined sugar causes blood sugar levels to soar and fall rapidly. This in turn leads to rotten moods and severe fatigue. High sugar intake also impairs estrogen metabolism, which can lead to excess levels of the hormone.

3. *Reduce dietary exposure to environmental estrogens.* Harmful chemicals, including pesticides, can enter the body and become lodged in fat cells. These chemicals—known as environmental estrogens—mimic the activity of estrogen in the body and may be a major factor in the growing epidemics of estrogen-related health problems, such as PMS and breast cancer. Avoid environmental estrogens whenever possible by choosing organic foods. Don't skimp on the fruits and veggies for fear of ingesting these compounds, however, since these foods contain antioxidants, which help your body neutralize toxins. Be aware, too, that the concentration of environmental estrogens is often higher in animal fats, meats, and dairy products than it is in plant foods. To remove surface pesticide residues, waxes, fungicides, and fertilizers, soak produce in a mild solution of additive-free soap, such as Ivory or pure castile soap. There are also all-natural, biodegradable cleansers available at most health food stores. Simply spray the produce with the cleanser, gently scrub, then rinse off. Alternatively, peel off the skin or remove the outer layer of leaves. The downside of peeling is that many of the nutritional benefits are concentrated in the skin and outer layers.

4. *Increase intake of soy foods.* Soy and soy foods contain phytoestrogens (plant estrogens). These substances are able to bind to the same cell receptors as the estrogen your body produces. That's a good thing, because when phytoestrogens occupy the "parking places," estrogen can't produce effects on cells. (Phytoestrogens are only about 2 percent as strong as the estrogen in your body.) By competing with estrogen, phytoestrogen causes a drop in estrogen effects, and are thus sometimes called antiestrogens.

5. *Eliminate caffeine.* Avoid caffeine, especially if you experience anxiety, depression, or breast tenderness as major PMS symptoms. Caffeine makes these problems worse.

6. *Keep salt intake low.* High salt intake, along with low potassium, makes it hard for your kidneys to maintain the fluid level your body needs. Specifically, salt causes your body to retain water, leading to bloating and swelling of the joints. Choose low-salt or no-salt foods, leave the salt shaker on the shelf, and eat high-potassium foods such as bananas and other fruits, vegetables, whole grains, and beans.

Supplemental Strategies

A good, high-potency vitamin and mineral supplement will provide you with the full range of micronutrients you need to minimize the symptoms of PMS. Pay special attention to vitamin B_6, magnesium, calcium, zinc, vitamin E, and essential fatty acids.

Vitamin B_6 and magnesium work as a team in many enzyme systems. Magnesium can't enter your cells unless it has plenty of vitamin B_6 as its "escort." Low magnesium is associated with depressed mood, mood swings, generalized aches and pains, breast tenderness, and weight gain.

Calcium supplementation has been shown to relieve PMS symptoms, especially low mood and poor concentration. It also helps reduce water retention and can boost neurotransmitter levels. While calcium supplementation is helpful, I recommend that women with PMS avoid dairy products. Dairy foods contain calcium, but they also contain vitamin D and phosphorus; when combined with calcium, these substances may interfere with your body's ability to absorb precious magnesium.

Zinc is necessary for sex hormones to function. It is also involved in controlling the secretion of hormones, especially prolactin. The more zinc you have on board, the lower your prolactin secretion, and the lower the risk of breast complaints associated with PMS.

Vitamin E is important for PMS primarily because it can reduce breast tenderness. It also improves fatigue, depression, nervous tension, and headache, and can help control weight gain.

Essential fatty acids are often low in women with PMS. Without adequate fatty acids, the prostaglandin system does not function normally, which can contribute to symptoms. The best way to get adequate levels of essential fatty acids is to take 1 tbsp of flaxseed oil daily.

———————— **Herbal Recommendations** ————————

Chasteberry extract is the number one herbal product for PMS, especially if you have acne, PMS-associated breast pain, infrequent periods, or a history of ovarian cysts. These conditions are characterized by corpus luteum insufficiency (lack of progesterone) or excess prolactin. Chasteberry extract is very effective at addressing such problems. In studies, 57 percent of women taking chasteberry extract reported significant improvement in their symptoms, while one-third experienced complete relief of symptoms. The usual dosage of chasteberry extract (standardized to contain 0.5 percent agnusides) in tablet or capsule form is 175 to 225 mg daily. If you use the liquid extract, the typical dosage is 2 ml daily.

Angelica (dong quai) is especially helpful if PMS is accompanied by painful menstruation (dysmenorrhea). Dong quai is widely referred to as "female ginseng" due to its popularity in Asia in the treatment of menstrual problems. When I recommend angelica for PMS, I tell my patients to take it beginning two weeks after menstruation stops and continue until menstruation starts again. If the patient also has a tendency for dysmenorrhea, I recommend that she keep taking it until menstruation has stopped. The dosage, to be taken three times per day, is:

- Powdered root or as tea: 1–2 g
- Tincture (1:5): 4 ml (1 tsp)
- Fluid extract: 1 ml (¼ tsp)

Licorice root appears to be most helpful for PMS relief when there is a great deal of fluid retention. It helps restore a healthier hormone balance by lowering estrogen and raising progesterone levels. It helps block the enzyme that breaks down progesterone. Licorice can also reduce water retention by blocking aldosterone. Here are dosage recommendations for the various forms of licorice, to be taken three times per day beginning on day 14 and stopping at the start of menstruation:

- Powdered root or as tea: 1–2 grams
- Fluid extract (1:1): 4 ml (1 tsp)
- Solid (dry powdered) extract (5 percent glycyrrhetinic acid content): 250–500 mg

Restoring Hormonal Balance After the Pill

Ellen, thirty-eight years old, wanted to get her hormones back in balance. She hadn't had a period in six years, ever since she stopped taking birth control pills. Her gynecologist told her that the pill was her only option for restoring hormonal balance. But Ellen didn't want to go back on the pill. She was worried because her mother had died from breast cancer, and Ellen didn't want to do anything that might increase her own risk of the disease. After working unsuccessfully with other doctors (including other naturopaths) for six years, she came to see me.

I explained to her that sometimes when women take birth control pills for a long time and then stop, prolactin levels may rise. Prolactin's chief function is to regulate development of the mammary glands and milk secretion during and after pregnancy. Elevated prolactin levels are the chief reason why nursing mothers usually do not get pregnant. In nonlactating women, elevated prolactin can cause absent or irregular cycles as well as PMS, ovarian cysts, breast tenderness, and acne. Ellen was experiencing all of these symptoms, so I was not surprised when her blood prolactin levels proved to be too high.

I prescribed the following: a high-potency multiple vitamin and mineral supplement, flaxseed oil, and chasteberry extract. It usually takes about three months for the effects of chasteberry to occur, so I tell women not to expect quick results. To my surprise, after only two weeks on my protocol, Ellen experienced her first period in six years.

If your periods are irregular or absent altogether, it is essential that you consult your doctor to find the cause. In my experience with patients, if the cause is an elevation in prolactin, chasteberry extract can help in most cases.

Excessive Menstrual Blood Loss

Many women experience heavy blood flow during their periods. If no medical cause can be found for the bleeding, such as fibroid tumors or endometriosis, the condition is known as *functional menorrhagia*. Often the problem can be prevented by adjusting the diet.

The first step, though, is to make sure that you don't have a serious underlying medical condition that may be causing the bleeding. *See your physician for an evaluation.*

It appears that in women with functional menorrhagia, the endometrium contains high levels of an essential fatty acid called arachidonic acid. Your body converts this substance into hormonelike substances called prostaglandins, which contribute to bleeding and menstrual cramps. During menstruation, release of arachidonic acid results in higher levels of prostaglandins. Most of the supply of arachidonic acid comes from animal fats in the diet, which is one reason I suggest reducing intake of animal products.

Other factors that may contribute to the problem are iron deficiency, vitamin A deficiency, and hypothyroidism. Bleeding causes loss of iron. By the same token, iron deficiency can contribute to bleeding problems. Low iron levels reduce enzyme activity in many tissues, including the lining of the uterus. Research has shown that taking 100 mg of supplemental iron a day can prevent excessive bleeding.

One study found that more than 90 percent of women had either complete relief or significant improvement in menorrhagia after taking vitamin A. Vitamin C also helps by strengthening blood capillaries and by increasing iron absorption. Antioxidants, including vitamin E, can reduce damage to uterine tissue caused by free radicals. Vitamin K and chlorophyll may also be useful, so be sure to increase your intake of dark green leafy vegetables like kale, spinach, mustard greens, and romaine lettuce.

CHECK YOUR THYROID FUNCTION!
Be sure to check your thyroid function if you suffer from PMS or excessive menstrual blood loss. Several studies have found that many women with PMS have low thyroid function and that treating these women with thyroid

hormone can lead to tremendous relief of PMS symptoms. Many of my patients with menorrhagia have also responded to thyroid hormone supplementation. (For more information, see pages 123–127).

In addition, hypothyroidism is one of the leading causes of infertility in women. The endometrium, the lining of the uterus, depends on good thyroid function to create a hospitable environment for the developing egg. It makes sense that a successful pregnancy would be tied to thyroid function, which in turn is linked to nutritional status. The mother must have an adequate supply of thyroid hormones and nutrients for her body to support the demands of a developing fetus.

If you are hypothyroid and are taking Synthroid or another thyroxine-only product but still are having trouble getting pregnant, consider switching to either natural thyroid or Thyrolar. These products contain both thyroxine and the other main thyroid hormone, T_3. Apparently these forms have better effects on the endometrium.

I have had several patients become fertile just by making this little switch. One patient, Joann, had tried everything for over eleven years. She had endured four stressful in vitro procedures, which had cost her $110,000 at fertility clinics—to no avail. Just two months after switching to natural thyroid, she got pregnant. She now introduces me to her friends as "the man who got me pregnant." Of course, I have to clarify that comment!

Tune-Up Tip: Female Fertility

The rate of infertility in the United States is on the rise. In about one-third of the cases the female is responsible, in another third it is the male, and in another third the cause is either unknown or involves both partners. For women, if no structural defect or disorder such as blocked fallopian tubes or endometriosis can be identified, I recommend trying four strategies before using any fertility drugs or hormones:

1. *Increase the quality of nutrition.* Eat a health-promoting diet and take a high-potency multiple vitamin and mineral formula.
2. *Rule out low thyroid function.* If you are taking Synthroid, switch to either natural thyroid or Thyrolar.
3. *Establish a regular menstrual cycle.* If necessary, use herbs such as chasteberry to help.
4. *Make fertility a "science project."* Read as much as you can. Ask your doctor for book suggestions. One of the best that I have seen is *Getting Pregnant: What Couples Need to Know Right Now,* by Niels H. Lauersen and Colette Bouchez (Fawcett Books, 1992).

Uterine Fibroids

Another condition associated with an increased estrogen-to-progesterone ratio is a benign growth in the uterus called a fibroid. Fibroids are bundles of smooth muscle and connective tissue that can be as small as a pea or as large as a grapefruit. Although they are sometimes called tumors, fibroids are not cancerous. However, because they disrupt the blood vessels and glands in the uterus, they can cause bleeding and loss of other fluids. Perhaps 20 percent of women over age thirty have at least one fibroid.

The treatment of uterine fibroids follows the same path as the treatment for PMS and fibrocystic breast disease, described above. For herbal support, I especially recommend black cohosh extract (see page 362). I have had several patients who improved dramatically by taking this herb and following the general dietary and nutritional supplement guidelines described above. One patient, Ruth, forty-one years old, had a fibroid the size of a softball. After she took black cohosh extract for three months, the fibroid shrank to the size of an egg, making it possible for her to cancel her scheduled hysterectomy.

Fibrocystic Breast Disease

FBD is a benign condition—not even a disease, really—that causes lumps and cysts to develop in breast tissue. Cysts are fluid-filled pockets; lumps are solid masses. These developments can lead to inflammation, causing the breast to swell and become painful. The pain can range from mild to severe. FBD is very common, occurring in perhaps 20 to 40 percent of women prior to menopause.

In some ways, FBD can be considered a feature of premenstrual syndrome, because it is the result of the hormonal changes during the menstrual cycle. Like PMS symptoms, FBD results from a high ratio of estrogen to progesterone, as well as from the presence of prolactin, the milk-producing hormone. These hormones stimulate cells in the milk ducts of the breast.

Also like PMS, FBD is cyclic. Lumps tend to develop in the days prior to the onset of menstruation, and they usually diminish soon afterward. Usually, though, before the breasts can return to their previous state, another menstrual cycle is under way. Over the years, as a result of this repeated stimulation and regression, most women's breasts have developed some degree of fibrocystic lumpiness. FBD does not usually occur in women after menopause.

The lumps associated with FBD are benign—that is, they are not cancerous. However, FBD is considered a risk factor for breast cancer. In other words, women who have FBD tend to be more likely to develop breast cancer later in life. Naturally, whenever a woman detects a lump in her breast, her first fear is that cancer has struck. Fortunately, most lumps are harmless. Still, it's important for you to consult with your doctor immediately if you notice any changes in your breasts.

Because FBD is associated with the menstrual cycle, the same dietary and supplemental strategies described above for PMS generally apply to the treatment of FBD. As in PMS, the goal is to restore a better balance between estrogen and progesterone (see pages 345–347).

It's especially important to eliminate caffeine from the diet. Caffeine stimulates overproduction of cellular products, such as fibrous tissue and cyst fluid. One study found that FBD symptoms improved in more than 97 percent of women who avoided caffeine entirely and in 75 percent of those who reduced their intake.

Low thyroid function also appears to play a role in FBD. Patients who take thyroid hormone often report less breast pain and swelling. In addition, lack of iodine in the diet may make breast tissue more sensitive to estrogen stimulation, so make sure you get enough iodine.

Tune-Up Tip: Elimination Is Essential

Women who have fewer than three bowel movements per week have a risk of fibrocystic breast disease 4.5 times greater than women who have at least one bowel movement a day. Reduced frequency of bowel movements means that more toxins are absorbed from the gut. It also means reduced elimination of estrogen. Try to establish good bowel habits, ideally leading to a daily bowel movement. To avoid constipation, increase the intake of high-fiber foods and make sure that you drink six to eight glasses of water per day.

FEMALE HEALTH ASSESSMENT • PART C:
Perimenopause and Menopause

Circle the number that best describes the intensity of your symptoms on the following scale:

- *0 = I do not experience this symptom*
- *1 = Mild*
- *2 = Moderate*
- *3 = Severe*

Hot flashes	0	1	2	3
Night sweats	0	1	2	3
Depression/mood swings	0	1	2	3
Insomnia	0	1	2	3
Sweating throughout day	0	1	2	3
Dryness of skin, hair, and vagina	0	1	2	3
Painful intercourse	0	1	2	3
Vaginal pain	0	1	2	3
Vaginal itching	0	1	2	3

Add the numbers circled and enter that subtotal here: _____

Circle the number of the answer that applies to you:

Hysterectomy before age 50	NO = 0	YES = 10
Osteoporosis (bone loss)	NO = 0	YES = 10

Add the numbers circled and enter that subtotal here: _____
Add the two subtotals and enter that total here: _____

Scoring   *9 or more: High priority*
        5–8: Moderate priority
        1–4: Low priority

Interpreting Your Score

At some point in life, usually between the ages of forty-five and fifty-five, the ovaries cease releasing eggs and begin producing far less estrogen. This is the menopause, a normal part of human aging. But without estrogen, the female body undergoes significant changes, which are addressed in the questions in Part C. Among the most common complaints of menopausal women are sudden episodes of overall body warmth, known as hot flashes. Many women also wake up at night drenched in sweat. The loss of estrogen causes dryness, pain, and itching in many tissues, including skin and the vagina. As a result, sexual intercourse may be a painful ordeal. One major concern is osteoporosis, since estrogen is needed to help maintain healthy bones.

Understanding Menopause and Perimenopause

Menopause is a natural stage in a woman's life at which the ovaries cease to function. They no longer release eggs and their production of ovarian hormones falls to minimal levels. Without hormones in circulation, the menstrual cycle ceases and the woman is no longer fertile. The average age of menopause is about fifty-one, but it can happen anytime from the age of 40 on. Six to twelve months without a period is the commonly accepted rule for diagnosing menopause. This time prior to the official designation of menopause is often referred to as perimenopausal, while the time after menopause officially occurs is referred to as postmenopausal. Women who have had their ovaries removed during an operation are said to be "surgically menopausal."

At menopause, the ovaries cease to produce estrogen and progesterone. As I explained earlier, estrogen signals the pituitary to stop producing FSH and LH. Without estrogen, the pituitary continuously pumps out high levels of FSH and LH in an effort to jump-start the ovaries. That's one reason why a blood test to measure FSH can establish whether menopause has occurred.

FSH and LH cause the ovaries and adrenal glands to step up production of androgens. Fat cells convert androgens into small amounts of estrogen. Still, women after menopause have only low levels of estrogen in their bodies. As you've learned, estrogen is important for the function of many tissues, including skin, mucous membranes, bones, and blood vessels.

Symptoms of menopause include hot flashes, headaches, vaginal dryness, frequent urinary tract infections, cold hands and feet, and changes in mental function.

Hot flashes result when the blood vessels in the skin dilate, causing a rise in temperature and reddening of the skin. The flash can last for a few seconds or several minutes, and may be accompanied by rapid heart rate, headaches, dizziness, weight gain, fatigue, and insomnia. Up to 80 percent of menopausal women in the United States report having hot flashes at menopause. In most cases, hot flashes subside over a few years as the body adjusts to its new hormonal status.

Lack of estrogen can cause the genital tissue to become thin, dry, and irritated, a condition known as atrophic vaginitis. As a result, many menopausal and postmenopausal women experience painful intercourse, increased risk of infection, and vaginal itching or burning. Bladder infections are also common, because at menopause there is a breakdown in the natural defense mechanisms that protect against bacterial growth in the urinary tract.

Mental changes at menopause, including forgetfulness and difficulty concentrating, can be very troubling. Often such problems arise as a result of age-related changes in the flow of oxygen and nutrients to the brain.

Dealing with Menopause

Typically, most conventional medical doctors regard menopause as a disease that must be treated with drugs and hormones. But in many cultures, menopause is seen as a normal part of life's process. In these societies, women often do not experience the same range or severity of symptoms associated with menopause, which makes me wonder whether menopause, as we know it in the West, is less a medical issue than a sociocultural phenomenon.

Medical treatment of menopause involves replacing the hormones that the ovary used to produce, especially estrogen. This practice is referred to as hormone replacement therapy, or HRT. Estrogen therapy controls hot flashes, restores vitality to the genitals and other tissues, and reduces risk of osteoporosis and cardiovascular disease.

But long-term use of estrogen replacement is associated with an increased risk of cancer of the breast or endometrium. To reduce the risk of endometrial cancer, progesterone (or its synthetic form, progestin) is usually added to the regimen because it protects the endometrium. If you have had a hysterectomy, you do not need to take progesterone. Women with diseases that get worse when estrogen is present, such as breast cancer, active liver disease, and pancreatitis, should not take hormones.

Other side effects of estrogen therapy include an increased risk of gallstones and formation of blood clots, nausea, breast tenderness, liver disorders, and fluid retention. Low-dose hormonal therapy is less likely to cause side effects than high-dose treatment, such as that used for oral contraception.

—— Strategies for Hormone Replacement ——

If you are considering HRT, here is a recap of some of the strategies used today.

One method is to take estrogen only—"unopposed estrogen"—for twenty-five days, followed by an estrogen-free interval of three to six days. Most doctors do not recommend this approach for women who still have a uterus because of the increased risk of uterine cancer.

Another approach, cyclic HRT, involves taking estrogen for twenty-five days, plus progestin for the last ten to twelve days of the cycle, followed by a three- to six-day hormone-free interval. For nine out of ten women, the cyclic HRT method causes predictable bleeding during the days without hormone.

A strong case can be made that the strategy known as continuous combined HRT offers the best benefit-to-risk ratio. This approach calls for taking both estrogen and progesterone every day, without an interval. This approach has several advantages:

- Avoidance of cyclical bleeding
- Avoidance of symptoms of premenstrual syndrome that often accompany estrogen
- Continuous protection of the endometrium against the cancer-causing effects of estrogen
- Greater convenience and patient compliance
- Lower daily and cumulative amounts of progestins required
- Prevention of rare conceptions by promoting endometrial atrophy
- Prolongation of the synergistic effects of estrogen and progesterone on bone integrity
- Regression of uterine fibroids

Tune-Up Tip: Replacing Hormones Naturally

If you take hormone replacements, you may choose from among natural and synthetic products. In my opinion, the preferred type of estrogen is a formulation called triple estrogen, or Tri-Est, which combines the three major natural forms of estrogen: estriol, estrone, and estradiol.

The preferred progesterone is micronized natural progesterone. *Micronized* means the hormone has been reduced to very small particles, which are easier to absorb. This form of the hormone is exactly the same as that produced by the body. My recommendation is to avoid synthetic progestins such as megestrol, norethindrone, and norgestrel as well as medroxyprogesterone acetate (such as Provera). Micronized progesterone is available in tablets as well as in creams.

Until there is more definitive research on the risks of HRT, I believe that most women should avoid it unless they are at risk of severe osteoporosis. (See pages 282–285 for my osteoporosis prevention program.) In my experience with hundreds of female patients over the years, diet, exercise, and lifestyle changes often relieve menopausal symptoms just as effectively as HRT and without the risks associated with long-term treatment.

——— Dietary and Supplement Strategies ———

As always, the most important dietary recommendation is to increase consumption of plant foods, especially those containing phytoestrogens such as soy, nuts, whole grains, apples, celery, parsley, and alfalfa. In countries where such foods are predominant in the diet, women have a lower incidence of hot flashes and other menopausal symptoms—not to mention a lower risk of breast and colon cancer.

Soy foods are especially important because they relieve hot flashes and vaginal atrophy. Soybeans contain isoflavones and phytosterols. One cup of soybeans can produce the same estrogenic effect as a tablet of Premarin, the most commonly prescribed form of estrogen therapy. Products made from whole soybeans, such as tofu and soy milk, are higher in isoflavonoids and are better for relief of menopausal symptoms than those produced from soy protein concentrates, such as meal-replacement formulas. Soy also reduces the risk of breast cancer and lowers LDL cholesterol, thus protecting against cardiovascular disease.

Certain supplements are also effective in relieving hot flashes and atrophic vaginitis:

- *Vitamin E* may help by increasing blood flow to genital tissue and by relieving dryness and irritation. It is available as an oil, cream, ointment, or suppository.
- *Bioflavonoids,* such as rutin and hesperidin, improve the strength and permeability of blood vessels. When taken with its metabolic partner *vitamin C,* hesperidin can help relieve hot flashes.
- *Gamma-oryzanol (ferulic acid)* is a growth-promoting substance found in grains. It enhances pituitary function and promotes the release of endorphins. Since the 1960s, gamma-oryzanol has been used effectively to treat menopausal symptoms, including hot flashes. One study found that 85 percent of women taking 300 mg per day experienced improvement in symptoms.

The herbs described on page 351 for treatment of PMS also work to relieve menopausal complaints. These include angelica (dong quai), licorice, chasteberry, and black cohosh, also known as Remifemin.

Tune-Up Tip: Black Cohosh Extract

The most widely used—and the only thoroughly studied—natural approach to treatment of the symptoms of menopause is a special extract of black cohosh *(Cimicifuga racemosa)* standardized to contain 1 mg of 27-deoxyacteine per tablet. The standard dose is two tablets twice daily. Over 1.5 million women have used black cohosh extract with great success. Clinical studies have shown that black cohosh extract relieves hot flashes as well as depression, night sweats, and vaginal atrophy. Black cohosh extract has been shown to produce symptomatic relief comparable to that of hormone replacement therapy without the risk of serious side effects.

Black cohosh extract offers a suitable natural alternative to HRT for menopause, especially where hormones are contraindicated, such as in women with a history of breast cancer, unexplained uterine bleeding, liver and gallbladder disease, pancreatitis, endometriosis, uterine fibroids, or fibrocystic breast disease.

Another valuable herb for menopausal women is *Ginkgo biloba* extract, which acts on the blood vessels. By improving circulation, ginkgo relieves cold hands and feet. It also enhances blood flow to the brain and enhances energy production by brain cells, improving the transmission of nerve signals. These effects can help reduce the memory problems and difficulty concentrating that affect many women at menopause. You may need to take ginkgo for as long as twelve weeks before noticing benefits.

Take 40 to 80 mg of the extract (standardized for 24 percent ginkgo flavon-glycosides) three times daily.

Lifestyle changes are crucial for effective menopause management. Exercising an average of thirty minutes per day reduces the frequency and severity of hot flashes. What's more, exercise also boosts mood and maintains muscle tone. Finally, weight-bearing exercise helps arrest the loss of bone due to osteoporosis—a crucial strategy for women as they age.

CASE HISTORY: Sue's Increased Libido

Sue, a forty-three-year-old insurance company employee, was typical of the many women I have treated who were going through perimenopause. More anxious than usual, Sue was experiencing hot flashes at times, and having very infrequent periods. However, her main complaint that brought her in to see me was a urinary tract infection. In the course of the interview, however, she admitted that she was also suffering from severe vaginal dryness. She told me that because of the dryness, sexual intercourse was not at all enjoyable even when they used lubricants. She was tempted to use HRT simply for the fact that she wanted to have her sex life back, but she was very fearful of its cancer-causing potential, since her mother had recently died of breast cancer.

I told Sue that in my experience the natural approach to menopause was extremely effective in dealing with vaginal dryness. In fact, in all of the cases where women have made the switch from HRT to the program that I have described above, they have reported to me that the relief was better with the natural approach compared with HRT.

In dealing with Sue's case, we had to first address the urinary tract infection (see page 367). A urine analysis was taken, and we began a course of uva ursi extract; I also encouraged her to drink cranberry juice. I explained to her that when we successfully reestablished proper moisture in the vaginal lining, her frequent bladder attacks would be eliminated. Sue was then placed on my standard program for menopause even though she was only perimenopausal, because her symptoms indicated low estrogen. I told her to increase her consumption of soy foods and then prescribed 1 tbsp of flaxseed oil daily, a high-potency multiple vitamin and mineral supplement, vitamin C with bioflavonoids (1,000 mg of each daily), 800 IU of vitamin E, and one tablet of Remifemin twice daily.

At her three-month checkup, Sue reported that her periods had returned. I had warned her that this might occur, as in my experience Remifemin tends to "milk" the ovaries for every last active follicle during perimenopause. She also reported restoration of the vaginal lining (this was confirmed by a vaginal exam by her gynecologist during her yearly Pap smear) and resumption of a more active sex life. She then proceeded to tell me that her libido was higher than it had ever been and wondered if it was the result of something that I'd given her. I explained to her that many of the patients that I had treated during perimenopause, menopause, and postmenopause with this program had also reported this effect. I cannot give an adequate explanation for it, but it is a consistent enough response that I believe it is real. My guess is that it is the Remifemin.

A Breast Cancer Prevention Plan

The rate of breast cancer is approximately five times higher among women in the United States than it is in certain other parts of the world. Recent research has shown most cases of breast cancer result from an unhealthy diet and lifestyle. Genetics plays a part, but many of the biggest risk factors are the ones that lie within your control. A list of factors linked to breast cancer appears in Table 10-1.

Table 10-1: Possible Risk Factors for Breast Cancer

Genetic factors
Hormonal factors (increased
estrogen exposure)
    Early onset of menstruation
    Pregnancy late in life or no
        pregnancy
    Late menopause
    Shorter menstrual cycles
Environmental factors
    Xenoestrogens (synthetic
        compounds that mimic
        estrogen)

    Pesticides, herbicides,
        halogenated compounds
    Lack of sunlight
    Power lines, electric blankets,
        radiation
Iatrogenic (resulting from medical
treatment)
    Oral contraceptives
    Hormone replacement therapy
    Radiation (diagnostic and
        therapeutic)
    Chemotherapy

Lifestyle factors
    Exposure to cigarette smoke
    Body weight (the more
        overweight you are, the
        greater the risk)
    Exercise level (women who
        exercise have a reduced rate)
    Alcohol and coffee consumption
Dietary factors linked to increased
risk
    Meats

Dairy
Total fat
Saturated fats
Refined sugar
Total calories
Alcohol
Low antioxidant intake
Low dietary fiber
Low intake of alpha-linolenic
    acid and omega-3 fatty acids
Decreased phytoestrogen intake

Diet affects breast cancer in two ways, one negative and one positive. Unhealthy foods—meats and dairy products, fats, refined sugar, alcohol—increase the risk; healthy foods—especially fish, whole grains, legumes, cabbage, and other vegetables, fruits, and nuts—can lower the risk.

Fish, particularly cold-water fish such as salmon, mackerel, halibut, and herring, are rich sources of the omega-3 fatty acids. In experimental studies, these fats have been shown to offer powerful protection against cancer, including breast cancer. In contrast, the omega-6 fatty acids found in most animal products, and in common vegetable oils such as corn and safflower oil, may promote breast cancer.

Supplementing the diet with flaxseed oil may increase your protection against breast cancer. Flaxseed oil contains twice the levels of omega-3 fatty acids as fish oils. A recent study of women with breast cancer found that those who had low levels of alpha-linolenic acid were at higher risk that the cancer would spread to other parts of the body. To put a positive spin on it: Supplementing the diet with flaxseed oil, which is approximately 58 percent alpha-linolenic acid, may help prevent breast cancer, invasive tumors, and metastasis.

In addition to containing fatty acids, flaxseed and flaxseed oils are abundant sources of lignans. These fiber compounds bind to estrogen receptors in your cells. By doing so, they interfere with the cancer-promoting effects of estrogen on breast tissue. Foods rich in phytoestrogens are also thought to protect against breast cancer because they too bind with estrogen receptors.

Lignans also work by stimulating production of sex hormone binding globulin, or SHBG. This protein attaches to molecules of estrogen to escort it out of the body. The more SHBG you have, the less active estrogen will be, and the lower your risk of breast cancer.

One of the key ways your body removes estrogen is by attaching glucuronic acid to the hormone in the liver and then excreting the complex in the bile. Unfortunately, some gut bacteria contain the enzyme glucuronidase. This enzyme uncouples (breaks) the bond between excreted estrogen and glucuronic acid. Excess glucuronidase activity in the gut is associated with an increased risk of cancer, particularly of estrogen-dependent breast cancer. The activity of this enzyme increases when the diet is high in fat and low in fiber. The level of glucuronidase activity may partly explain why certain dietary factors contribute to breast cancer and why other dietary factors are preventive.

The activity of glucuronidase can be reduced by establishing proper bacterial flora. The method is to eat a diet high in plant foods and supplement the diet with the beneficial bacteria *Lactobacillus acidophilus* and *Bifidobacterium bifidum*. Other dietary factors that can dramatically reduce the activity of this enzyme are the consumption of onions and garlic and foods high in glucaric acid such as apples, Brussels sprouts, broccoli, cabbage, and lettuce. Glucaric acid is also available in pill form.

Table 10-2: Dietary Factors That May Prevent Breast Cancer

Fish	Vegetables
Whole grains	Nuts
Legumes	Fruits
Cabbage	

NEW HOPE FOR BREAST CANCER PREVENTION

Calcium D-glucarate, a pill form of glucaric acid, may turn out to be the "magic bullet" in the prevention of breast cancer, especially in women who have already had the disease. Preliminary research is quite encouraging. Currently, women with a history of breast cancer are prescribed the drug tamoxifen. This drug is associated with numerous side effects and its overall effectiveness is still a matter of controversy. In contrast, calcium D-glucarate is completely safe and, if preliminary results hold true, is more effective than tamoxifen. Calcium D-glucarate is currently being investigated at the Memorial Sloan-Kettering Cancer Center in New York. It is just entering the health food market as well.

Given the epidemic nature of breast cancer, it is essential that every woman in America take steps to learn how they can prevent this often deadly disease. Primary prevention involves reducing controllable risk factors, adhering to a healthful lifestyle, eating a diet consisting primarily of protective factors (see Table 10-2), consuming 1 tbsp of flaxseed oil daily, and taking additional antioxidant nutrients (especially vitamin C, a minimum of 500 mg per day, and vitamin E, a minimum of 400 IU per day). I would also recommend that high-risk women take a high-quality *L. acidophilus* and *B. bifidum* product (approximately 2 billion live bacteria per day) and calcium D-glucarate (200 to 400 mg three times daily).

Bladder Infections (Cystitis)

At least once a year, nearly one woman in five—of all ages—suffers from the urinary tract discomfort that results from a bladder infection. The problem may increase during perimenopause. Symptoms include a burning pain on urination, increased urinary frequency, and pain in the lower abdomen. The urine itself is often cloudy, dark, or foul-smelling. Untreated bladder infections can have serious complications. If you experience these symptoms, consult a physician immediately. Here are other recommendations that can help.

The first strategy is to increase urine flow. The technique is simple: Drink more liquids. The best choices are pure water, fresh juices diluted with an equal amount of water, and herbal tea. Drink at least 64 ounces of liquid a day, at least half of which should be water. Avoid soft drinks, concentrated fruit drinks, coffee, and alcoholic beverages.

Cranberry juice (16 ounces per day) is particularly valuable as a strategy to prevent and relieve infections of the bladder and urinary tract. It may be that cranberry juice works by increasing the acidity of urine or because it contains a substance, hippuric acid, that destroys bacteria. However, I am more convinced by the research that cranberry juice reduces the ability of bacteria to stick to the mucous lining of the urinary tract. If the bacteria can't gain a toehold, then the risk of infection is minimal. Blueberry juice may work in similar fashion. However, other juices (grapefruit, guava, mango, orange, and pineapple) do not appear to offer protection.

Pure unsweetened cranberry juice is too strong for most people's taste. Most of the cranberry juices available in grocery stores are actually "cocktails" consisting of only one-third juice mixed with sugar and water. However, sugar can severely lower your immunity to infection (see page 154). If possible, select cranberry juice blended with apple or grape juice, or use blueberry juice. Cranberry extracts are also available in pill form.

If you opt to take a pill, I recommend upland cranberry (uva ursi) over regular cranberry. Uva ursi (*Arctostaphylos uva ursi*) contains arbutin, which has long been used as a diuretic and for relief of urinary tract complaints, especially those caused by *E. coli*—the most common cause of bladder infections. In the body, arbutin is converted to a substance called hydroquinone. However, arbutin by itself can be destroyed by intestinal bacteria. Taking the whole plant or extracts prevents this problem, allowing for improved absorption of the arbutin molecule, thus leading to higher levels of hydroquinone. Here are the dosages for uva ursi in various forms to be taken three times daily with a glass of water:

Dried leaves or as a tea: 1.5 to 4.0 g (approximately 1–2 tsp)
Freeze-dried leaves: 500–1000 mg
Tincture (1:5): 4–6 ml (1–1½ tsp)
Fluid extract (1:1): 0.5–2.0 ml (¼–½ tsp)
Powdered solid extract (10 percent arbutin content): 250–500 mg

THE ACID TEST?

In treating urinary infections, health care experts have long debated whether it's better to increase the acid quality of urine or to increase its alkali levels. Increasing acidity can be difficult; you'd need to drink at least a quart of cranberry juice at one time to do the trick.

In my opinion, alkalinization appears to be easier and more effective. Citrate salts are best, because they are rapidly absorbed and metabolized without affecting pH in the digestive tract or producing a laxative effect. They are excreted as carbonate, thus raising the pH of the urine. (pH levels higher than 7 are alkaline; lower than 7 are acidic.) Studies show that citrate can relieve pain and reduce infection in up to 80 percent of cases. Take calcium citrate at a dosage that supplies 125 to 250 mg of calcium three to four times daily to alkalinize the urine.

There's another advantage to alkalinizing the urine: Many of the herbs used to treat UTI, such as uva ursi, contain antibacterial components that work better in an alkaline environment.

Summary: Tune-Up for Women

- Eat a healthy diet—rich in plant foods (especially soy), fish, and fiber (30–40 g per day), low in fat, sugar, salt, and caffeine.
- Exercise at least thirty minutes three times a week.
- Improve detoxification of estrogen through use of B vitamins, magnesium, and, if needed, lipotropic factors (1,000 mg of choline plus 500 mg of methionine or cysteine or both).
- Take a high-potency multiple vitamin and mineral supplement.
- Take 1 tbsp flaxseed oil a day.
- Take extra antioxidants: vitamin C, minimum 500 mg per day; vitamin E, minimum 400 IU per day.
- Try to have a bowel movement every day.

Lifestyle Tune-Up #10:
Become a "Good Finder"

In order for people to be really happy with themselves and life, I believe that they must become what Zig Ziglar refers to as "good finders"—people who look for the good in other people or situations.

A classic experiment illustrates just how powerful an effect looking for the good can have on others. The study, conducted at Harvard University by Dr. Robert Rosenthal, involved three groups of students and three groups of rats. He informed the first group of students, "You're in luck. You are going to be working with genius rats. These rats have been bred for intelligence and are extremely bright. They will perform the tests like running through a maze with great ease."

The second group was told, "Your rats are just average. They are not too bright, not too dumb, just a bunch of average rats. Don't expect too much from them."

The third group was told, "Your rats are really dumb. If they find the end of the maze, it will be purely by accident."

For the next six weeks, the students conducted experiments with the rats involving having individual rats run through a maze. Their performance was timed. Not surprisingly, the genius rats behaved like geniuses and had the lowest times. The average rats were average and the dumb rats were really dumb.

So what is so amazing about this study? Well, it turns out that all of the rats were from the same litter. There were no genius, average, or dumb rats. The only difference between them was the direct result of the difference in attitude and expectations of the students conducting the experiments.

Does the same thing happen with humans? Most definitely. Studies conducted with teachers and children produced the same kind of results as the studies with the rats. Remarkable as it may seem, it has been shown many times in controlled experiments that parents, teachers, managers, and others will get exactly what they expect. A name has been given to this phenomenon: the Pygmalion effect.

According to Greek mythology, Pygmalion was a sculptor and king of Cyprus who fell in love with one of his creations. The ivory statue came to life after Pygmalion's repeated prayers to the goddess of love, Aphrodite. Pygmalion's vision was so powerful and his faith so strong, his vision became his reality. The myth exemplifies the truth that what we see reflected in many objects, situations, or persons is what we put there with our own expectations. We create images of how things should be, these images tend to become self-fulfilling prophecies.

If we expect only the worst from people, that is exactly what we see. If we can focus our attention on the positives, if we can look for the good in people and situations, that becomes our reality. In addition, if we are constantly criticizing and looking for the negatives in people, especially our loved ones, this attitude is reflected, and we too are harshly judged and criticized.

To be happy and have positive relationships, you absolutely must become a good finder. You must look for the good in people. You must expect the best from people. And you must reinforce the good that you see. You must also demonstrate your love and appreciation.

It is not enough to simply feel love in our friendships and intimate relationships; we must express these feelings. We must demonstrate to our loved ones just how important they are to us. We must continually find ways to communicate our deepest feelings through our actions, whether they are verbal, written, through touch, or by our behavior. We all need to see, hear, and physically feel loved and appreciated. I strongly urge you to seek out ways to continually tell those around you how much you love and appreciate them. It creates a powerful feedback cycle that raises your feelings of self-worth.

CHAPTER 11

Tune-Up for Men

Rightly or wrongly, sex is often at the center of a man's sense of identity. Perhaps that's because testosterone, the hormone responsible for the sex drive, is considered the "male" hormone (although, as discussed in Chapter 10, women have testosterone too).

When a man suffers from sexual problems, such as impotence, premature ejaculation, or infertility, he may feel unmanly. The thought of being unable to perform sexually is at odds with his image of himself. In fact, decreased sexual performance is a concern for nearly one man out of four over the age of fifty. As men age, other health problems, such as poor circulation, can make the problem worse. What's more, changes in the prostate gland, an organ found only in men, can interfere not only with sex but with urination. Cancer of the prostate is a leading killer of males, especially in the later decades of life. Fortunately, many of these problems can be addressed through the same tune-up strategies that promote general good health and well-being.

In this chapter I'll describe steps you can take to maintain sexual vitality throughout your lifespan. If you're concerned about fertility, you can take advantage of natural strategies to increase your chances of conceiving a child with your partner. You'll also learn how to reduce the risk or severity of prostate disorders and infections of the genital organs that can severely disrupt the quality of life.

First, to get you oriented, here's a quick guided tour of the male body.

The Male Sexual System

The male sexual system includes the penis, testicles (also called the testes, the plural form of testis), the prostate gland, and the various ducts and vessels that carry fluids during ejaculation.

The penis contains erectile tissue, blood vessels, nerves, and the urinary tube (the urethra), all surrounded by skin. Men who have not been circumcised have a sheath of skin (the foreskin) that covers the tip of the penis (the glans). The glans is rich in the nerves that respond to sexual stimulation.

Inside the penis are three cylindrical chambers that are responsible for erection. Two of these, lying on either side of the shaft, are called the corpora cavernosa. The third, the corpus spongiosum, lies below and between the others. The urethra passes through the corpus spongiosum.

When a man becomes sexually aroused, nerves signal the arteries to increase blood flow into these chambers. At the same time the veins, which normally drain blood away from the penis, clamp down. Because blood flows in faster than it can drain away, the pressure in the penis builds, expanding and firming up the chambers until the erection is complete. After orgasm, the nerves signal the veins to reopen. Blood drains out, the chambers deflate, and the penis returns to its flaccid state.

The testicles are two oval glands that are responsible for the production of sperm and androgens (male hormones), especially testosterone. They lie inside the scrotum, a thin sac that hangs below the base of the penis. Each testicle is surrounded by a thick, protective capsule of connective tissue.

Inside the testicle are numerous tiny tubes where immature sperm cells are born. The cells migrate to the epididymis, a coiled tube that lies alongside each testicle. (If you unrolled the tube, it would be about twenty feet long.) The journey through the epididymis takes several weeks, during which the sperm cells mature. The sperm are stored in tubes called seminal vesicles, awaiting ejaculation. During orgasm, the sperm cells travel out of the testicles through a tube called the vas deferens. *Vas* is the Latin word for "duct"; a vasectomy—the operation that makes a man infertile—involves cutting this tube so sperm can't escape.

KEEPING COOL

As every man knows, the testicles are very sensitive to pain. You may wonder why, then, they exist outside the body in such a vulnerable spot. There's a logical answer: Sperm formation cannot occur effectively at normal body temperature (98.6 degrees Fahrenheit). By placing the testicles outside the body, nature keeps them a degree or two cooler. The testicles are also equipped with muscles so they can be drawn closer to the body when they get too cold—as every man who has ever stepped out of a swimming pool on a chilly day can verify.

Sperm produced by the testicles are just one component of semen, the fluid that spurts out of the penis during orgasm. Other organs in the male system, known as the accessory glands, contribute different components to the semen. These components are designed to preserve the sperm, facilitate its journey, and make fertilization of the egg more likely.

- The bulbourethral glands are located inside the body, behind the root of the penis and before the prostate. They contribute a mucus that neutralizes any acidic urine that remains in the urethra.
- The seminal vesicles, found on the wall of the bladder, produce a yellowish fluid that helps maintain the proper consistency of semen. The fluid also contains sugar, which the sperm use to fuel their frantic swim upstream. About 60 percent of the ejaculate consists of fluid from the seminal vesicles.
- The prostate gland releases prostatic fluid, which is highly alkaline and which thus protects sperm as they travel through the acid environment of the female reproductive tract. The urethra also passes through the prostate gland. The prostate acts as a valve that allows sperm and urine to flow in one direction. It also functions as a pump that forces semen along the urethra and out through the penis.

The Stages of the Male Sexual Act

For men, as for women, sex can begin with the slightest stimulation: a light touch, a favorite smell, a whispered word, an arousing image. Even the mere thought of sex can get the blood stirring. In response, nerve signals flash back and forth between the brain and the organs. One such signal causes the blood vessels to release a gas, nitric oxide, which causes the muscles in the vessels to relax and become wider. (The 1998 Nobel Prize for physiology or medicine was awarded to the American scientists who discovered the role of nitric oxide in the body.) Blood flows in, producing the erection. Expansion of the penis causes pressure on the veins, trapping the blood and allowing the erection to be sustained. Meanwhile other nerve signals stimulate the bulbourethral glands to release fluid that lubricates the urethra and the glans.

The pleasant friction of sexual activity sends signals along nerve pathways. When the stimulation becomes extremely intense, the reflex centers of the spinal cord trigger a massive discharge of nerve impulses. The heart rate, breathing, and blood pressure rise. The reproductive ducts and glands contract, emptying their contents into the urethra. Muscles in the penis contract and propel semen. Feelings of pleasure wash over the body. This technical description does not do justice to the event itself, which we call the climax or orgasm.

Almost immediately after orgasm, the muscles and nerves of the body relax. Blood leaves the penis, causing it to return to its flaccid state. Most men need to rest for a period of time—ranging from a few minutes to several hours—before they can achieve orgasm again.

Tune-Up Tip: Exercise for a Better Sex Life

You know that regular exercise is important, but will it improve your sex life? Absolutely. According to a recent study, exercise not only boosts cardiovascular fitness, it increases interest and ability to participate in sex. The study examined the impact of exercise on sexuality in seventy-eight sedentary but healthy men, whose average age was forty-eight. They exercised an hour a day, three or four times per week, for three months. During the first and last months of the study, they kept daily diaries. By the end of the study, the diaries showed that, compared with a control group, these men had a higher frequency of sexual activity, more reliable physical function during sex, and a greater percentage of satisfying orgasms. The higher the degree of physical fitness, the better the sexuality.

ASSESSING ERECTILE FUNCTION AND LIBIDO

Circle the number that best describes the intensity of your symptoms on the following scale:

0 = I do not experience this symptom
1 = Mild
2 = Moderate
3 = Severe

Difficulty attaining and/or maintaining an erection	0	1	2	3
Anxiety or fear of sexual intimacy with women	0	1	2	3
Premature ejaculation	0	1	2	3
Pain/coldness in genital area	0	1	2	3

Add the numbers circled and enter that subtotal here: _____

Circle the number of the answer that applies to you:

Infertility	NO = 0	YES = 10
Varicose veins in scrotum (varicocele)	NO = 0	YES = 10
Low sperm count	NO = 0	YES = 10

Add the numbers circled and enter that subtotal here: _____
Add the two subtotals and enter that total here: _____

Scoring   *8 or more: High priority*
3–7: Moderate priority
1–2: Low priority

Interpreting Your Score

This questionnaire covers the issue of reduced sexual drive and function. Despite the stereotype, men are not always interested in having sex. Sometimes, though, the spirit may be willing but the flesh may be weak. A drop in libido can be the result of many factors: a poor diet, hormonal disruptions, or a disease or other physical ailment. Emotional concerns, such as anxiety about performance or a fear of intimacy, may also play a role.

Impotence (Erectile Dysfunction)

Impotence is defined as the inability to achieve and sustain an erection adequate for sexual intercourse. Recently medical experts have started to use the more precise term *erectile* (or *male sexual*) *dysfunction*. This helps distinguish problems with erection from other disorders, such as infertility (inability to produce sperm capable of fertilizing an egg), loss of sex drive (libido), premature ejaculation (having orgasm too soon), or inability to achieve orgasm.

As many as twenty million men in the United States suffer from erectile dysfunction. That number will rise dramatically as our population ages. One recent study found that 52 percent of men between the ages of forty and seventy reported a problem with erections. Although the frequency of erectile dysfunction increases with age, such problems are not necessarily the inevitable result of aging. Many men in their seventies, eighties, and older remain virile and sexually active, while younger men may be frustrated and upset by their lack of sexual ability.

In about 85 percent of cases, erectile dysfunction results from a physiological cause, such as a problem with blood circulation, use of medications or alcohol, or a metabolic disorder such as diabetes. Abdominal surgery, such as prostate surgery, can sever the nerves responsible for erection. For one man in ten, the cause is psychological, arising due to stress, depression, or anxiety. In some cases, the cause is unknown.

The first step in correcting the problem is to determine whether you have a physical condition that is causing or contributing to erectile dysfunction. See a physician, particularly a urologist, for a physical exam. There are special tests that can be performed to evaluate your situation. In one test, called nocturnal penile monitoring, you attach a band around your penis before going to sleep. If you have an erection during the night, the band breaks. This simple method indicates that you are indeed able to have an erection. You may also need to undergo tests to evaluate the blood vessels and nerves. Psychological tests can determine whether harmful thoughts and feelings are getting in the way of your ability to enjoy sex.

Nearly half of men with erectile dysfunction have atherosclerosis— hardening of the arteries, especially (but not exclusively) the blood vessel that serves the penis. Thus the problem with erections may be a sign of a more dangerous cardiovascular condition that could lead to a potentially fatal heart attack or stroke. For a complete discussion of atherosclerosis, and what to do to prevent or reverse it, see Chapter 6. Pay particular attention to the discussion on pages 212–213 about vitamin B_3 (niacin), especially the form known as inositol hexaniacinate. Besides being an effective strategy for reducing the risk of atherosclerosis, inositol hexaniacinate improves blood flow. It is widely used in Europe as an aid to circulation.

Many prescription medications can interfere with sexual function. The biggest culprits are the drugs that lower blood pressure (antihypertensives), including diuretics, beta-blockers, calcium channel blockers, and ACE inhibitors. If your blood pressure is only mildly or moderately elevated, you probably don't need these drugs. Talk to your doctor about your regimen and see if you can quit using medication. As you've learned from this book, there are many natural remedies for a wide range of conditions, including high blood pressure, that do not pose a risk of side effects.

Long-term use of alcohol or tobacco also contributes to impotence. Excessive drinking can cause the testicles to shrink, thus reducing the supply of testosterone. Smoking cigarettes can inhibit the ability to achieve erection.

Since much of our sexuality is under the control of hormones, it is not surprising that endocrine disorders can interfere with sexual ability. Normally, as men reach middle age, testosterone production drops by about 1 percent each year. A more rapid decline may be a sign of a condition called hypogonadism, or low activity by the sexual organs. This problem may result from a disease affecting the testicles, such as cancer, or changes in the way hormonal signals travel to and from the brain.

People with diabetes are at higher risk of impotence due to atherosclerosis and nerve damage. Hypothyroidism is a concern, because thyroid hormones are crucial for effective functioning by virtually every cell in your body. You may want to consider taking supplemental doses of thyroid hormones. Other endocrine-related causes include high levels of prolactin (which in women stimulates production of milk by the breasts). See Chapter 4 for a more complete discussion of metabolic disorders.

Diseases of, or injury to, the male sexual organs can cause erectile dysfunction. Peyronie's disease causes the connective tissue within the penis to thicken, making the penis bend at an angle when erect. Intercourse is often difficult and painful. The condition sometimes improves without any treatment. However, I recommend an enzyme called bromelain, a protein-digesting enzyme from pineapple that prevents the buildup of connective tissue. Take 750 mg of bromelain three times daily on an empty stomach. Take bromelain along with a concentrated extract of *Centella asiatica* (gotu kola). This herb contains triterpenic acids that can normalize connective tissue. I have recommended this approach to several patients, who report substantial improvement within two to six weeks.

If the problem of erectile dysfunction persists, there are several effective medical options available to you. Low hormone levels can be corrected by taking testosterone injections every two to four weeks (or more frequently, depending on your individual needs). A skin patch is available that can be attached to the arm or a shaved area of the scrotum. Although this method delivers steadier doses of testosterone, the patch can sometimes irritate the skin and is more expensive than injections.

Instead of testosterone, I recommend using DHEA to boost testosterone levels. On page 137 I told you the story of Fred and how we based his dosage of DHEA on his testosterone levels. I think this approach is safer and more beneficial than testosterone therapy. If for some reason the DHEA does not boost testosterone, I would recommend androstenedione as the next best choice at a dosage of 50 mg daily. You may remember that this compound was the subject of some debate during Mark McGwire's assault on Roger Maris's home run record. Androstenedione is only one step away from testosterone, while a few more steps of conversion are needed to turn DHEA into testosterone.

The popular drug Viagra, taken an hour before anticipated intercourse, works by improving blood flow into the penis. Other drugs are available that can be injected into the penis or inserted through a tube into the urethra. At this writing, pharmaceutical companies are developing a cream that can be applied and that may produce quick results; such an approach, if it is found to work, may be the most acceptable. It is also possible to undergo surgery to correct faulty blood vessels or to implant "balloons" that inflate and produce erection. Vacuum pumps work by drawing blood into the organ; a ring applied around the base of the penis holds the blood in place until after orgasm. Psychotherapy may be important for men who are wrestling with stress, frustration, and anxiety.

ANDROSTENEDIONE IS NO "HOME RUN" PILL While there is some evidence that androstenedione can raise testosterone levels in adult females and males, it should definitely not be used for this purpose in people below the age of thirty years, especially young men. Due to the body's normal metabolic pathways when testosterone levels are high, additional androstenedione gets converted into estrogen.

A 1999 article that appeared in the *Journal of the American Medical Association (JAMA)* clearly demonstrated that androstenedione should *not* be taken by young men and teenagers. It offers no benefit and carries with it significant health risks. The study, conducted at the University of Iowa, involved thirty healthy men age nineteen to twenty-nine years with normal testosterone levels. Twenty of the men performed eight weeks of whole-body resistance training. During weeks one, two, four, five, seven, and eight, ten of the men were given 300 mg of androstenedione a day, and the others were given a placebo.

The researchers discovered that muscle strength did not differ between the placebo and androstenedione groups before training or after four and eight weeks of resistance training and supplementation. They also found that testosterone levels in the blood were not affected by the supplement intake, but that estrogen levels increased dramatically. There were also slightly higher levels of LDL ("bad") cholesterol and slightly lower levels of HDL ("good") cholesterol in the subjects who took androstenedione. The bottom line is that androstenedione provides no benefit to this age group, but carries with it significant health risks.

The Natural Approach to Erectile Dysfunction

Achieving an erection depends on a mix of factors: proper levels of male sex hormones, sensory stimulation, and a good blood supply. In turn, all of these factors depend upon adequate nutrition.

Diet

The diet and nutritional guidelines discussed throughout this book will help you function at your sexual best. A diet rich in whole foods, particularly vegetables, fruits, whole grains, and legumes, is extremely important. Adequate protein is also a must. Be sure you consume high-quality protein from fish, chicken, turkey, and lean cuts of beef (preferably hormone-free) rather than from fat-filled sources such as hamburgers, roasts, and pork.

Special foods that may enhance virility include liver, oysters, nuts, seeds, and legumes. All of these foods are good sources of zinc. Zinc is perhaps the most important nutrient for sexual function. Because zinc is concentrated in semen, frequent ejaculation can greatly diminish your body's supply. Zinc deficiency, in turn, can lead to reduced sexual drive, since the body will try to conserve its supply of this important trace mineral. Daily intake should be 30 to 60 mg.

Others key nutrients for sexual function include essential fatty acids, vitamin A, vitamin B_6, and vitamin E. A high-potency multiple vitamin and mineral formula ensures adequate intake of these nutrients as well as others important in health and sexual function.

—— Enhancing Sexual Function with Herbs ——

Herbal medicines are often used in the natural treatment of erectile dysfunction. The goal is to select herbs that improve the activity of the male glandular system, improve the blood supply to erectile tissue, and enhance the transmission of nerve signals.

- Potency wood or muira puama (*Ptychopetalum olacoides*) has long been used by natives of Brazil as an aphrodisiac and nerve stimulant. A recent study at the Institute of Sexology in Paris found that taking a daily dose of 1 to 1.5 g of extract raised libido in more than 60 percent of patients and helped more than half of those who complained of erection failure.
- *Ginkgo biloba* extract is extremely beneficial in treating vascular insufficiency in many tissues, including the brain. Recent evidence indicates *Ginkgo biloba* extract appears to be effective in the treatment of erectile dysfunction caused by lack of blood flow. Select a product that is standardized to contain 24 percent ginkgo heterosides (flavonglycosides) and take 40 mg three times a day. Long-term therapy—at least twelve weeks—is usually necessary before you see results.
- Damiana (*Turnera diffusa*) has been used in the United States for more than a century as an aphrodisiac and for improving sexual ability, but I know of no clinical studies to support this claim. Damiana slightly irritates the urethra, thereby producing increased sensitivity in the penis. A cup of damiana tea should be sufficient to produce urethral

irritation. Damiana is usually not taken alone but is combined with other herbs.

- *Panax ginseng* (Korean or Chinese ginseng), the most widely used and most extensively studied ginseng, is generally regarded as having the most potent effects of all the ginsengs. Many people claim it is a sexual rejuvenator, but human studies to support this belief have not been performed. However, ginseng has been shown to promote growth of the testes and to increase sperm formation and testosterone levels. In animals, ginseng appears to increase sexual activity and mating behavior. Siberian ginseng may have similar effects. Ginseng also reduces stress, fights fatigue, and boosts energy levels, which can contribute to sexual vitality. The typical dosage for *Panax ginseng* root powder or extract containing 5 percent ginsenosides is 100 mg, one to three times daily. Start with low doses and increase gradually, depending on response.

WARNING: Barking Up the Wrong Tree   Yohimbe bark *(Pausinystalia johimbe)* is the source of a powerful prescription drug called yohimbine, which increases blood flow to erectile tissue and is used in the treatment of impotence. In my opinion, and in that of the FDA, yohimbe bark, available in health food stores, can be unsafe and should be used only under supervision of a physician. I am concerned about both the risk of side effects and the quality of yohimbe products available over the counter, since most of these products do not state the amount of yohimbine they contain per dose.

Male Infertility

In a way, every physiological function I've described throughout this book exists for one purpose only: to create an adult human being capable of reproducing itself and thus preserving the species for another generation. Unfortunately, about 15 percent of couples who want children have trouble conceiving. In about one-third of cases of infertility, the problem lies with the male; in another third, the female is responsible, and in the rest both partners are responsible. All told, perhaps 6 percent of men between the ages of fifteen and fifty are infertile.

Most infertile males produce low numbers of sperm or they produce sperm that is of poor quality. Although it takes only one sperm to fertilize an egg, a man ejects nearly 200 million sperm during a single ejaculation. The female reproductive tract puts up barriers so that only about 40 sperm actually reach the egg, and only one is able to penetrate the egg's outer shell. The more sperm entering the race, the greater the chances of fertilization.

Nine times out of ten, the cause of male infertility is low sperm count. Sometimes a physical cause can be identified: an obstruction in the sperm ducts, problems with ejaculation, or a problem with the accessory glands that contribute various fluids to semen. Often, too, disease, stress, or abuse of chemicals can temporarily lower sperm count (see Table 11.1). But 90 percent of the time, doctors can't find out why the man does not produce enough sperm. In this section I'll discuss natural strategies for tuning up sperm production.

Table 11-1: Causes of Temporary Low Sperm Count

- Increased scrotal temperature
- The common cold, the flu, other infections
- Increased stress
- Lack of sleep
- Overuse of alcohol, tobacco, or marijuana
- Many prescription drugs
- Exposure to radiation
- Exposure to solvents, pesticides, and other toxins

SPERM COUNTS: A BRIEF DISCUSSION

In recent decades there has been a drop in both the average quantity and quality of sperm. In 1940 the average sperm count was 113 million per ml, but half a century later the count plummeted to 66 million per ml. The amount of seminal fluid also fell by 20 percent. Put another way: Today's man produces only about 40 percent as many sperm per ejaculation as a man did just prior to World War II. Experts attribute the decline to a variety of factors: poor diet, unhealthy lifestyle, dangerous chemicals in the environment. Wearing briefs as opposed to boxers can also be a factor, since tight underpants hold the scrotum closer to the body and may keep the testicles too warm to produce enough viable sperm.

But quantity isn't the only factor. A high sperm count means nothing if most of those sperm are unhealthy or abnormal. Sperm that are oddly shaped, that have damaged tails, or that lack the swimming stamina they need to reach the egg are likely to die during their arduous journey through the female reproductive tract. Tests are available that measure sperm function, including their motility and ability to penetrate the egg. Another test detects the presence of antisperm antibodies, which indicate a past or present infection in the male reproductive tract.

Medical treatment is often effective when the cause of low sperm count can be identified. For example, surgery can relieve blocked sperm ducts or varicoceles (varicose veins in the testicle). Use of antibiotics can cure infections. Changing or eliminating prescription medications can reduce the sex-related side effects. Since use of tobacco, alcohol, or illicit drugs—especially marijuana—can interfere with sperm production (among other damaging effects), it makes sense to avoid these substances.

One of the simplest things you can do to raise your fertility is maintain a low scrotal temperature. Ideally, the scrotum keeps the testicles at a temperature between 94 and 96 degrees Fahrenheit. Higher temperatures can cause sperm production to slow or stop completely. Scrotal temperature is higher in men who wear tight-fitting underwear (especially underwear made from synthetic fabrics) or jeans. Other causes include soaking in hot tubs, jogging, or using exercise machines such as treadmills, rowing machines, or cross-country ski simulators. After exercising, a man should allow his testicles to hang free to recover from heat buildup during exercise. Cool showers (even ice, if you can stand it) can help. A device called a "testicle cooler" is available. It looks like a jockstrap and contains a pump with tubes through which cool water circulates.

—— A Natural Approach to Increased Fertility ——

Scrotal temperature is a key factor in sperm production, but so is nutritional status. For optimal fertility, it makes sense to eat a healthy diet that supports potency. Certain nutrients deserve special mention. Let's start with the antioxidants.

Free radicals can damage cells in the body, and sperm cells are no exception. High levels of free radicals have been found in 40 percent of infertile men. Cigarette smoking in particular is associated with decreased sperm counts and lower sperm motility. Exposure to heavy metals such as lead, cadmium, arsenic, and mercury may also be involved. Sperm are sensitive to free radicals because they depend on the integrity and fluidity of their cell membranes for proper function. Free radicals shoot through the membrane and rip it to shreds. Unlike other cells in the body, sperm are low in the enzymes needed to repair oxidative damage. What's more, sperm generate their own free radicals as a strategy for breaking down barriers to fertilization.

The key antioxidants, vitamin C, beta-carotene, selenium, and vitamin E, play critical roles in sperm formation and protect the cells against free radical damage.

Vitamin C is especially important protecting the sperm's precious cargo, its DNA, from damage. Ascorbic acid levels are much higher in seminal fluid than in other body fluids, including the blood. One study showed that reducing dietary vitamin C from 250 mg to a mere 5 mg per day in healthy human subjects lowered ascorbic acid levels in semen by 50 percent; at the same time, the number of sperm that had damage to their DNA increased by 91 percent. Smoking cigarettes greatly reduces vitamin C levels, which is one reason smokers are more likely to be infertile. Another study found that taking 1,000 mg of vitamin C per day increased sperm count, reduced agglutination (attachment of harmful antibodies to sperm), and increased chances of pregnancy.

Vitamin E is a crucial antioxidant for protecting against damage to the unsaturated fatty acids that make up part of the sperm cell membrane. Vitamin E does not appear to increase sperm counts or motility, but it may play an essential role in enhancing the ability of sperm to penetrate eggs. I usually recommend that my infertile male patients take 600 to 800 IU of vitamin E per day.

The *right balance of fats and oils* is important. Avoid saturated fats, found primarily in animal products such as butter and lard. Watch out for hydrogenated plant oils, particularly coconut oil and palm oil. Besides containing toxic residues, cottonseed oil is a rich source of a substance called gossypol, which is known to inhibit sperm function. In fact, gossypol is being investigated as a possible basis for a "male birth control pill."

At the same time, increase your intake of polyunsaturated oils, especially from nuts and seeds. These oils are important for sexual function including sperm formation and activity.

Zinc is perhaps the most critical trace mineral for male sexual function. It is involved in virtually every aspect of male reproduction, including hormone metabolism, sperm formation, and sperm motility. Decreased testosterone levels and low sperm counts are among the key signs of zinc deficiency. Zinc is also important for sexual vitality. The best sources of zinc are whole grains, legumes, nuts, and seeds. A high-potency multivitamin and mineral supplement will also contain appropriate doses of zinc.

Vitamin B$_{12}$ is crucial for making new cells, so it is logical that a deficiency of the vitamin leads to reduced sperm count and lower sperm motility. Studies have found that taking 1 to 6 mg of B$_{12}$ a day can significantly increase sperm count.

The amino acid *arginine* also is required for the replication of cells. If other nutritional measures fail to work for men with very low sperm counts, supplementing with arginine (at least 4 grams a day for at least three months) may be effective.

Carnitine is a vitaminlike compound that stimulates the breakdown of long-chain fatty acids within your cells' energy-producing factories (the mitochondria). A deficiency in carnitine decreases fatty acid concentrations and leads to low energy. Carnitine concentrations are especially high in the epididymis and sperm. Research shows that the more carnitine present in sperm, the better they are able to swim. The optimal dosage is 300 to 1,000 mg of L-carnitine three times per day. However, this strategy can be expensive, and I usually recommend its use only as a last resort after other nutritional measures fail.

Certain herbs may also be valuable. As noted earlier, *Panax ginseng* promotes growth of the testicles and may increase sperm formation and testosterone levels. Another Chinese herb, *Astragalus membranaceus,* enhances the immune system and may work to enhance sperm motility, especially following an infection. Typical dosage is 500 mg three times per day.

The Dangers of Environmental Estrogens

One of the main problems contributing to male infertility is exposure to excessive levels of estrogen, the so-called female hormone. Men's bodies contain estrogen too, but high levels can interfere with normal function. The biggest danger results from exposure of a male fetus to estrogens in the womb and at puberty. The hormone can interfere with development of the sexual organs, including the testicles. Estrogens appear to prevent certain cells (Sertoli cells) from multiplying during testicular development, both in the womb and at puberty. These cells support, protect, and regulate the nutrition of developing sperm. The more Sertoli cells you have, the more healthy sperm you can produce.

One main culprit in former years was exposure in the womb to diethylstilbestrol (DES). Between 1945 and 1971, this synthetic form of estrogen was prescribed to millions of pregnant women to prevent spontaneous abortion and premature labor. However, we now know that DES caused many cases of abnormal development of the reproductive tract, decreased semen volume, and low sperm count. It also caused devastating damage to the daughters of DES mothers, who have an extremely high risk of structural defects in the uterus and uterine cancer. DES is no longer used in pregnant women, but its damaging legacy persists.

Estrogens that come from our food, water, or air supply are called environmental estrogens. For thirty years the livestock industry used DES and other synthetic estrogens to fatten animals for market. Though this strategy is now banned, the beef and poultry industry in the United States still uses growth hormones, and cow's milk still contains substantial amounts of estrogen. The rise in dairy consumption since the 1940s parallels the drop in sperm count noted in men in the United States. In my opinion, it is essential for men to avoid consuming products from animals raised on hormones, especially if they already have a low sperm count or low testosterone levels.

Some reports indicate that estrogens may also be found in drinking water. In theory, these hormones enter the water supply having been excreted in urine by women taking birth control pills. Apparently filtering by water treatment facilities does not completely remove the estrogens. These hormones are particularly potent because they do not bind to sex hormone binding globulin (SHBG), the blood protein that "escorts" estrogen out of the body. Instead, the estrogen remains unbound, or free, so it circulates in the blood and causes effects on various tissues. To reduce the risk, I recommend drinking purified or bottled water.

Many of the poisons in our environment can cause weak estrogen activity in the body. Examples include PCBs and dioxin. These toxic chemicals interfere with sperm formation and can seriously disrupt sexual development during puberty. (For a whole host of reasons, it makes sense to avoid exposure to these substances.)

If your testosterone levels are low or marginal, or if your estrogen level is high, try to eat a diet rich in nuts, seeds, and legumes (beans), especially soy. As a source of isoflavonoids, soy foods are considered phytoestrogens (plant estrogens). In the body, phytoestrogens exert weak estrogenic effects. That is, they bind to estrogen receptors on cells, thus blocking binding by environmental estrogens as well as the body's own powerful estrogens that can interfere with testosterone. Although phytoestrogens have estrogenic activity, it is only a tiny fraction of the activity that estrogen has, so the net effect is reduced estrogen activity. Phytoestrogens may further reduce estrogen effects by stimulating production of SHBG.

The more SHBG you have, the faster you excrete estrogen in the feces and the less impact estrogen has on your cells and tissues.

CASE HISTORY: The Miracle Baby

Jim and Anita had been trying to conceive a child for over four years with no success. The problem was Jim's sperm. He not only had a low sperm count, but there was a high percentage of abnormal sperm, and even the few that were normal did not swim very well. His sperm also failed to penetrate hamster eggs. Most fertile men have 100 percent penetration, and a penetration of less than 10 percent is usually indicative of infertility. Jim's result was 0 percent—not a good sign. Jim and Anita told me I was their last stop before going for in vitro fertilization, where Anita would be given drugs to increase the number of active follicles in her ovaries and then have the eggs removed surgically. Jim's sperm would literally be injected into the eggs. After fertilization the eggs would be implanted into Anita's uterus. This process was going to be extremely expensive—about $30,000.

Jim's diet and lifestyle were extremely healthy. However, I was amazed to find out all of the things that he did that increased testicular temperature. He wore briefs even while sleeping, he wore an athletic supporter when exercising, he typically rode an exercise bike for thirty minutes a day, and he loved to spend time in the hot tub. What was really amazing to me was that none of the fertility experts they had consulted over the years ever told him these practices may be the cause of his low sperm count.

I told Jim that I wanted him to avoid overheating of the testicles and to apply ice to them every night for twenty minutes before going to bed naked. I also had him on the full gamut of nutritional and botanical supplements to boost fertility because they only gave me two months. Jim had another sperm count and hamster egg penetration test after being on the program for two months. The results showed a 50 percent increase in sperm count, a 33 percent reduction in abnormal sperm, and a hamster egg penetration rate of 3 percent. However, in all of these areas Jim's values were still well below what is considered necessary to be fertile. The fertility expert told Jim that he would never get Anita pregnant on his own. But about two weeks after Jim had informed me of the test results, and just before Anita was to start the fertility drugs, Jim and Anita showed up at my office unexpectedly to tell me that Anita was pregnant. I am happy to tell you that they gave birth to a very healthy little boy, Dylan. They call him their miracle baby.

I do not know if what I recommended was directly responsible, but I do believe that it helped increase their odds of conception.

Prostate Health

PROSTATE HEALTH ASSESSMENT

Circle the number that best describes the intensity of your symptoms on the following scale:

>   *0 = I do not experience this symptom*
>   *1 = Mild*
>   *2 = Moderate*
>   *3 = Severe*

Difficulty urinating	0	1	2	3
A sense of bladder fullness	0	1	2	3
Increased straining with smaller amounts of urine passed	0	1	2	3
Need to wake up to urinate at night	0	1	2	3
Dripping after urination	0	1	2	3
Pain or fatigue in the legs or back	0	1	2	3
Lack of sex drive	0	1	2	3

Add the numbers circled and enter that total here: _____

Scoring   *6 or more: High priority*
                    3–5: Moderate priority
                    1–2: Low priority

Interpreting Your Score

This assessment reflects the kinds of problems that can develop in the prostate gland. Because it is located so near the urinary organs, a swollen prostate can block the flow of urine and cause such complications as painful urination or a dribbling urine stream. In most cases, prostate enlargement is a benign condition—that is, it is not cancerous. However, cancer of the prostate is a common, potentially fatal disease among men. In the early stages prostate cancer may not cause symptoms, but later the tumor may spread and cause pain in the back or legs. The hormonal disruption of prostate cancer may cause a drop in sexual drive.

Proper prostate function is essential for normal reproductive function. Unfortunately, disorders of the prostate are extremely common in American men. The main concerns are enlargement of the prostate (benign prostatic hyperplasia, or BPH), prostate infection (prostatitis), and prostate cancer. BPH is virtually inevitable in men if they live long enough—the same may also be true for prostate cancer.

BPH results when testosterone is converted to a highly active form called dihydrotestosterone (DHT), which stimulates prostate cells to grow larger. The *benign* in BPH is an important aspect of the condition. BPH is not cancer and in most cases is not dangerous. Enlargement can begin as early as age forty, but it may not cause symptoms until later in life. Because the prostate surrounds the urinary tube (the urethra), enlargement of the prostate can pinch the tube and cause problems with urination, including increased urinary frequency (more trips to the bathroom), waking up often at night to urinate, and reduced force in the stream of urine (dribbling).

Prostatitis is an inflammation of the prostate gland, usually the result of bacterial infection that has spread from the urethra. In some cases, but not all, prostatitis is sexually transmitted. It can also result from use of a urinary catheter, a plastic tube inserted in the urethra to facilitate urination. Symptoms include pain on urination and increased frequency. Some men experience fever and a discharge from the penis. In more severe cases, abdominal pain is present and blood may appear in the urine.

Prostate cancer is a serious illness. Like other cancers, it occurs when cells in the gland begin to grow in an out-of-control fashion. The tumor grows in size, producing a nodule that can sometimes be felt during a rectal examination. Left unchecked, the tumor can penetrate outside the wall of the gland and can spread to other organs and tissues. In the earliest stages, the man may not notice any symptoms. Later the symptoms resemble those of BPH: difficulty starting urination, poor urinary flow, and increased frequency. If the disease spreads, urine flow may stop completely and pain, often severe, may develop. Prostate cancer typically grows very slowly. Most men who get prostate cancer will not die because of it; indeed, they may never know they have it. Even so, prostate cancer is a leading killer of men. About one in ten men will develop prostate cancer during their lifetimes (see Table 11.2). The disease is fatal in about one-fourth of cases. The earlier it is diagnosed and treated, the greater the chances of survival.

Table 11-2: Prostate Cancer Risk Factors

- *Age:* By the time a man is 50, he has a 30 percent chance of developing prostate cancer. The older a man gets, the more likely he is to develop the disease.
- *Ethnicity:* African Americans have the highest rate of prostate cancer.
- *Family history:* Men with a family history (at least one first-degree relative, such as a father or brother) have a risk two to three times greater.
- *Diet:* A diet high in animal fats doubles the risk while a diet high in carotenes, particularly lycopene, and other antioxidants may cut the risk in half.
- *Smoking:* A major risk factor, smoking depletes antioxidant defenses and is high in cadmium, a mineral that interferes with zinc's role in the healthy prostate.
- *Sexual history:* There is evidence that the human papillomavirus, a sexually transmitted virus, increases the risk of prostate cancer.

Although scientists are not yet sure what causes prostate cancer, diet is clearly a factor. The rate of prostate cancer is higher among men who eat a typically Western diet, high in refined sugar and animal fat and protein, low in fiber and carotenes from plant foods. Some studies suggest that low intake of carotene may be among the most significant risk factors for prostate cancer. The best sources of carotenes are dark green leafy vegetables (kale, collards, and spinach), and yellow-orange fruits and vegetables (apricots, cantaloupe, carrots, sweet potatoes, yams, and squash). In the past few years lycopenes, the red pigments found in tomatoes, have come to be regarded as an important dietary weapon in the fight against prostate cancer.

WARNING Prostate disorders can only be diagnosed by a physician. Do not self-diagnose. If you are experiencing any symptoms associated with BPH or prostate cancer, see your physician immediately for proper diagnosis.

Diagnosing Prostate Disorders

Every man over the age of forty should have an annual physical checkup that includes a digital rectal exam. In this procedure, the doctor inserts a gloved lubricated finger into the rectum and feels the prostate. An enlarged prostate feels bigger than normal; if prostatitis is present, the prostate may feel tender or painful; in some cases of cancer, the doctor can detect an abnormal growth. The digital rectal exam isn't always enough, because sometimes, even when BPH is present, the prostate may not have grown enough to reveal an abnormality. Likewise, a cancerous tumor may be too small, or may be in the wrong position, for the physician to detect it.

If the doctor suspects a problem, further tests will be conducted. BPH can be detected with the aid of ultrasound. In prostatitis, a sample of urine or prostatic fluid will reveal signs of infection or inflammation. A biopsy (tissue sample) is needed to confirm a diagnosis of cancer. Cancerous prostate cells secrete a unique molecule called prostate-specific antigen (PSA). Blood tests can measure the level of PSA present. Generally, PSA levels of greater than 4 nanograms per milliliter (ng/ml) indicate cancer may be present and biopsy is needed; levels of greater than 10 ng/ml are considered proof of cancer. All men over age fifty should have both a digital rectal exam and a PSA test every year. Because African-American men are at higher risk of prostate cancer, they should have these two tests beginning at age 40. Also, because prostate cancer can run in the family, the tests should begin at age forty if you have a father or brother with the disease.

—— Medical Treatment of Prostate Conditions ——

Left untreated, BPH can progress to the point where it completely blocks the outflow of urine from the bladder. As a result, urine can back up into the blood, posing a potentially life-threatening condition called uremia. To prevent this, and to relieve the annoying symptoms of BPH, treatment is usually needed. A drug called finasteride (Proscar) is available. This drug works by blocking the activity of an enzyme that converts testosterone into highly active DHT, the form of the hormone that triggers excess growth of prostate cells.

If the drug doesn't work, surgical methods can reduce the amount of prostate tissue. One procedure called transurethral resection of the prostate (TURP) involves inserting a tiny tool through the urethra and whittling away chunks of prostate tissue. Such a procedure is uncomfortable at best, painful at worst. It can also cause long-term complications, including erectile dysfunction or incontinence, and may not be a permanent solution. Lately, a new technique has been developed involving the use of heat to reduce the size of the prostate.

Doctors treat prostatitis with antibiotics. However, these drugs don't always work and the condition tends to recur frequently.

Treatment options for prostate cancer include surgery, radiation, implantation of radioactive seeds in the gland, and cryosurgery ("freezing"). Because the disease is so slow-growing in most cases, and because it may not develop into a life-threatening condition, one option is to do nothing. Doctors refer to this strategy as "watchful waiting," because they will continue to monitor the progress through regular blood tests and repeat biopsies. Of course, doing nothing can give the cancer a chance to grow and spread. But the risks of other forms of prostate cancer treatment are also high. Many men experience loss of control over their urine (urinary incontinence) following surgery or radiation. What's more, it may be necessary to remove nerves near the prostate if the cancer has spread into them. Those nerves are the ones that trigger erection. Thus medical treatment for prostate cancer leaves many men permanently impotent.

In my opinion, watchful waiting is the best approach for most slow-growing prostate tumors. However, if the cancer has already spread or is especially aggressive, traditional surgical or radiation treatment is usually needed. A 1998 study found that the survival rate in men with fast-spreading prostate cancer was much higher when patients were treated with surgery and radiation rather than radioactive seed implants. At this time, trying to choose the best treatment for prostate cancer is confusing and frightening. The best advice I can give is to consult several doctors, especially urologists, who specialize in different treatments for prostate cancer and choose the one in whom you have the most confidence. In other words, choose the doctor, not the therapy.

— The Natural Approach to Prostate Disorders —

It shouldn't surprise to you learn that diet appears to play a critical role in the health of the prostate. It's especially important to avoid pesticides, increase the intake of zinc and essential fatty acids, and keep your cholesterol low. These steps often lead to clinical improvement in BPH and prostatitis.

Pesticides are a concern because once they enter the body, they can concentrate in prostate tissue. Their presence may then trigger the cells to become enlarged. In animal studies, synthetic hormones that are used to fatten up food animals before slaughter have also caused changes in prostate tissue. In my view, the increase in occurrence of BPH over the past few decades reflects the growing impact of toxic environmental chemicals on our health. Choosing a diet rich in natural, organic, whole foods prevents excess intake of these toxins. In particular, minerals (calcium, magnesium, zinc, and selenium), plant pigments (flavonoids, carotenes, lycopenes, and chlorophyll), fiber, and sulfur-containing compounds (such as those found in garlic and onions) all possess actions that help the body remove harmful chemicals and heavy metals. (See Chapter 3 for more information on detoxification.)

Zinc is essential for prostate health and is especially valuable for preventing BPH. As mentioned earlier, zinc is also crucial for making testosterone and for developing healthy, active sperm. The prostate has the highest concentration of zinc of any body tissue. During ejaculation, the prostate secretes a zinc-rich fluid that helps sperm swim. The fluid also works as an antibiotic. Low zinc levels may be a risk factor for frequent prostate infection and low fertility. Zinc supplementation has been shown to shrink the prostate and to relieve symptoms in most patients. Foods rich in zinc include nuts and seeds.

Such foods also are excellent sources of essential fatty acids, which are important for healthy prostate function. An old folk remedy for BPH is to eat $1/4$ to $1/2$ cup of pumpkin seeds each day. Taking just 1 tsp per day of oil from flaxseed, sunflower seed, evening primrose, or soy is another good way to make sure you get enough of the essential fatty acids. And, just as women are encouraged to increase their intake of soy foods and other phytoestrogens to prevent breast cancer, I also recommend that men do the same to prevent prostate cancer.

The breakdown products of cholesterol metabolism have been shown to accumulate in prostate tissue. As they build up, these metabolites may cause cell damage leading to prostate enlargement or possibly cancer. Drugs that lower cholesterol levels have been shown to reduce BPH. Tips on reducing cholesterol through natural strategies are discussed in more detail on pages 203–217.

Sorry to tell you, guys, but another important strategy for reducing BPH is to avoid drinking beer. Beer increases release of the hormone prolactin by the pituitary gland. This hormone increases the rate at which testosterone is converted into DHT, which stimulates the growth of prostate cells. It is possible to reduce prolactin levels and control BPH by taking a drug called bromocriptine, but this method poses a risk of severe side effects and is not widely used. I recommend instead passing up a mug of suds and taking supplemental zinc and vitamin B_6, which can reduce prolactin levels without side effects.

Botanical Strategies for BPH

One of the most valuable natural strategies is the use of *saw palmetto berry extract*. The saw palmetto is a small scrubby palm tree native to the West Indies and the southern Atlantic seaboard. Its berries have long been prized as an aphrodisiac and sexual rejuvenator, and for centuries they have been used as a treatment for prostate conditions. Like Proscar, saw palmetto extract appears to work by inhibiting production of DHT, but it goes further by actually blocking the binding of DHT at cell receptor sites. In more than a dozen double-blind clinical studies, purified fat-soluble extract of the berries, containing 85 to 95 percent fatty acids and sterols, has been shown to improve signs and symptoms of BPH in nearly nine out of ten patients within four to six weeks. In contrast, Proscar may work for less than half of those who take it for as long as a year. As a bonus, saw palmetto extract is significantly less expensive than Proscar and is without side effects. The standard dosage is 160 mg twice daily.

An extract of flower pollen, known as Cernilton, has been used in Europe for more than twenty-five years as a treatment of prostatitis and BPH. It is particularly valuable as a strategy for prostatitis, because it reduces inflammation and infection. It also promotes urine flow by helping the bladder contract and by relaxing the urethra. The standard dosage of flower pollen products is 2 tablets taken three times per day.

CASE HISTORY: The Urologist

Ron was not your typical fifty-six-year-old man coming to see me because of an enlarged prostate. He was also a urologist—a medical doctor who deals with problems in the urinary tract. Ron's first visit was in 1987, well before herbal treatments for BPH were as well known as they are today and also before drug therapies such as Proscar or Hytrin were available as well. Back in 1987, there was little that conventional medicine had to offer for BPH. In fact, the only real treatment was transurethal resection of the prostate (TURP), a surgical procedure in which a larger opening through the bladder is chiseled out. Ron knew firsthand the problems with this surgery—he had performed thousands of them. One of his patients was slated to have a TURP, but then canceled when his symptoms of BPH improved so much after seeing me and following my recommendations.

Ron wanted to learn more, especially since he was developing BPH himself. I was very surprised when Ron told me he was a urologist, but I was also really excited, because I knew that if I was able to help him, he in turn might start using some of these natural approaches instead. Ron was a perfect candidate because his BPH was in the early stages. My experience is that saw palmetto extract alone is effective in nearly 100 percent of early cases within two months. In more moderate BPH, it is effective in about 70 percent of cases, while in more severe cases, it is not that effective on its own.

Ron was getting up only one or two times a night on the average. But after just two weeks of using saw palmetto extract he was sleeping through the night. Ron went on to be a great promoter of saw palmetto extract in his own practice. His open-mindedness and integrity in being a doctor who puts his patients first should be commended.

Tune-Up Tip: Sitz Yourself Down

Some men find relief of urinary blockage by taking hot sitz baths. The warmth works to relax and open the urinary pathways. There are specially designed tubs available for this purpose, but you can also take a sitz bath in your regular bathtub. Heat the water to between 105 and 115 degrees Fahrenheit. Immerse the pelvic region for three to ten minutes, then sponge the region with a cool cloth.

Note: Hot sitz baths are not indicated for acute inflammation or infection of the prostate.

Tune-Up Tip: E for Effort?

Recent research in Finland found that a daily dose of 50 IU of vitamin E reduced the risk of prostate cancer by 32 percent among men who smoked cigarettes. Apparently the vitamin works by preventing small inactive (latent) tumors from burgeoning into full-blown active cancers. Scientists are not sure yet whether use of vitamin E is of value in cancer prevention among nonsmokers, but it certainly seems likely.

PC-SPES: WHAT'S THE STORY?

Many men have taken a product called PC-SPES, a combination of eight herbs, for treatment or prevention of prostate cancer. *PC* stands for prostate cancer, and *SPES* comes from the Latin word for "hope." The combination was developed by Sophie Chen, Ph.D., a Chinese-born scientist educated in the United States, as a remedy to help a friend with prostate cancer. In studies, about 70 percent of more than 1,700 men with prostate cancer reported improvement after taking PC-SPES.

Recently a report in the *New England Journal of Medicine* has clouded this issue a bit. The authors of the study validated many of the positive aspects of PC-SPES, such as its ability to reduce testosterone concentrations and reduce levels of PSA, the blood marker for prostate cancer. But in patients with the disease they reached a rather bizarre conclusion: "Our results suggest that PC-SPES may prove useful in the treatment of hormonally sensitive prostate cancer; but when used concurrently with standard or experimental therapies, PC-SPES may confound the results." What the authors appear to be saying is: "PC-SPES probably works, but don't use it if you're being treated because doctors may not be able to tell if it's the drugs or the herbs that are providing the benefit."

In my experience, men with prostate cancer do not really care *what* is working as long as *something* is working (and so long as the side effects are not too unpleasant). If you have prostate cancer, my recommendation is to make sure that your doctors have read the report in the *New England Journal of Medicine* thoroughly and reached their own conclusions. If you choose to use PC-SPES, ask them to monitor you carefully. For more information on PC-SPES, contact the Education Center for Prostate Cancer Patients at www.ecpcp.org or call them at 1-516-942-5000.

Genital Infections

GENITAL INFECTION ASSESSMENT

Circle the number that best describes the intensity of your symptoms on the following scale:

    0 = I do not experience this symptom
    1 = Mild
    2 = Moderate
    3 = Severe

Discharge from penis	0	1	2	3
Past or present rash on penis	0	1	2	3

Swollen genitals	0	1	2	3
Swelling in groin	0	1	2	3
Rose-colored (bloody) urine	0	1	2	3
Pain or burning while urinating	0	1	2	3
Pain upon ejaculation	0	1	2	3

Add the numbers circled and enter that subtotal here: _____

Circle the number of the answer that applies to you:

Venereal disease (gonorrhea,
syphilis, herpes) now or
in the past   NO = 0   YES = 10

Enter the number circled as a subtotal here: _____
Add the two subtotals and enter that total here: _____

Scoring   *5 or more: High priority*
3–4: Moderate priority
1–2: Low priority

Interpreting Your Score

This questionnaire addresses the possibility of a genital infection. Viruses, bacteria, and fungi can all cause troubling symptoms such as rash, swelling, or pain. Infection can develop in the prostate, epididymis, seminal vesicles, bladder, and urethra. Even though such infections are often so mild as to cause no symptoms, they may often cause infertility and reduced sexual vitality.

If you suspect an infection, it is important that you see a doctor immediately for a comprehensive exam. Signs of trouble include any unusual discharge from the penis, pain or burning sensation with urination or ejaculation, pain in the scrotum or pelvic region, or abnormal growths or patches on the genitalia. A number of organisms, including bacteria, viruses, and fungi, can produce infection.

One of the most common causes of urinary infection is *Chlamydia trachomatis,* an organism that, biologically speaking, is kind of a cross between a virus and a bacterium. Considered a sexually transmitted disease, chlamydia causes pelvic inflammatory disease (PID) in women and is a major factor in female infertility. In men, chlamydia is a major cause of acute prostatitis and urethritis (inflammation of the urethra). Symptoms include pain or burning during urination or ejaculation. In serious cases, the infection can spread to tissues within the testicle, possibly resulting in scarring and blockage of sperm-carrying vessels. Usually infection of these tissues or the prostate does not cause symptoms. However, chlamydia can lead to infertility. Perhaps as many as 70 percent of infertile men have evidence of chlamydial infection.

Medical treatment calls for the use of antibiotics, especially tetracycline and erythromycin. Often, though, the stubborn little chlamydia organism can hide out in cells, avoiding the barrage of drugs and waiting for the day when it can reemerge to cause further trouble. While antibiotics may keep the bug in check, such treatment does not appear to boost sperm count or improve sperm quality. Ideally, because chlamydia can be passed during intercourse, both partners should take antibiotics when the condition is diagnosed in one of them. I do not recommend antibiotics as a fertility aid. Instead, such drugs should be taken if there is reason to believe that a chronic infection is present and after the fertility strategies discussed above have been tried.

If antibiotics are used, I would recommend taking bromelain, an enzyme derived from pineapple. Bromelain enhances the immune system and exerts direct antimicrobial effects. I strongly recommend using bromelain along with conventional antibiotics as well as herbal antibiotics. Studies show bromelain can boost the absorption of antibiotics and increase their ability to do the job. The standard dose is 400 to 500 mg three times daily, taken on an empty stomach. I would also recommend that you take *L. acidophilus* and *B. bifidum* according to the guidelines on page 53.

Summary: Tune-Up for Men

- A healthy diet and lifestyle, including plenty of sleep, exercise, limited use of alcohol, and no use of tobacco, are important for maintaining male sexuality and fertility.
- Increase consumption of foods containing carotenes and lycopenes, such as dark green leafy vegetables and yellow, orange, and red fruits and vegetables, especially tomatoes. Also eat plenty of fiber and sulfur-containing foods, such as garlic and onions, for better detoxification.
- Reduce exposure to environmental estrogens by drinking bottled water, avoiding exposure to pesticides and other chemicals, eating organic foods, and increasing consumption of foods rich in phytoestrogens such as soy, nuts, seeds, and beans.

- Take a high-potency multivitamin and multimineral supplement.
- Take extra doses of antioxidants: vitamin C, 500 mg three times per day; vitamin E, 400–800 IU per day.
- Be sure to get adequate zinc; take at least 30 mg daily.
- Take 1 tbsp of flaxseed oil daily.
- Consider DHEA supplementation:
  - Age 40–50: 15–25 mg per day
  - Age 50–70: 25–50 mg per day
  - Over 70: Higher doses may be needed
- Develop an effective time management program (see Lifestyle Tune-Up Tip #11).

Lifestyle Tune-Up #11:
Learn to Manage Your Time

One of the biggest stressors in modern life is poor time management. It is a major reason men and women are most likely to display type A behavior—the type of behavior (linked to a higher risk of heart disease) characterized by an extreme sense of time urgency, competitiveness, impatience, and aggressiveness. People with type A personalities simply do not feel they have enough time. As a result, they are more likely to be very impatient, always in a hurry, and even a bit rude at times. Here are some tips on time management:

- *Set priorities.* Realize that you can only accomplish so much in a day. Decide what is important, and limit your efforts to that goal.
- *Organize your day.* There are always interruptions and unplanned demands on your time, but create a definite plan for the day based on your priorities. Avoid the pitfall of always letting the immediate demands control your life.
- *Delegate authority.* Delegate as much authority and work as you can. You can't do everything yourself. Learn to train and depend on others.
- *Tackle tough jobs first.* Handle the most important tasks first, while your energy levels are high. Leave the busywork or running around for later in the day.
- *Minimize meeting time.* Schedule meetings to bump up against the lunch hour or quitting time; that way they can't last forever.
- *Avoid putting things off.* Work done under pressure of an unreasonable deadline often has to be redone. That creates more stress than if it had been done right the first time. Plan ahead.
- *Don't be a perfectionist.* You can never really achieve perfection anyway. Do your best in a reasonable amount of time, then move on to other important tasks. If you find time, you can always come back later and polish the task some more.
- *Take time off to smell the roses.* Don't be so involved with your work and timetable that it interferes with your ability to enjoy the simple things in life.

Epilogue:
A Question of Magic

At the end of Lifestyle Tune-Up #1, I stated that the quality of your life is equal to the quality of the questions you ask yourself. My all-time favorite question came to me one night when I was giving a speech to an audience of over two thousand people at the Disneyland Hotel. Disneyland holds a special place in my heart and soul. My parents took my sisters and me there when I was twelve years old. It was one of the highlights of my childhood—a very special memory.

Now, twenty-six years later, I was able to bring my parents, my wife, and my daughter, Alexa, to Disneyland. She was two and a half at the time. To say the experience was overwhelming is putting it mildly. The most magical moment of my life to that time was holding my daughter when she spotted Mickey Mouse while my wife and parents looked on. I no longer had to imagine what it felt like to hold pure joy and excitement in my very arms. Perhaps you have had a similar experience. I hope so. I am not embarrassed to tell you that tears were streaming down my face. I cannot express in words the feeling that I experienced. All that I can tell you is that it was wonderful—truly magical. (I think it fitting to tell you that the night of September 17, 1996, was also the night that our son, Zachary, was conceived. Hey, after all, they do call it the "Magic Kingdom." It certainly was for us.)

Anyway, as I was finishing my speech to this group that night, I shared my Disneyland story and encouraged each of them to ask the question "How can I make my life more magical?" Almost as soon as I got the question out of my mouth, the answer occurred to me: *by making the lives of those around me more magical.*

How can you make your life more magical? Think about it. I cannot imagine a better way to tune up your life than finding the answer to that question.

Index

Michael Murray, N.D., is a doctor of naturopathy, which seeks to harness the power of nature to prevent illness and achieve the highest level of health possible. He received his doctorate in naturopathic medicine from Bastyr University in Seattle, Washington. His particular focus is clinical nutrition and herbal medicine. Dr. Murray teaches medical students at Bastyr University, has published many books and articles, appears frequently on radio and television, and lectures to doctors and lay people around the world on the subject of naturopathic healing.

Dr. Murray can be reached through his website:

www.doctormurray.com